Self-Assessment for Vascular and Endovascular Specialists

Including over 500 multiple choice questions covering a wide range of vascular disorders to test the skills of all vascular specialists. Suitable for postgraduate trainee vascular medicine internists, interventional radiologists, vascular surgeons, and endovascular therapists as they prepare for exams or ensure that they remain up to date.

Divided into 21 subject-specific sections and meticulously written and researched, the questions and their accompanying rationales are enhanced by explanatory illustrations and supported by key references. Students and experienced clinicians will be prepared for both testing and teaching in all aspects of clinical practice.

Advances in the treatment of vascular disease have played a significant role in rising life expectancy over the past 70 years, resulting in lower morbidity, mortality, and quicker recoveries. However, there remains an urgent challenge in controlling risk factors such as obesity, sedentary lifestyles, and tobacco abuse. As explosive growth in endovascular technology continues, it is more important than ever for vascular specialists to remain proficient and stay up to date.

T0315175

Self-Assessment for Vascular and Endovascular Specialists

Sachinder Singh Hans, MD, FACS, FRCS(C)

Medical Director
Vascular and Endovascular Services
Henry Ford Macomb Hospital Clinton TWP (MI)
Clinical Assistant Professor of Surgery
Wayne State University School of Medicine, Detroit, Michigan
Board Certified in Vascular Surgery, Surgical Critical Care and General Surgery

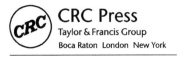

CRC Press
Taylor & Francis Group
Boca Raton London New York

CRC Press is an imprint of the
Taylor & Francis Group, an **informa** business

Designed cover image: Shutterstock 181632251

First edition published 2024
by CRC Press
2385 NW Executive Center Drive, Suite 320, Boca Raton, FL 33431

and by CRC Press
4 Park Square, Milton Park, Abingdon, Oxon, OX14 4RN

CRC Press is an imprint of Taylor & Francis Group, LLC

© 2024 Sachinder Singh Hans

Library of Congress Cataloging-in-Publication Data
Names: Hans, S. S. (Sachinder Singh), author.
Title: Self-assessment for vascular and endovascular specialists /
Sachinder Singh Hans.
Description: First edition. | Boca Raton, FL : CRC Press, 2023. | Includes
bibliographical references and index. | Summary: "Including over 500
multiple choice questions covering a wide range of vascular disorders to
test the skills of all vascular specialists. Suitable for postgraduate
trainee vascular medicine internists, interventional radiologists,
vascular surgeons, and endovascular therapists as they prepare for exams
or ensure that they remain up to date. Divided into 21 subject specific
sections and meticulously written and researched, the questions and
their accompanying rationales are enhanced by explanatory illustrations
and supported by key references. Students and experienced clinicians
will be prepared for both testing and teaching in all aspects of
clinical practice. Advances in the treatment of vascular disease have
played a significant role in rising life expectancy over the past 70
years, resulting in lower morbidity, mortality, and quicker recoveries.
However, there remains an urgent challenge in controlling risk factors
such as obesity, sedentary lifestyles, and tobacco abuse. As explosive
growth in endovascular technology continues, it is more important than
ever for vascular specialists to remain proficient and stay up to
date"-- Provided by publisher.
Identifiers: LCCN 2023023082 (print) | LCCN 2023023083 (ebook) | ISBN
9781032486123 (hardback) | ISBN 9781032485553 (paperback) | ISBN
9781003389897 (ebook)
Subjects: MESH: Vascular Diseases | Vascular Surgical Procedures | Problems
and Exercises
Classification: LCC RC691 (print) | LCC RC691 (ebook) | NLM WG 18.2 |
DDC 616.1/3--dc23/eng/20230907
LC record available at https://lccn.loc.gov/2023023082
LC ebook record available at https://lccn.loc.gov/2023023083

ISBN: 9781032486123 (hbk)
ISBN: 9781032485553 (pbk)
ISBN: 9781003389897 (ebk)

DOI: 10.1201/9781003389897

Typeset in Utopia Std
by KnowledgeWorks Global Ltd.

Dedication

This book is dedicated to the memory of my late brother,
Dr. Jagjit Singh Hans, MD, Professor of Internal Medicine, Government Medical College
Patiala (Pb), India.
He was inspirational to me for pursuing surgery as my career.

Contents

Preface

Vascular disease affects a large segment of Western populations and results in serious complications if not managed appropriately. During the past seven decades, the treatment of vascular disease has progressed from medical management to open reconstruction. More recently, the explosive growth of endovascular technologies has resulted in lower morbidity, mortality, and quicker recoveries.

In spite of the availability of recent advances and technological successes, there remains an urgent challenge in controlling risk factors causing vascular disease. These include obesity, sedentary lifestyles, unhealthy diets, and tobacco abuse, as well as increasing incidence of diabetes mellitus and uncontrolled hypertension in patients of low socioeconomic status, resulting in renal failure and kidney replacement therapy.

The complexity of vascular diseases has meant that some vascular specialists are limiting their practice in many categories of vascular pathology, including complex aortic disease, limb salvage, venous disease, thoracic outlet syndrome, and vascular access procedures for end-stage kidney disease. In order to remain proficient as a vascular specialist, one has to keep up with the knowledge of the current literature; specialists must thus engage in self-assessment of their skills. Additionally, throughout the world vascular specialists must become certified and pass maintenance or certification examinations.

This book thus provides the tools for self-assessment, with over 500 questions (each with four possible answers, an explanation for the best answer, and one to two references). This book is not a substitute for a textbook in vascular surgery, leading vascular journals, and experience gained during clinical practice. It should primarily be considered a primer for taking the vascular examinations and a quick reference for a clinical problem. As the literature advances and technology evolves, some answers may become out of date, and the reader is advised to consult the latest literature.

Acknowledgments

First and foremost, I wish to thank Miranda Bromage, Senior Medical Editor, CRC Press/Taylor & Francis, for providing unrelenting support starting from acceptance of the proposal to the final publication of this work. I appreciate the support of Hudson Greig, Editorial Assistant at CRC Press/Taylor & Francis. My sincere thanks to Juliet Mullenmeister, MLIS, AHIP, and Melanie Bednarski, MLIS, AHIP, from the Library Department of Henry Ford Macomb Hospital for their diligent medsearch and editorial support. Miss Kait Fecteau helped in transcription, and Dr. Shyamal Pansurya, surgery resident at Henry Ford, provided IT support to complete the submission to CRC Press. Dr. Scott Dulchavsky, MD, PhD, Chairman of Surgery, Henry Ford Health, provided the leadership in getting this project completed, as well as the financial support from the department for which I will always be grateful. My thanks to my wife, Dr. Bijoya Hans, for attending to the tasks in my absence because of the time commitment for preparation of this work and to my son, Gautam Hans, JD, MS, for proofreading and editing the Preface.

Author

Dr. Sachinder Singh Hans is a vascular surgeon in Clinton Township, Michigan. He received his medical degree from Government Medical College, Patiala, Internship (January–December 1969) and House Officer Surgery (1970) from Rajindra Hospital, Patiala (Pb.) India. He has been in practice for more than 45 years. Board certifications include:

- American Board of Surgery – Surgery
- American Board of Surgery – Surgical Critical Care
- American Board of Surgery – Vascular Surgery
- Education includes:
  - Postgraduate Institute of Medical Education, Chandigarh, India with Master in Surgery (MS) June 1972
  - Registrar of Surgery Chandigarh, India June 1972–1973
  - Government Medical College of Patiala, MI, 1969
  - Internships & Residencies Ascension Macomb–Oakland Hospital, Surgery, MI, 1977
  - Fellowship in Vascular Surgery, Beaumont Hospital-Royal Oak, Vascular Surgery, MI, July 1979–June 1980

SECTION 1: ANATOMY, PHYSIOLOGY, AND HEMODYNAMICS

MCQs 1–18

Q1. A common origin of the brachiocephalic artery and left common carotid artery (bovine aortic arch) is present in:
A. Under 10% of individuals
B. 11%–20% of individuals
C. 21%–30% of individuals
D. Greater than 30% of individuals

Q2. Dysphagia lusoria is caused by:
A. Aberrant aneurysmal left subclavian artery
B. Aberrant aneurysmal right subclavian artery
C. Double aortic arch
D. Right-sided aortic arch

Q3. The most common persistent embryogenic connection between the carotid and vertebrobasilar system persists in the form of:
A. Persistent hypoglossal artery
B. Persistent trigeminal artery
C. Persistent otic artery
D. Proatlantal intersegmental artery

Q4. The left vertebral artery may arise from the arch of the aorta in between the origins of the left common carotid artery and left subclavian artery in:
A. 0.4% of individuals
B. 5%–7% of individuals
C. 8%–11% of individuals
D. 12%–15% of individuals

Q5. Brachial artery variations occur in:
A. 5% of individuals
B. 6%–10% of individuals
C. 11%–15% of individuals
D. 16%–20% of individuals

Q6. The high origin of the anterior tibial artery from the popliteal artery occurs in:
A. 1%–4% of individuals
B. 5%–7% of individuals
C. 8%–10% of individuals
D. Greater than 10% of individuals

Q7. Cerebral autoregulation is the response of cerebral vessels to a change in arterial blood pressure. The threshold and saturation points of systemic mean blood pressure are approximately:
A. 60 mmHg and 150 mmHg
B. 70 mmHg and 140 mmHg
C. 80 mmHg and 130 mmHg
D. 90 mmHg and 120 mmHg

Q8. Resistance refers to the direct ratio of decrease in pressure to flow in a given vascular territory. The vascular territory that is responsible for the largest contribution to resistance is the:
A. Aorta
B. Arterioles
C. Capillaries
D. Venules

Q9. The largest contributor to vascular resistance is:
A. Vessel length
B. Blood viscosity
C. Radius of the vessel
D. Hematocrit

Q10. The wall shear stress for a given vessel radius is directly related to:
A. Larger viscosity
B. Larger velocity
C. Larger viscosity and larger velocity
D. Arterial wall strengthening

DOI: 10.1201/9781003389897-1

Q11. According to Laplace law, circumferential stress is inversely proportional to:
A. Pressure load on the vessel
B. Vessel radius
C. Wall thickness
D. Viscosity

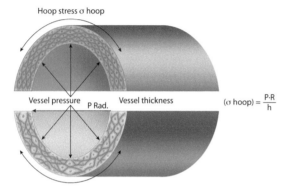

Laplace Law

Hoop stress σ hoop

Vessel pressure P Rad.   Vessel thickness

$$(\sigma \text{ hoop}) = \frac{P \cdot R}{h}$$

Q12. At low strains and pressures, the burden of bearing the stress is carried out by:
A. Elastin fibers
B. Collagen fibers
C. Endothelium
D. Blood components

Q13. All of the following statements about fibromuscular dysplasia (FMD) are true except:
A. Result of atherosclerosis
B. Result of non-inflammatory process
C. Primarily affects midsize vessels
D. Most often asymptomatic

Q14. A typical value of the pulse wave velocity is in the range of:
A. 0–4 m/s
B. 5–10 m/s
C. 11–15 m/s
D. Greater than 15 m/s

Q15. Fibromuscular dysplasia most often presents as:
A. Medial hyperplasia
B. Medial fibroplasia
C. Intimal fibroplasia
D. Perimedial fibroplasia

Q16. Just superior to the right renal artery the suprarenal aorta is separated from the interior vena cava by the:
A. Right crus
B. Median arcuate ligament
C. Left crus
D. Cisterna chyli

Q17. Vascular stiffness is determined by the ratio of elastin to collagen and by the thickness of the vessel wall and is expressed as:
A. More elastin causes more stiffness, with a thicker wall
B. More collagen and a thinner wall
C. More collagen and a thicker wall
D. Less elastin and a thinner wall

Q18. Laminar flow ceases when the Reynolds number is:
A. Less than 1000
B. 1001–1500
C. 1501–2100
D. Greater than 2000

RATIONALE 1–18

1. RATIONALE

The three main arteries of the head and neck supplying the cerebral arterial bed arise from the most proximal segment of the arch or the distal portion of the ascending aorta. Their origins may be quite separate or very close, as there may be a common origin of the brachiocephalic trunk with the left common carotid artery in 10% of the population. This variation has clinical significance, as the proximal landing zone is increased by such a variation during performance of thoracic endovascular aortic repair (TEVAR). During transfemoral left carotid artery stenting, access to the left common carotid artery may pose technical challenges. Occasionally, there is "V-shaped origin" of both common carotid arteries from a single short trunk before the continuation on each side of the neck.

Correct Answer **A** Under 10% of individuals

Reference
Berguer, R. (2014). Anatomy and function of the carotid and vertebral systems. In R. Berguer (Ed.), *Function and surgery of the carotid and vertebral arteries* (pp. 1–31). Philadelphia, PA: Lippincott, Williams and Wilkins.

2. RATIONALE

The aberrant right subclavian artery was first described in 1725 as arising from the descending thoracic aorta, is one of the most common congenital anomalies of the aortic arch and occurs in 0.05%–1% of the population. Symptoms of the aberrant right subclavian artery are mostly related to the development of aneurysmal disease, which occurs at its origin. The aneurysm can develop in nearly 60% of cases of aberrant right subclavian artery and is known as Kommerell diverticulum. Dysphagia may develop in early childhood or later in life due to aneurysmal changes. The course of the artery is usually posterior to the esophagus. The ideal method of diagnosis is barium esophagogram with confirmatory CT or MR angiography.

Correct Answer **B** Aberrant aneurysmal right subclavian artery

Reference
Levitt, B., & Richter, J. E. (2007). Dysphagia lusoria: a comprehensive review. *Dis Esophagus, 20*(6), 455–460. PMID: 17958718.

3. RATIONALE

Carotid basilar anastomoses are rare arterial anomalies in which embryonic connections between the carotid and vertebral arterial system persist. The persistent trigeminal artery is the most common and the most cephalad-located embryological anastomosis between the developing carotid artery and the vertebrobasilar system to persist into adult life. Its incidence ranges from 0.1% to 0.6% by MRA and CTA imaging. The persistent primitive hypoglossal artery has been reported in 0.03%–0.26% of cases undergoing cerebral arteriography. A persistent hypoglossal artery arises from the internal carotid artery between the cervical first and cervical second vertebral body levels and traverses through the hypoglossal canal to join the vertebrobasilar circulation.

Correct Answer **B** Persistent trigeminal artery

Reference
Meckel, S., Spittau, B., & McAuliffe, W. (2013). The persistent trigeminal artery: development, imaging anatomy, variants, and associated vascular pathologies. *Neuroradiology, 55*(1), 5–16. PMID: 22170080.

4. RATIONALE

After arising from the first part of subclavian artery, the vertebral artery ascends through the foramen in the transverse process of the sixth cervical vertebra into the first cervical vertebra and then it courses laterally, entering the skull through the foramen magnum and joins the opposite vertebral artery to form the basilar artery. Vertebral arteries are often (80%–85%) variable in their size. In many instances, one vertebral artery may be large and dominant with the contralateral vertebral artery hypoplastic or in rare circumstances even absent. The origin of the vertebral artery can be variable. They may arise from the second portion of the subclavian artery and may have a duplicate origin. The left vertebral artery may arise from the arch of the aorta between the left common carotid artery and left subclavian artery in 5%–7% of cases, and the vertebral artery may enter the fourth. fifth, or seventh cervical vertebra.

Correct Answer **B** 5%–7% of individuals

Reference
Satti, S. R., Cerniglia, C. A., & Koenigsberg, R. A. (2007). Cervical vertebral artery variations: an anatomic study. *AJNR Am J Neuroradiol, 28*(5), 976–980. PMID: 17494682.

5. RATIONALE

Anatomically, the axillary artery becomes the brachial artery at the lateral border of the teres major muscle and terminates by dividing into the radial and ulnar artery about 1 cm below the elbow joint. The brachial artery may occasionally divide proximally (in the middle of the upper arm) and then reunite. The brachial artery may course superficially in front of the median nerve and then behind the nerve (3.6%–9%). High bifurcation of the brachial artery into the radial and ulnar artery occurs in 8% of cases. Most often in this variant, the radial artery then becomes the brachioradial artery and courses on a superficial plane, while the ulnar artery and the common interosseous artery continue as a common trunk. Variations in the brachial artery have implications in clinical practice this may result in complications during vascular interventions and open reconstructions. High bifurcation of the brachial artery is important during performance of an arteriovenous graft for permanent hemodialysis access. Some studies have demonstrated inferior patency of arteriovenous grafts in patients with high bifurcation of the brachial artery.

Correct Answer **D** 16%–20% of individuals

Reference
Anbumani T. L., Anthony Ammal S. and Thamarai Selvi A. (2016). An anatomical study of variations in termination of brachial artery, with its embryological basis and clinical significance. *Int J Med Res Health Sci, 5*(3), 85–89. https://www.ijmrhs.com/medical-research/an-anatomical-study-on-the-variations-of-short-saphenous-vein-and-its-termination.pdf

6. RATIONALE

The popliteal artery terminates into anterior tibial artery and tibioperoneal trunk at the inferior border of the popliteus (4–5 cm below the knee joint line). The high origin of the anterior tibial artery or its aberrant course may increase the risk of iatrogenic arterial injury during knee surgery. In a review of femoral arteriograms in 1,242 patients, 89.2% had a normal branching pattern of the popliteal artery, hypoplastic or aplastic posterior tibial artery in 5.1%, hypoplastic or aplastic anterior tibial artery in 1.7%, true bifurcation in 1.4%, and high origin of the anterior tibial artery in 1.2%. When the branching pattern of the popliteal artery is normal in one extremity, there is a 13% probability that the contralateral side will have a variable pattern. When the branching pattern is variant in an extremity, there is a 28% probability that the opposite side will have a variant pattern.

Correct Answer   A 1%–4% of individuals

Reference
Kil, S. W., & Jung, G. S. (2009). Anatomical variations of the popliteal artery and its tibial branches: analysis in 1242 extremities. *Cardiovasc Intervent Radiol, 32*(2), 233–240. PMID: 18982387.

7. RATIONALE

The autoregulatory response to changes in blood pressure helps to maintain a constant and stable cerebral blood flow despite wide fluctuations in mean blood pressure. Decrease in blood pressure leads to cerebral vasodilation and increase in blood pressure leads to cerebral vasoconstriction. This autoregulation is much less effective at maintaining constant blood flow at mean pressures below 60 mmHg or mean pressure above 150 mmHg. This autoregulation is modulated by the activity of the autonomic nervous system renin-angiotensin system in the vessel wall, via CO_2, by vasoactive and morphologic changes in the vessel walls. This autoregulatory range is shifted toward the right in patients with long-standing hypertension. This autoregulatory response is also present in the coronary and renal vasculature, but not in the peripheral vasculature. Cerebral blood flow can be measured noninvasively by vascular Doppler sonography, magnetic resonance imaging, and near-infrared spectroscopy.

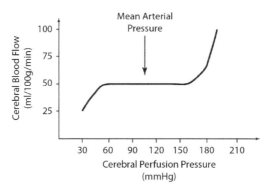

Correct Answer   A 60 mmHg and 150 mmHg

Reference
Willie, C. K., Tzeng, Y. C., Fisher, J. A., & Ainslie, P. N. (2014). Integrative regulation of human brain blood flow. *J Physiol, 592*(5), 841–859. PMID: 24396059.

8. RATIONALE

The arterioles constitute the vascular territory with the largest contribution to the resistance, as a maximum drop in pressure occurs in them. Arterioles are also known as resistive arteries. Mean arterial pressure is relatively constant in the aorta and the muscular, as well as elastic arteries with pulsatile flow. Pulsatility disappears greatly in the arterioles and is absent in capillaries and venules. Peripheral vascular resistance or systemic vascular resistance (SVR) is the resistance in the circulatory system that is used to create blood pressure and the flow of blood. When the blood vessels constrict, it leads to an increase in SVR and a decrease in SVR when blood vessels dilate. Vascular resistance is used to maintain organ perfusion, and in shock there is a decrease in SVR causing decreased organ perfusion. SVR is mediated by local metabolites and neurohormonal factors.

Correct Answer   B Arterioles

Reference
Delong, C., & Sharma, S. (2022). Physiology, peripheral vascular resistance. In *StatPearls*. Treasure Island (FL): StatPearls Publishing.

9. RATIONALE

It is apparent that the arterioles constitute the vascular territory with the largest resistance, as they experience the largest drop in pressure. These vessels are known as *resistive* arteries. The resistance is determined by several factors, including vessel length and diameter. *Poiseuille* flow is a useful concept from fluid mechanics to understand the relationship between flow, pressure, and resistance. The pressure gradient (ΔP) drives flow through the vessel, which moves from a point of higher pressure (pressure proximal) to a point of lower pressure (pressure distal). The flow has a parabolic shape, with a maximum velocity (velocity max) at the center of the lumen and zero velocity at the interface with the endothelial surface.

In the Hagen–Poiseuille flow equation, the relationship between flow (Q), pressure drop (ΔP), and resistance are:

$$Q = \frac{\pi R^4}{8\mu L} \Delta P$$

$$\text{Resistance} = \frac{8\mu L}{\pi R^4}$$

where μ is the blood viscosity, L is the vessel length over which the given pressure drop (ΔP) takes place, and R is the vessel radius. It is thus apparent that the vessel radius plays a much larger role in terms of vascular resistance than the vessel length due to its power-of-4 exponent. This explains why relatively small changes in vascular tone significantly alter vascular resistance (e.g., a 10% vasoconstriction results in an increase of 50% in vascular resistance).

Correct Answer   C Radius of the vessel

Resistance: Resistance refers to the ratio of the drop in pressure to flow in a vascular territory:

$$\text{Resistance}(R) = \frac{\text{Change in Pressure}}{\text{Flow}} = \frac{\Delta P}{Q}$$

Reference
Klabunde, R. E. (2012). *Cardiovascular physiology concepts*. Wolters Kluwer Health.

10. **RATIONALE**

The wall shear stress expresses the force per unit area exerted by the wall on the fluid in a direction on the local tangent plane. The fluid in the human body is represented by the blood. The typical value of the wall shear stress in the arterial system is 10–100 dynes/cm². Acting tangentially to the endoarterial surface, pressure is much larger (1000 times). Wall shear stress ($\tau = \mu$ velocity divided by R). It is obvious from this equation that a larger viscosity and velocity will lead to larger wall shear stress. High wall stress is the most important factor in the development of high-risk plaque. In a thoracic endograft, the wall shear stress acts tangentially to the surface of the endograft, whereas the pressure is perpendicular to the surface of the endograft.

$$\text{Wall shear stress } (\tau) = \mu \; \frac{\text{Velocity}_{max}}{R}$$

Correct Answer   C Larger viscosity and larger velocity

Reference
Figueroa, C. A., Taylor, C. A., & Chiou, A. J., et al. (2009). Magnitude and direction of pulsatile displacement forces acting on thoracic aortic endografts. *J Endovasc Ther, 16*(3), 350–358. PMID: 19642798.

11. **RATIONALE**

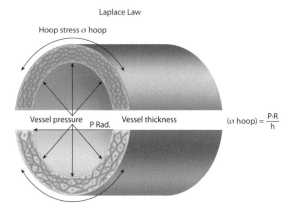

Laplace law for the gauge pressure inside a cylindrical membrane is given by $\Delta P = Y$ divided by r (Y/r), where Y is the surface tension and r is the radius of the cylinder. Therefore, there is an inverse relationship between the pressure and the radius. Hoop stress is the stress that occurs along the pipe's circumference when pressure is applied and acts perpendicular to the axial direction. Three principal stressors are measured when the ends are closed and the cylinder and the pipe are subjected to internal pressure: Hoop stress, longitudinal stress (L), and radial stress (r). In a thin-walled pipe with a wall thickness less than the diameter, radial stress is negligible. The hoop stress increases the pipe's diameter, whereas the longitudinal stress increases the pipe's length. Hoop stress is usually twice the size of the longitudinal stress. Hoop stress is also called tangential or circumferential stress. According to Laplace law, given equal end pressures and wall morphology, the wall of a larger-diameter blood vessel experiences greater tension than that of a smaller-diameter pipe (blood vessel).

$$\text{Wall tension follows Laplace's law:}$$
$$\text{Wall tension} = \text{Pressure} \times \text{Radius}$$
$$\text{Wall stress} = \frac{\text{Pressure} \times \text{Radius}}{2 \times \text{Wall thickness}}$$

Correct Answer **C** Wall thickness

Reference
Schmidt-Nielsen, K. (1990). *Animal physiology: adaptation and environment.* Cambridge University Press.

12. RATIONALE

The elastin matrix has a low stiffness value. At higher stress, the collagen fibers cause the vessel to become stiffer. The shape and compliance curves as well as stiffness curves for two different blood vessels are distinct, due to the axes of stress/pressure and strain/volume varying. Compliance is the change in the volume (Δv) imposed on the blood vessel by a given change in the pressure (ΔP) as the pulse pressure between the systole and diastole. The larger the pressure, the smaller the compliance. Distensibility (D) is equal to the ratio of changes in the luminal area between the systole and the diastole divided by the pulse pressure. Distensibility is therefore a similar metric to compliance obtained via changes in the luminal area of the vessel rather than via changes in volume. At low strains and pressures, elastin fibers bear the burden of stress, which has low values of stiffness.

Correct Answer **A** Elastin fibers

Reference
Ferruzzi, J., Collins, M. J., Yeh, A. T., et al. (2011). Mechanical assessment of elastin integrity in fibrillin-1-deficient carotid arteries: implications for Marfan syndrome. *Cardiovasc Res, 92*(2), 287–295. PMID: 21730037.

13. RATIONALE

Most patients with cerebrovascular FMD are asymptomatic middle-aged women who are otherwise healthy. The cause of FMD is unknown. Approximately 10% of patients with FMD have an affected family member as well. Patients may present with headaches or dizziness, and a carotid bruit may be detectable on physical examination. The incidence of ischemic cerebral events is quite low at long-term follow-up. Occasionally, cerebral ischemia secondary to a thromboemboli originating from a diseased arterial segment or from a low-flow state occurs. Patients may present with arterial dissection. There is a higher incidence of intracranial aneurysms in patients with internal carotid artery or vertebral artery FMD. Duplex ultrasound is a standard first-line modality in diagnosing FMD. However, Doppler velocity diagnostic criteria applicable to atherosclerotic disease are not reliable in the diagnosis of FMD. CTA or MRA of the neck are useful techniques in diagnosing FMD. CTA is preferable, but MRA may be helpful in diagnosing concurrent arterial dissection through simultaneously acquired T1-fat saturation images with a time-of-flight or gadolinium-enhanced imaging. Low-dose aspirin is indicated. Duplex surveillance to rule out aneurysmal degeneration should be obtained on a yearly basis. In selected cases balloon angioplasty is indicated in patients who fail medical management and in whom the lesion is progressive.

Correct Answer **A** Result of atherosclerosis

Reference

Kadian-Dodov, D., Gornik, H. L., & Gu, X., et al. (2016). Dissection and aneurysm in patients with fibromuscular dysplasia: findings from the U.S. registry for FMD. *J Am Coll Cardiol*, *68*(2), 176–185. PMID: 27386771.

14. RATIONALE

Pulse wave velocity represents the velocity at which the pressure and flow waves propagate through the circulatory system and indicates the speed at which a wave travels down an elastic vessel with typical values in the 5–10 m/s range. The speed is faster in the stiffer vessel. Pulse wave velocity is a biomarker of arterial stiffness, which is a known independent predictor of all-cause cardiovascular mortality in patients with hypertension. Pulse wave velocity increases with age for every blood pressure category, denoting an overall stiffness of the aorta with increasing age.

Correct Answer **B** 5–10 m/s

Reference

Xiao, N., Humphrey, J. D., & Figueroa, C. A. (2013). Multi-scale computational model of three-dimensional hemodynamics within a deformable full-body arterial network. *J Comput Phys*, *244*, 22–40. PMID: 23729840.

15. RATIONALE

Fibromuscular dysplasia is classified according to the affected segment of the arterial wall. The same classification is used for all the arteries affected by fibromuscular dysplasia. Medial fibroplasia is the most common (80%–90%), with a "string-of-beads" appearance secondary to alternating thinned and thickened medial ridges. This appearance on arteriography is secondary to stenotic webs that cause sequential stenosis and dilatations in the arterial wall. These dilatations may lead to aneurysmal degeneration. Intimal fibroplasia is responsible for about 10% cases of fibromuscular dysplasia, resulting in a long concentric stenotic lesion secondary to intimal collagen deposits. The differential diagnosis includes atherosclerosis, vasculitis, and connective tissue disorder.

Correct Answer **B** Medial fibroplasia

Reference

Poloskey, S. L., Olin, J. W., & Mace, P. (2012). Fibromuscular dysplasia. *Circulation*, *125*(18), e636–e639. PMID: 22566353.

16. RATIONALE

The right crus separates the suprarenal aorta from the inferior vena cava (IVC). During transperitoneal exposure of the juxtarenal aorta, the left renal vein may need to be divided close to the IVC to preserve collateral venous flow from the left kidney via the gonadal and adrenal vein. After division of the medial crus, the suprarenal aorta is carefully exposed and mobilized. The adrenal artery often needs to be ligated and divided before application of a suprarenal aortic clamp during transperitoneal repair of the juxtarenal abdominal aortic aneurysm. Mobilization of the left renal vein and placement of a silastic vessel loop around the left renal vein may provide adequate exposure for suprarenal artery clamping. It is important to decide which technique (mobilization or division) to use because preservation of these branches is critical to provide collateral venous outflow if the left renal vein needs to be ligated. The 5-year survival after open juxtarenal abdominal aortic aneurysm repair is 70%, even at centers of excellence with low perioperative mortality.

Correct Answer　**A** Right crus

Reference
Shepard, A. D. (2017). Open nonruptured infrarenal aortic aneurysm repair. In S. S. Hans, A. D. Shepard, & H. R. Weaver (Eds.), *Endovascular and open vascular reconstructions: a practical approach* (pp. 197–204). Boca Raton, FL: CRC Press.

17. RATIONALE

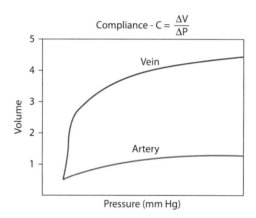

Vascular compliance and stiffness of the arterial wall influence the pulsatility of the pressure waveforms. Stiffness (E) is the ratio between increments in stress and strain. Vascular stiffness (E) is determined by the ratio of elastin to collagen fibers, with more collagen resulting in a thicker wall, which results in stiffer vessels. Vascular stiffness is a metric of vascular health, as it plays an important role in dampening the pulse of pressure as it propagates from the arterial tree. Compliance (C) is the change in volume (ΔV) imposed on the vessel by a given change in pressure (ΔP), such as the pulse pressure (PP) between the systole and diastole.

$$C = \frac{\Delta V}{\Delta P} = \frac{\Delta V}{\Delta PP}$$

The compliance of an artery depends on the pressure that it endures. The larger the pressure, the smaller the compliance. Distensibility (D) refers to the ratio of changes in the luminal area between systole and diastole divided by the pulse pressure. Viscosity is an important contributor to resistance. In fluids like plasma, the viscosity is constant, but whole blood has a complex viscosity pattern due to the mixture of plasma, cells, and proteins. Hematocrit levels have a profound effect on blood viscosity, with higher hematocrit greatly increasing the viscosity for all shear rates.

Correct Answer　**C** More collagen and a thicker wall

Reference

Xiao, N., Humphrey, J. D., & Figueroa, C. A. (2013). Multi-scale computational model of three-dimensional hemodynamics within a deformable full-body arterial network. *J Comput Phys*, *244*, 22–40. PMID: 23729840.

18. RATIONALE

Flow in a liquid pipeline (blood vessels in most instances) may be a smooth, laminar flow, also known as viscous flow. A visualization of laminar flow can be seen in the figure. Delaminar flow is characterized by a gradient of flow lines representing different blood velocities at different locations in a tube (blood vessels). These differences in blood flow velocities are due to shear stress. Because of friction, there is a decrease in the velocity of the blood closest to the wall. As the liquid (blood) flow rate is increased, the blood velocity increases, and the flow will change from laminar to turbulent flow with eddies. The Reynolds number is a value for a given fluid (blood), the conditions at which flow will remain laminar. Blood viscosity (cells and protein) is a variable affecting the Reynolds number. Laminar flow ceases when Reynolds number is greater than 2000.

Correct Answer D Greater than 2000

Reference

Falkovich, G. (2018). Basic notations and steady flows. In G. Falkovich (Ed.), *Fluid mechanics* (2nd ed., pp. 1–62). United Kingdom: Cambridge University Press.

SECTION 2: VASCULAR LABORATORY

MCQs 1–27

Q1. The ideal angle of insonation when interrogating the carotid artery during carotid duplex imaging is:
A. 30 degrees
B. 45 degrees
C. 60 degrees
D. 90 degrees

Q2. Echogenicity on a B-mode imaging is based on a comparison with a reference structure of a plaque. Select the appropriate combination for comparison:
A. Blood for hyperechoic
B. Bone for hypoechoic
C. Strap muscles for hypoechoic
D. Sternocleidomastoid muscles for isoechoic

Q3. The following flow pattern is identified in subclavian steal syndrome:
A. Reversal of flow in the ipsilateral carotid artery
B. Reversal of flow in the ipsilateral vertebral artery
C. Reversal of flow in the internal mammary artery
D. Reversal of flow in the subclavian artery

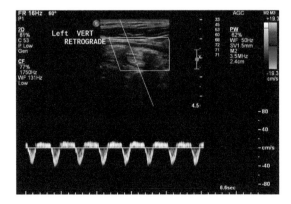

Q4. Transcranial Doppler evaluation is technically not feasible in:
A. Less than 5% of patients
B. 5%–15% of patients
C. 20%–30% of patients
D. Can be performed in all patients

Q5. A toe-brachial index is considered abnormal when the value is:
A. 0.9
B. 0.8
C. 0.7
D. 0.63 or less

Q6. Aliasing with carotid color duplex examination is most likely to occur with all of the following except:
A. Tortuous vessels
B. Low PRF settings
C. High PRF settings
D. Severe (hemodynamically significant) carotid stenosis

Q7. A 64-year-old man has classic symptoms of left hip claudication on walking 100 yards with the relief of the pain at rest. Peripheral pulses in the right lower extremity are normal. In the left lower extremity, pulses are slightly diminished but palpable. Ankle-brachial index is 1.0 on both sides. There is no history of back pain, and neurogenic claudication is ruled out by normal MRI of the lumbar spine.

The next course of action is:
A. CTA of abdomen and lower extremities
B. MRA of abdomen and lower extremities
C. Exercise testing
D. Catheter-based lower extremity arteriography

DOI: 10.1201/9781003389897-2

Q8. Flow signal is least dependent on Doppler angle with:
A. Gray-scale imaging
B. Color Doppler imaging
C. Power Doppler imaging
D. Pulsed Doppler spectral analysis

Q9. The limitations of carotid duplex examination include all of the following except:
A. Excessive carotid plaque calcification
B. Contralateral carotid occlusion
C. Excessive tortuosity or looping of ICA
D. Detection of intimal flap

Q10. The main advantage of MR angiography is:
A. Lower cost compared to other imaging modalities
B. Use of contrast medium is not necessary
C. Greater exposure to ionizing radiation
D. Better resolution than catheter-based arteriography

Q11. Multidetector CTA for cerebrovascular imaging is superior to MRA, as it is faster, easier to acquire, and less expensive than MRA. In terms of resolution, CTA has:
A. Same resolution as MRA
B. Better resolution than MRA
C. Inferior resolution than MRA
D. Less radiation

Q12. The best imaging technique for evaluation of the vertebral arteries is:
A. DSA
B. Duplex ultrasound
C. MRA
D. CTA

Q13. How does lower extremity CT angiography compare to catheter-based angiography?
A. Less contrast and lower radiation exposure
B. Less contrast but more radiation exposure
C. More contrast and more radiation exposure
D. More contrast and lower radiation exposure

Q14. A 60-year-old man has typical symptoms of bilateral hip claudication. His baseline ankle-brachial index (ABI) at rest is 0.98 on the right and 0.97 on the left. Post-exercise on a treadmill, ABI drops to 0.78 on the right and 0.72 on the left, with a return to baseline values after 15 minutes. What level of disease is most likely present in this patient?
A. Multilevel
B. Iliac artery occlusive disease
C. Femoral-popliteal occlusive disease
D. Neurogenic claudication

Q15. A dampened waveform with a delay to peak systole is seen in the common femoral artery. This type of pattern is seen in which of the following vascular pathologies?
A. Pseudoaneurysm
B. Distal occlusion
C. Aortoiliac occlusive disease
D. Arterial venous fistula

Q16. Which statement best reflects a hemodynamically significant stenosis in an artery?
A. An increase in the velocity at the site of stenosis
B. A decrease in the velocity at the site of stenosis
C. Increased pressure gradient across the stenotic segment
D. An increase in the velocity at the site of stenosis and increased pressure gradient across the stenotic segment

Q17. Volume flow in a brachiocephalic arteriovenous fistula for hemodialysis access is:
A. 500–600 mL/min
B. 601–700 mL/min
C. 701–800 mL/min
D. Greater than 800 mL/min

Q18. Plethysmography pulse-volume recordings are preferable to Doppler segmental pressures in patients with suspected lower extremity arterial occlusive disease in:
A. Type II diabetes mellitus
B. Peripheral neuropathy
C. Calcified arteries
D. Cases where the specific type or location of the lesion needs to be determined

Q19. **Flow reversal that is positive for superficial venous reflux is:**
A. >0.05 second
B. >0.5 second
C. >0.005 second
D. >5 seconds

Q20. **A phasic spectral waveform within the right subclavian vein and a pulsatile spectral Doppler waveform within the left subclavian venous flow suggests:**
A. An obstruction proximal to the left subclavian vein
B. An obstruction proximal to the right subclavian vein
C. An obstruction distal to the left subclavian vein
D. An obstruction distal to the right subclavian vein

Q21. **A monophasic fasting superior mesenteric artery signal is suggestive of which of the following complications:**
A. Median arcuate ligament syndrome
B. Superior mesenteric artery stenosis
C. Portal hypertension
D. A normal waveform

Q22. **For diagnosis of significant renal artery stenosis, an abnormal renal-to-aortic ratio is:**
A. <2
B. 2–2.5
C. 2.5–3.4
D. >3.5

Q23. **During the duplex evaluation of the femoral-popliteal in situ arterial bypass, the velocity at the proximal anastomosis is 80 cm/s. Doppler signal within 2 cm of the distal anastomosis detects a velocity of 220 cm/s. These findings are indicative of:**
A. <20% stenosis of the in situ bypass
B. Normal flow in the bypass
C. 20%–50% stenosis in the bypass
D. >50%–99% stenosis in the bypass

Q24. **The cold water immersion test results in a greater than 20% decrease in peak systolic pressure, which is suggestive of:**
A. Thoracic outlet syndrome
B. Primary Raynaud disease
C. Scleroderma with finger ulceration
D. Systemic lupus erythematosus

Q25. **A 70-year-old woman underwent SMA stenting and celiac artery stenting angioplasty for severe celiac artery stenosis and >70% stenosis of the SMA for symptoms of intestinal angina 5 years ago. On follow-up, peak systolic velocity (PSV) of the SMA is 402 cm/s with symptoms of vague abdominal discomfort. The PSV of the celiac artery is 260 cm/s. These findings suggest:**
A. >70% in-stent restenosis (ISR) of the celiac artery but <70% ISR of the SMA
B. >70% ISR of the SMA and <70% ISR of the celiac artery
C. <70% ISR of the celiac artery and SMA
D. >70% ISR of celiac artery and SMA

Q26. **A 76-year-old woman underwent carotid stenting for symptomatic greater than 70% stenosis of the right internal carotid artery. A follow-up carotid duplex at 2 years demonstrates a peak systolic velocity of 346 cm/s and IC/CC ratio of 4.20. This is suggestive of what degree of in-stent restenosis:**
A. ICA occlusion
B. Equal to or greater than 80% reduction
C. Equal to or greater than 50% reduction
D. Equal to or greater than 20% reduction

Q27. **The best noninvasive diagnostic imaging study for the diagnosis of vertebral artery dissection is:**
A. Duplex ultrasonography
B. CTA
C. MRA
D. Catheter-based arteriography

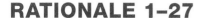

RATIONALE 1–27

1. RATIONALE

Carotid duplex scanning combines B-mode imaging, pulsed Doppler spectral analysis, and color-flow imaging. B-mode imaging helps in the evaluation of the carotid plaque morphology according to its echogenicity, with hypoechoic-like soft plaques, hyperechoic-like calcific plaques, or isoechoic. It can also determine if the plaque is homogeneous or heterogeneous. That may be attributed to intraplaque hemorrhage. Using B-mode imaging as a guide to the precise placement of the pulse Doppler gate velocity measurements and spectral sound analysis of the Doppler signals can be used to determine the degree of stenosis. An angle of 60 degrees between the axis of the artery and the sample volume should be maintained for velocity measurements. In patients with severe angulation or tortuosity, an angle of less than 60 degrees should be used. An angle greater than 60 degrees should never be used, as small errors in angle measurements will cause large errors in the calculation of velocity measurements.

Correct Answer   C 60 degrees

Reference
Gaiser, R., & Fox, T. B. (2016). *Vascular technology examination PREP* (1st ed.). New York: McGraw Hill.

2. RATIONALE

Echogenicity reflects the overall brightness of the plaque, with hyperechoic referring to echogenic (white) and hypoechoic referring to echolucent (dark or black) plaques. The reference structure to which echogenicity of the plaque should be compared is the blood for hypoechoic and bone for hyperechoic. Complicated carotid plaques that are more often associated with ipsilateral focal neurological symptoms are commonly echolucent and heterogenous with an irregular ulcerated surface in contrast to uncomplicated plaques often seen in asymptomatic patients that are usually hyperechoic homogeneous with a smooth surface. The reference structure for isoechoic plaque is the sternomastoid muscle.

Correct Answer   D Sternocleidomastoid muscles for isoechoic

Reference
Kremkau, F. W. (2020). Principles and instruments of ultrasonography. In J. S. Pellerito & J. D. Pollack (Eds.), *Introduction to vascular sonography* (pp. 23–55). Philadelphia, PA: Elsevier.

3. RATIONALE

Normally, the flow in the vertebral artery is toward the cranium. Demonstration of absent flow indicates occlusion. In patients with asymmetric flow in both vertebral arteries with symptoms of ischemia, upper extremity arterial Doppler is used to determine the difference between blood pressure in both arms. In most instances, subclavian steal syndrome is a hemodynamic entity. The so-called alternating flow (bunny rabbit) or total reversal of flow at rest demonstrates the stages of subclavian steal. It is called a syndrome if clinical symptoms of posterior ischemia develop.

Spectral Doppler showing a "bunny rabbit" waveform indicating latent or occult subclavian stenosis.

Correct Answer **B** Reversal of flow in the ipsilateral vertebral artery

Reference
Khan, S., Rich, P., Clifton, A., & Markus, H. S. (2009). Noninvasive detection of vertebral artery stenosis: a comparison of contrast-enhanced MR angiography, CT angiography, and ultrasound. *Stroke*, *40*(11), 3499–3503. PMID: 19762707

4. RATIONALE

Transcranial Doppler is helpful in evaluating blood flow in the circle of Willis in the brain through an intact skull. A 2-MHz pulsed Doppler is used to evaluate the intracranial MCA, ACA, PCA, and distal ICA, as well as the ophthalmic, vertebral, and basilar arteries through trans-temporal, transorbital, submandibular, and transforaminal windows in the skull. The temporal windows needed for evaluation are absent in 5%–15% of patients. The machine emits the sound pulse and waits for the time needed to make a round trip to and from the specific depth and then senses the reflected signal so that the direction of flow, pulsatility index, and velocity based on Doppler pulsatility can be determined. Each intracranial vessel can be insonated through a specific bone window and at a specific depth. Typically, the MCA is insonated through a temporal window at a depth of 30–60 mm with a flow toward the probe and a mean velocity of 55 ± 12 cm per second. Diagnosis of intracranial stenosis and occlusion is based on an increase in the velocity, post-stenotic turbulence, discrepancy between the two sides, and reversal of flow.

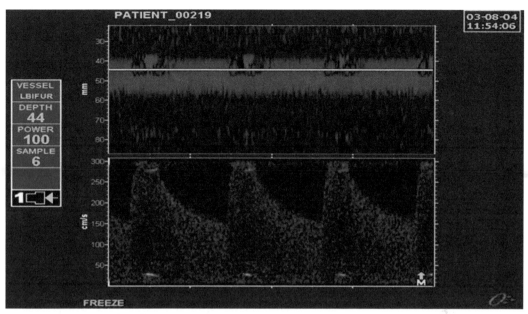

Left middle cerebral artery (MCA) stenosis showing elevated velocity in the left MCA as well as post-stenotic turbulence.

Correct Answer   **B** 5%–15% of patients

Reference
Ribo, M., & Alexandrov, A. (2007). Vertebral artery ultrasonography. In A. F. AbuRahma & J. J. Bergan (Eds.), *Noninvasive vascular diagnosis: a practical guide to therapy* (pp. 97–102). London: Springer-Verlag.

5. RATIONALE

A normal ankle-brachial index is 0.93–1.3, mild disease equals 0.8–0.9, moderate disease equals 0.4–0.8, and severe disease is less than 0.4. For the toe-brachial index, normal is equal to or greater than 0.63, mild disease is 0.4–0.62, moderate disease is 0.20–0.39, and severe disease is 0.19.

Ankle-Brachial Index	Toe-Brachial Index
Normal 0.93–1.3	Normal ≥0.63
Mild 0.8–0.92	Mild 0.4–0.62
Moderate 0.4–0.8	Moderate 0.20–0.39
Severe <0.4	Severe 0.19

Toe pressure measurement is performed in a similar fashion as arm and ankle pressure measurements. A mini cuff is placed around the base of the digit (commonly the first digit, but occasionally the second) and attached to the standard monometer. The most commonly used probes are photoplethysmography (PPG) probes and continuous-wave Doppler flow detectors placed on the distal phalanx. In patients with diabetes mellitus and chronic kidney disease, the tibial arteries are incompressible due to calcification and the ankle-brachial index is not obtainable. Toe pressures are sensitive to a decrease in arterial flow to the plantar arch and digital arteries.

In patients with calcification and non-compressibility of the digital arteries, transcutaneous oxygen measurements are more useful. Toe pressure and toe-brachial index are predictive of cardiovascular mortality and amputation-free survival in patients with peripheral arterial disease.

Correct Answer   D 0.63 or less

Reference
Rooke, T. W., Hirsch, A. T., & Misra, S., et al. (2012). 2011 ACCF/AHA focused update of the guideline for the management of patients with peripheral artery disease (updating the 2005 guideline): a report of the American College of Cardiology Foundation/American Heart Association Task Force on Practice Guidelines: developed in collaboration with the Society for Cardiovascular Angiography and Interventions, Society of Interventional Radiology, Society for Vascular Medicine, and Society for Vascular Surgery. *Catheter Cardiovasc Interv, 79*(4), 501–531. PMID: 21960485

6. RATIONALE

Pulsed wave spectral Doppler sends a pulse, and the machine waits until the return of that pulse before the next pulse is sent. Pulse repetition frequency (PRF) is the number of pulses transmitted in 1 second. Aliasing is a wraparound of the spectral waveform as it is out of insufficient sampling speed. If a sampling speed is low, the displayed waveform is incorrect, causing positive shift information to be displayed as negative. Aliasing is the result of the Doppler shift exceeding one half the PRF (Nyquist limits). In order to eliminate aliasing, the frequency shift needs to decrease and PRF needs to increase. Increasing the PRF can be achieved by increasing the Doppler PRF or decreasing the depth. The Doppler shift can be reduced by lowering the operating frequency of the transducers. A tortuous ICA, significant ICA stenosis, and low PRF have the potential to cause aliasing. Increasing the Doppler angle will also eliminate aliasing.

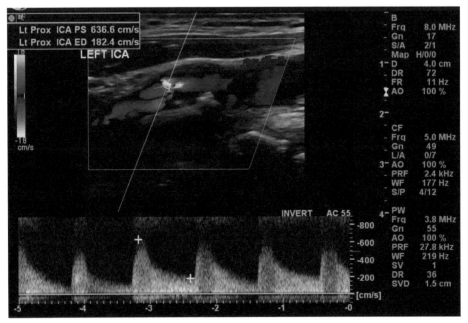

Color-flow and spectral Doppler image of the left internal carotid artery showing peak systolic velocities of 636 cm/s and end-diastolic velocities of 182 cm/s consistent with a 70%–99% stenosis. The color image also shows color "aliasing" indicating a high-grade lesion.

Correct Answer   C High PRF settings

Reference
Kremkau, F. W. (2020). Principles and instruments of ultrasonography. In J. S. Pellerito & J. D. Pollack (Eds.), *Introduction to vascular sonography* (pp. 23–55). Philadelphia, PA: Elsevier.

7. RATIONALE

Most patients with symptoms of intermittent claudication have a decreased ankle-brachial index (ABI) at rest. Exercise testing is performed in the select group of symptomatic patients with normal ABI. After measurements of resting ABI, BP cuffs are kept at both ankles and upper extremities and the patient walks on a treadmill 2 miles/hour at a 12-degree inclination for 5 minutes or the patient must stop because of pain. After resting, ankle and arm pressures are measured every 2 minutes for 10 minutes. If there is no decrease in ABI or there is an absence of symptoms, arterial occlusion can be ruled out. Patients with peripheral arterial disease but normal ABI at rest experience a mild drop in ABI after exercise that returns to baseline within minutes. Patients with moderate disease have a persistent decrease in ABI for 10–15 minutes post-exercise. The exercise test is more helpful in the diagnosis of iliac artery as compared to femoral artery occlusive disease. In patients who cannot tolerate walking on a treadmill, flow can be increased by reactive hyperemia using torniquet occlusion of a proximal cuff above the systolic blood pressure for 5 minutes.

Correct Answer   C Exercise testing

Reference
Stivalet, O., Paisant, A., Belabbas, D., et al. (2019). Exercise testing criteria to diagnose lower extremity peripheral artery disease assessed by computed-tomography angiography. *PLos One*, *14*(6), e0219082. PMID: 31247050

8. RATIONALE

Arterial duplex test interpretation is based on both normal B-mode gray-scale imaging and Doppler findings varying from normal to an increasing degree of stenosis. The velocity spectrum of the aorta, iliac, femoral-popliteal-tibial, and external carotid artery is triphasic with high outflow resistance with a systolic flow component, early reversal of flow in diastole, and a late diastolic forward flow. Low-resistance arterial flow as in renal, celiac, vertebral, and the ICA is continuous throughout the pulse cycle with a systolic flow component resulting in a monophasic pulsed Doppler signal. Color Doppler imaging refers to pixel encoding of blood flow (away or toward the transducer) and mean velocity. When the blood flow velocity is greater than the mean peak velocity, a threshold of the color bar (color aliasing) will occur as the pulse repetition frequency is no longer sufficient. Increasing the Doppler angle and pulse repetition frequency is used to reduce the aliasing artifact. Pulse Doppler imaging is based on the amplitude of a backscattered Doppler signal. The sensitivity of the flow direction increases three to five times as compared to color Doppler imaging. This technique is used for the evaluation of small-sized vessels and detection of slow or thicker flow associated with high-grade stenosis. Flow direction cannot be determined with power Doppler imaging, and the flow signal is less dependent on the Doppler angle. B-flow imaging reveals blood flow and a gray scale with different shades of gray and is most useful to demonstrate complex flow abnormalities in the bypass graft anastomosis and AV fistulas, as Doppler artifacts can obscure flow patterns.

Correct Answer **C** Power Doppler imaging

Reference
Moneta, G. L., Yeager, R. A., Antonovic, R., et al. (1992). Accuracy of lower extremity arterial duplex mapping. *J Vasc Surg, 15*(2), 275–283; discussion 283–274. PMID: 1735888

9. **RATIONALE**

Certain clinical situations, such as contralateral carotid occlusion, are associated with increased compensatory flow in the ipsilateral ICA resulting in overestimation of the degree of stenosis. In the presence of excessive tortuosity of the ICA, there is difficulty in insonating the artery at a 60-degree angle. Carotid plaque calcification results in certain areas of the vessel being hidden, which may be the most stenotic with underestimation of the degree of stenosis. The presence of tandem carotid lesions causes decreased flow due to proximal lesions or increased resistance with distal lesions. In cases of proximal brachiocephalic or proximal CCA lesions, the waveforms in the distal CCA and ICA can be dampened and have a delayed systolic rise time or a low slope-to-peak systole as compared to the contralateral side, leading to underestimation of the stenosis. In cases of significant distal disease in the ICA, the waveforms can become more of a high-resistance signal, where there is a sharp systolic rise time and significant reduction in diastolic flow that can go down to zero in cases of distal ICA occlusion. Decreased cardiac output may result in dampening of the waveforms on both sides. The presence of hypertension or tachycardia may result in increased pulsatility in the absence of carotid stenosis. Diffuse cerebrovascular disease may result in bilateral high-resistance waveforms in the absence of cervical disease. The presence of an intimal flap in a patient with spontaneous or traumatic ICA dissection can be easily diagnosed on carotid duplex study.

Correct Answer **D** Detection of intimal flap

Reference
El-Sayed, H. F., Mouawad, N. J., Satiani, B. (2018). Noninvasive vascular lab testing for carotids, vertebrals and transcranial Doppler. In S. S. Hans (Ed.), *Extracranial carotid and vertebral artery disease: contemporary management* (pp. 68–83). Cham, Switzerland: Springer Verlag.

10. **RATIONALE**

MRA is the only vascular imaging technique that can be performed without the injection of contrast media—a technique referred to as time-of-flight (TOF) MRA. In contrast to routine MRI, TOF MRA expresses a signal from stationary tissues instead of using the movement of blood in the lumen of the blood vessels to create a signal referred to as flow-related enhancement. In order to isolate flow in the arteries, venous flow enhancement is excluded by the use of saturation bands above the imaging volume, thus saturating flow from the cranial to caudal direction. TOF MRA can be performed using both 2D and 3D acquisition modes. An advantage of the 2D mode is a shorter imaging time and better sensitivity to slow flow, and it can visualize long segments of blood vessels. The disadvantages include decreased sensitivity to in-plane flow and decreased special resolution. A stair-step artifact worsened by patient motion can be seen. 3D TOF MRA is more commonly used to evaluate the head and circle of Willis and a smaller area where imaging is needed. In addition, 3D TOF MRA has superior resolution. Disadvantages include insensitivity to slow flow and longer acquisition time.

Contrast-enhanced MRA (CE MRA) relies on an intravascular contrast agent to directly generate a signal within the vessel lumen. CE MRA is able to acquire the same imaging volume in a shorter period of time using a single breath-hold, even for imaging a larger field. CE MRA is also acquired in the coronal plane, so that aortic arch disease can be assessed. CE MRA is more accurate than TOF MRA in the settings of slow-flow or high-grade stenosis, which can be overestimated with TOF MRA. TOF MRA is not limited in the setting of vascular calcification and should be preferred when calcification limits duplex imaging or CTA. Phase contrast MRA, a non-contrast imaging technique, is more often used for MR venography.

Correct Answer   **B** Use of contrast medium is not necessary

Reference

Brott, T. G., Halperin, J. L., Abbara, S., et al. (2011). 2011 ASA/ACCF/AHA/AANN/AANS/ACR/ASNR/CNS/SAIP/SCAI/SIR/SNIS/SVM/SVS guideline on the management of patients with extracranial carotid and vertebral artery disease: executive summary: a report of the American College of Cardiology Foundation/American Heart Association Task Force on Practice Guidelines, and the American Stroke Association, American Association of Neuroscience Nurses, American Association of Neurological Surgeons, American College of Radiology, American Society of Neuroradiology, Congress of Neurological Surgeons, Society of Atherosclerosis Imaging and Prevention, Society for Cardiovascular Angiography and Interventions, Society of Interventional Radiology, Society of NeuroInterventional Surgery, Society for Vascular Medicine, and Society for Vascular Surgery. *J Am Coll Cardiol, 57*(8), 1002–1044. PMID: 21288680

11. RATIONALE

Selective catheter-based arteriography using digital subtraction angiography (DSA) remains the gold standard in cerebrovascular imaging. Selective catheter-based DSA imaging of the cerebral vascular circulation is an invasive technique and carries a small risk (<1%) of neurological complications. CTA is performed following the rapid intravenous infusion of iodinated contrast with proper bolus timing to obtain an accurate assessment. CTA is obtained in the axial plane, and these axial images can be reformatted in the coronal and sagittal planes. Advanced postprocessing techniques allow for acquisition of 3D volume and surface-rendered images as well as segmentation techniques helping to isolate vessels from surrounding structures like bone and soft tissues. CTA allows for evaluation of the vessel lumen and vessel wall along with visualization of surrounding anatomical structures. Disadvantages include potential risk of contrast and exposure to ionizing radiation and preparation with steroids and antihistamines in patients with iodinated contrast allergies. Appropriate timing of imaging in relationship to the contrast bolus administration can be affected by cardiac output, speed of CT the scanner, and blood volume status of the patient. This may result in a lower-quality examination.

Correct Answer   **B** Better resolution than MRA

Reference

Lell, M., Fellner, C., Baum, U., et al. (2007). Evaluation of carotid artery stenosis with multisection CT and MR imaging: influence of imaging modality and postprocessing. *AJNR Am J Neuroradiol, 28*(1), 104–110. PMID: 17213434

12. **RATIONALE**

Posterior circulation strokes account for 15%–20% of all strokes, and 20%–25% of those are due to vertebral artery occlusive disease. Evaluation of the vertebral arteries is most challenging by CTA, MRA, and DUS due to their smaller size. One-half of patients will present initially with stroke, and 26% of patients present with TIA symptoms followed by stroke in a rapid fashion. The mortality associated with posterior circulation stroke is 20%–30%, which is much higher than an anterior circulation ischemic event. Up to one-third of vertebrobasilar ischemic episodes are caused by embolization from a plaque or mural lesions of the subclavian, vertebral, and basilar arteries.

The most common site of disease is at the origin of the vertebral artery that may not be well imaged by DUS or MRA. The best imaging modality for evaluation of vertebral disease is catheter-based angiography using the DSA technique in an oblique projection.

Correct Answer **A** DSA

Reference

Berguer, R., Flynn, L. M., Kline, R. A., & Caplan, L. (2000). Surgical reconstruction of the extracranial vertebral artery: management and outcome. *J Vasc Surg, 31*(1 Pt 1), 9–18. PMID: 10642704

13. **RATIONALE**

Lower extremity CT angiography (CTA) is indicated in the evaluation of peripheral arterial disease (PAD), trauma, congenital malformation, vasculitis, arterial variants, and surgical or endovascular planning. Three phases of imaging are generally performed: Precontrast imaging, arterial phase imaging, and venous delayed phase imaging. Arterial phase imaging is performed typically with either a fixed scan delay or bolus tracking. A fixed scan delay of 40 seconds enables imaging to automatically commence after the delay. Bolus tracking relies on achieving a predetermined attenuation (usually 100–120 Hounsfield units) within the area of interest in the infrarenal aorta, and imaging is initiated after a fixed time period. Typically, 100 cc of iodinated contrast is used, but this quantity may be increased to image larger patients or diminished if the patient is scanned on newer equipment with a faster speed table. Lowering the X-ray tube voltage and increasing the pitch with a helical CT scan decreases radiation exposure. Three-dimensional postprocessing with maximum intensity projection (MIP) multi-planar reformatted, 3D VR images and shaded surface displays can be used to augment analysis of the reconstructed cross-sectional axial images. Imaging the entire course of the vessel in a single plane (centerline) is useful in evaluating vascular density and planning for sizing of the endografts. In the presence of arterial calcification, the evaluation of arterial stenosis does compromise diagnostic accuracy with limited spatial resolution of CT, with partial volume averaging of different densities in a single voxel and high-density calcification increasing the density of tissues within the same voxel and adjacent voxels. This can exaggerate the size of the calcified plaque, causing a blooming artifact. Use of dual-energy CT (DECT) allows for the automatic reduction of CT luminograms by removing calcium and bone.

Correct Answer **A** Less contrast and lower radiation exposure

Reference

Ofer, A., Nitecki, S. S., & Linn, S., et al. (2003). Multidetector CT angiography of peripheral vascular disease: a prospective comparison with intraarterial digital subtraction angiography. *AJR Am J Roentgenol, 180*(3), 719–724. PMID: 12591682

14. RATIONALE

The normal response to exercise is either no change or an increase in the ABI following exercise. A reduction in the ABI following exercise indicates the presence of arterial occlusive disease. The greater the decrease in ABI, the more severe the disease. The recovery time to baseline ABI also provides information about the disease; if the recovery time is more than 12 minutes, multilevel disease is more likely. The treadmill test tends to be more positive with proximal disease since the aortoiliac vessels supply all the musculature of the lower extremities such as large gluteal muscles and muscles of the thigh, so that the effect of lesions in aortoiliac vessels is greater than those with isolated occlusion of the inferior femoral arteries. Exercise testing is not of any value for the diagnosis of infrapopliteal artery occlusive disease.

Correct Answer   A Multilevel

Reference
Stein, R., Hriljac, I., & Halperin, J. L., et al. (2006). Limitation of the resting ankle-brachial index in symptomatic patients with peripheral arterial disease. *Vasc Med*, *11*(1), 29–33. PMID: 16669410

15. RATIONALE

A dampened waveform with a delay to peak systole, also referred to as tardus parvus, in the common femoral artery is suggestive of significant proximal stenosis or occlusion (aortoiliac). This phenomenon is observed downstream to the site of stenosis and is the result of the magnitude of blood flow to the narrowed vessels during ventricular systole. This characteristic pattern is also useful in assessing for renal artery stenosis.

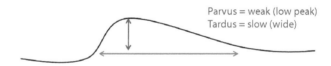

Correct Answer   C Aortoiliac occlusive disease

Reference
H., K., Jabaz, D. F., & Weerakkody, Y., et al. (2023, 1/20/2023). Tardus Parvus. Retrieved from https://radiopaedia.org/articles/tardus-parvus?lang=us

16. RATIONALE

In a normal artery, blood flow velocity and the pressure do not show any significant change. In the presence of hemodynamically significant stenosis within an artery, the pressure gradient increases across the segment of stenosis. There is an increase in the velocity of the blood flow within the stenosis. There is turbulent flow past the area of stenosis, resulting in a decrease in pressure distal to the stenosis as compared to the pressure proximal to the stenotic segment. This pressure change is referred to as the pressure gradient. The absolute value of blood pressure at this point is not relevant to blood flow.

Correct Answer   D An increase in the velocity at the site of stenosis and increased pressure gradient across the stenotic segment

Reference
Pellerito, J. (2019). Doppler flow imaging and spectral analysis. In *Introduction to vascular ultrasonography E-book* (pp. 56–84). Elsevier Health Sciences.

17. RATIONALE

A 7–12-MHz linear transducer is used to evaluate hemodialysis access. 2D gray-scale images, color Doppler images, pulse-wave spectral Doppler waveforms, volume flow measurements, and peak systolic velocity measurements are obtained. Volume fluid is calculated by the ultrasound machine. Diameter measurement is required to determine the area, and pulse-wave spectral Doppler measures the time averaged mean velocity.

Volume flow in the fistula equals the time average velocity multiplied by the area multiplied by 60, where area is the cross-sectional area of the vessel in square centimeters (since the vessel is cylindrical, its section is a circle whose area is calculated as the square of the radius.

Findings in normal hemodialysis access include:

1. Peak systolic velocity (PSV) between 150 and 300 cm/s
2. High diastolic flow with low-resistance waveform
3. High volume flow (greater than 500 mL/min)

Low volume flow (less than 500 mL/min) is indicative of severe stenosis. A focal increase in PSV >100% indicates severe stenosis, and these two findings may necessitate a fistulogram.

Correct Answer   **D** Greater than 800 mL/min

Reference
Gaiser, R., & Fox, T. B. (2016). *Vascular technology examination PREP* (1st ed.). New York: McGraw-Hill.

18. RATIONALE

When interpreting the segmental systolic limb pressures of the extremities, the following criteria are utilized to consider if the examination is normal:

1. Equal to or less than 30 mmHg difference between any two adjacent lower limb segmental systolic pressures
2. High thigh systolic pressure recordings equal to or greater than 30 mmHg above the higher brachial systolic pressure

In general, if the high thigh pressure is 30 mmHg or less when compared to high brachial pressure, this is indicative of iliac artery occlusive disease, and if similar findings are present on both sides, it may indicate bilateral iliac or aortic (infrarenal) stenosis. If the pressure gradient is 30 mmHg or higher between the thigh and calf, it indicates femoral-popliteal disease and between the calf and ankle indicates infrapopliteal disease. Pulse volume recordings (PVRs) are performed using the same cuffs as the segmental pressures, so the PVR waveforms are acquired at the same levels. PVR waveforms represent the entire amount of perfusion through the underlying segment of the limb, including collateral flow. PVR waveforms cannot distinguish between collateral flow and regular flow, with the possibility of underestimating the severity of the disease. PVR waveforms are not influenced by cuff artifact or arterial calcification, thus making them more reliable in arterial flow assessment. A cuff artifact may occur when the width of the blood pressure cuff is either too large or too small for the limb. If the width of the cuff is less than 20% of the limb diameter, it will result in a falsely elevated peak systolic pressure. If the width of the cuff is too large, it can result in a peak systolic pressure that is artificially lower.

Correct Answer   **C** In patients with calcified arteries

Reference
Gaiser, R., & Fox, T. B. (2016). *Vascular technology examination PREP* (1st ed.). New York: McGraw-Hill

19. **RATIONALE**

Pulse-wave (PW) spectral Doppler should be used to identify and quantify flow reversal in the caudal direction following distal compression. The normal response of blood flow in the deep and superficial veins following distal compression should have no reversal of blood flow or very little reversal. When the reversal of blood flow exceeds 0.5 second in the standing position, it is considered significant for venous reflux. Some literature suggests that for deep venous reflux, it should be 1.0 second because of the larger size of the deep veins. The extended reversal of blood flow that occurs when the distal compression is released is considered significant and a positive sign for venous insufficiency. Venous reflux can also be evaluated by performing proximal compression or having the patient perform a Valsalva maneuver. The normal response should be cessation of flow followed by augmentation and resumption of flow in the correct (cephalad) direction upon release. When venous reflux is present, there will be a reversal of blood flow (caudal direction) and the normal cephalad direction will be resumed when released.

Correct Answer   **B** >0.5 second

Reference
Gaiser, R., & Fox, T. B. (2016). *Vascular technology examination PREP* (1st ed.). New York: McGraw-Hill

20. **RATIONALE**

On spectral analysis, the veins that are farther away from the heart will have waveforms like that of the lower extremity. Veins with spontaneity, augmentation in response to distal compression, and with phasic flow as demonstrated in the axillary, basilic, and brachial veins. The veins closer to the heart such as internal jugular; brachiocephalic (difficult to insonate); and subclavian veins demonstrate cardiac pulsations and respiratory patterns. Any change from each vein's normal waveform may be indicative of proximal obstruction. Lack of spontaneity and phasicity indicates distal and proximal obstructions, respectively, for the veins farther from the heart, as in veins of the lower extremity. A continuous waveform with loss of pulsatility in the central veins is usually indicative of a proximal obstruction. That is the reason behind obtaining a venous study on both sides. If a normal pulsatile waveform is demonstrated in the right subclavian vein and on the left side a phasic waveform with minimal pulsatility is seen, it may suggest a proximal obstruction on the left side.

Correct Answer   **B** An obstruction proximal to the right subclavian vein

Reference
Gaiser, R., & Fox, T. B. (2016). *Vascular technology examination PREP* (1st ed.). New York: McGraw-Hill

21. **RATIONALE**

Mesenteric duplex imaging is typically performed with a low frequency (2–8 MHz) curvilinear transducer in a fasting state (at least 8–10 hours). The study is repeated about 30 minutes after eating a meal if the fasting waveforms are normal. Gray-scale images of the celiac axis, SMA, and rarely IMA followed by color and spectral Doppler study is obtained. In a fasting state, the celiac axis (main supply to the liver and spleen) has a low-resistance distal bed. The SMA should have a high-resistance waveform due to constricted arterioles distally in the resting state. After a meal, there is arteriolar dilatation to increase the blood supply to the intestines, with a change to a low-resistance flow pattern with forward flow in all phases of the cardiac cycle. If in the fasting state the SMA flow pattern is low resistance (monophasic), then a postprandial study is not necessary, as distal arterioles are abnormally persistently dilated due to hypoxia. For a diagnosis of mesenteric ischemia, velocity measurements are diagnostic. For the celiac artery, normal peak systolic velocity is 50–160 cm/s, and peak systolic velocity greater than 200 cm/s predicts 70% diameter stenosis. For the SMA, normal PSV (110–177 cm/s) with peak systolic velocity greater than 275 cm/s predicts greater than 70% stenosis. If significant celiac axis stenosis/occlusion is suspected, the gastroduodenal artery should be imaged to evaluate for retrograde flow, as the gastroduodenal artery becomes an important collateral circulation source to the liver and spleen via the pancreaticoduodenal arteries from the SMA in the presence of celiac axis occlusion.

Correct Answer   **B** Superior mesenteric artery stenosis

Reference
AbuRahma, A. F., Stone, P. A., Srivastava, M., et al. (2012). Mesenteric/celiac duplex ultrasound interpretation criteria revisited. *J Vasc Surg*, *55*(2), 428–436.e426; discussion 435–426. PMID: 22195765

22. **RATIONALE**

The renal-to-aortic ratio is not accurate when the peak systolic velocity (PSV) of the aorta is less than 40 cm/s or greater than 90–100 cm/s. Normal PSV is less than 180 cm/s at the origin, proximal, mid, and distal renal artery. PSV of greater than 180–200 cm/s along with post-stenotic turbulence is suggestive of equal to or greater than 60% diameter reduction of the renal artery. An abnormal resistive index (equal to or greater than 0.7) is indicative of renal artery stenosis; the resistive index is calculated by PSV minus EDV divided by PSV. Acceleration time and index are measured by calipers along the systolic slope. The normal acceleration time is less than 0.1 second. A delay in the acceleration slope, also known as tardus parvus, present as a rounding of the systolic peak, is suggestive of an obstruction proximal to the point of sampling.

Correct Answer   **D** >3.5

Reference
Neumyer, M. M. (2000). Native renal artery and kidney parenchymal blood flow duplex examination with and without color flow imaging. In C. Rumwell & M. McPharlin (Eds.), *Vascular technology: an illustrated review* (pp. 101–103). Davies Pub.

23. **RATIONALE**

Duplex surveillance of the lower extremity bypass (femoral-popliteal/tibial) in conjunction with ankle-brachial indices are extremely useful for detecting occult stenosis in the bypass. A 10- to

12-MHz or 5- to 7-MHz linear transducer is used depending on the type (vein or prosthetic) and depth of the bypass. Duplex surveillance of the infrainguinal bypass includes 2D gray-scale imaging, color Doppler images, and a pulse-wave spectral Doppler waveform with measurements of peak systolic velocity at the:

1. Inflow artery

2. Proximal anastomosis

3. Proximal bypass

4. Mid-bypass

5. Distal bypass

6. Distal anastomosis

7. Outflow artery

A significant stenosis manifests as doubling of the peak systolic velocity between the adjacent segments and represents greater than 50% stenosis (hemodynamically significant). In addition, there is evidence of post-stenotic turbulence just distal to the stenosis and a reduced peak systolic velocity value with a delayed rise farther distal to the area of stenosis. In patients undergoing in situ vein bypass reconstruction, there remains a possibility of a retained venous branch resulting in an arteriovenous fistula.

Correct Answer   D >50%–99% stenosis in the bypass

Reference
Tinder, C. N., Chavanpun, J. P., Bandyk, D. F., et al. (2008). Efficacy of duplex ultrasound surveillance after infrainguinal vein bypass may be enhanced by identification of characteristics predictive of graft stenosis development. *J Vasc Surg, 48*(3), 613–618. PMID: 18639428

24. RATIONALE

The cold immersion test is performed to confirm the diagnosis of primary Raynaud disease with intermittent symptoms of numbness and cold in response to cold temperatures or stress in the fingers and, uncommonly, the toes. Areas of the skin turn white and then blue. The digital arteries supplying the skin develop vasospasms, limiting blood flow. Testing for primary Raynaud disease is completed by first obtaining digital photoplethysmogram (PPG) waveforms and pressures at rest in a normal-temperature environment followed by immersion of the hands or feet in a basin of ice water for 1–3 minutes. Once the hands and feet are taken out of the ice water, they are dried and digital waveforms and pressures are obtained at 2 minutes, 5 minutes, and 10 minutes. Resting digital pressures should be near 90% of the higher brachial pressure. The PPG waveform is normally similar to the PVR waveform – a rapid upstroke, sharp peak, and a dicrotic notch. In patients with:

1. Raynaud disease, a peak pulse waveform may be seen on the pre-immersion PPG waveform where the dicrotic notch is higher than normal

2. Decrease in systolic pressure of greater than 20% pre-immersion

3. Waveform resumes pre-immersion waveform pattern within 5–10 minutes of being removed from ice water

In thoracic outlet syndrome, there is a reduction in flow in certain maneuvers as noted by the PPG waveform. These maneuvers consist of:

A. Military position (palms facing forward and elbows posteriorly)

B. Overhead abduction of 180 degrees

C. Arms at 90 degrees abduction posteriorly

D. Adson maneuver with arms abducted out to the sides (90 degrees) with the head turned to either side

Correct Answer **B** Primary Raynaud disease

Reference
Gaiser, R., & Fox, T. B. (2016). *Vascular technology examination PREP* (1st ed.). New York: McGraw-Hill.

25. RATIONALE

The ability of native duplex ultrasound criteria to accurately predict ISR continues to be the focus of further studies. It has been demonstrated that native vessel criteria overestimate the degree of in-stent stenosis. Patients with superior mesenteric artery and celiac artery stents tend to have an increased peak systolic velocity, and therefore native peak systolic velocity criteria are unreliable for the determination of in-stent restenosis. The PSV criteria of ≥70% stenosis is higher for ISR than for native visceral stenosis. The velocity criteria that define equal to or greater than 70% in-stent restenosis of the SMA is equal to or greater than 445 cm/s and equal to or greater than 289 cm/s for a stented celiac artery.

Correct Answer **C** <70% ISR of the celiac artery and SMA

Reference
Soult, M. C., Wuamett, J. C., Ahanchi, S. S., et al. (2016). Duplex ultrasound criteria for in-stent restenosis of mesenteric arteries. *J Vasc Surg*, 64(5), 1366–1372. PMID: 27633165

26. RATIONALE

Receiver operating characteristic analysis demonstrated the following optimal threshold criteria: residual stenosis > or = 20% (PSV > or = 150 cm/s and ICA/CCA ratio > or = 2.15), in-stent restenosis > or = 50% (PSV > or = 220 cm/s and ICA/CCA ratio > or = 2.7), and in-stent restenosis > or = 80% (PSV 340 cm/s and ICA/CCA ratio > or = 4.15).

Progressively increasing PSV and ICA/CCA ratios correlate with evolving restenosis within the stented carotid artery. Ultrasound velocity criteria developed for native arteries overestimate the degree of in-stent restenosis encountered. These changes persist during long-term follow-up and across all grades of in-stent restenosis after CAS. The proposed new velocity criteria accurately define residual stenosis > or = 20%, in-stent restenosis > or = 50%, and high-grade in-stent restenosis > or = 80% in the stented carotid artery.

Correct Answer **B** Equal to or greater than 80% reduction

Reference
Lal, B. K., Hobson, R. W., 2nd, Tofighi, B., et al. (2008). Duplex ultrasound velocity criteria for the stented carotid artery. *J Vasc Surg*, 47(1), 63–73. PMID: 18178455

27. RATIONALE

Conventional catheter-based arteriography is seldom necessary for the diagnosis of extracranial dissection despite being the most sensitive diagnostic study because of its invasive nature. The classic signs for dissection seen on neuroimaging are an enlarged artery with a crescent-shaped rim of hyperintense signal from the hematoma that is surrounding the decreased lumen. In 41%–75% of cases, dissection may present with the radiographic "rat's tail or string sign," which represents a tapered stenosis on neuroimaging. CTA has a high sensitivity and specificity; however, it is associated with radiation exposure and can pose a technical challenge in obtaining the high-quality imaging of the vertebral arteries. CTA offers more advantages over MR angiography in visualization of the vertebral arteries due to bony artifacts on MRI being unable to provide a clear visualization of the vertebral arteries. Catheter-based arteriography is unable to visualize intramural hematomas.

Correct Answer   B CTA

Reference

Debette, S., & Leys, D. (2009). Cervical-artery dissections: predisposing factors, diagnosis, and outcome. *Lancet Neurol, 8*(7), 668–678. PMID: 19539238

SECTION 3: RADIATION SAFETY

MCQs 1–5

Q1. The threshold effective single dose of radiation resulting in dermal necrosis is:
A. 10 Sv
B. 11–19 Sv
C. 20–24 Sv
D. 25 Sv

Q2. A statistically significant increase in cancer risk has not been proven in populations exposed to doses of less than:
A. 100 mSv
B. 200 mSv
C. 300 mSv
D. 400 mSv

Q3. Per ICRP recommendations, the annual whole-body dose limit for physicians in 1 year should not exceed:
A. 20 mSv
B. 30 mSv
C. 40 mSv
D. 50 mSv

Q4. The typical effective dose in computed tomography of the abdomen is:
A. 5 mSv
B. 10 mSv
C. 20 mSv
D. 25 mSv

Q5. What amount of scattered radiation dose will decrease if the square of the distance of the operator doubles?
A. Twofold
B. Fourfold
C. Sixfold
D. Eightfold

DOI: 10.1201/9781003389897-3

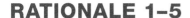

RATIONALE 1–5

1. RATIONALE

The deterministic effects of radiation are dose dependent resulting in cell death; loss of hair follicles; and effects on the skin, bone marrow, gonads, and lens of the eye. These acute events take place when the threshold level of radiation has been exceeded. The dose required to produce these determinative effects often exceed 1–2 Sv. Symptoms develop when a significant proportion of cells are killed by radiation with a subsequent inflammatory response and eventual fibrosis, resulting in further organ damage. The effective threshold of a single dose (Sv) resulting in temporary sterility is 0.1, permanent sterility is 3–6, cataracts is 0.5, bone marrow depression is 0.5, transient erythema of the skin is 2, desquamation is 2–10, temporary hair loss is 4, dermal necrosis is 25, and skin atrophy is 10 (Sv).

Correct Answer   D 25 Sv

Reference
National Research Council. (2006). *Health risks from exposure to low levels of ionizing radiation: BEIR VII phase 2*. Washington, DC: National Academies Press.

2. RATIONALE

The stochastic effects of radiation cause cell mutations resulting from DNA damage to a single cell and are unrelated to the dose. Mutations may lead to cancer and heritable genetic defects. Radiation doses of less than 100 mSv/year in terms of stochastic effects is very low. Leukemia and other cancers have been associated with radiation exposure. The probability of fatal cancer developing as a result of radiation exposure is 4% per 1 Sv of a lifetime dose equivalent. Among atomic bomb survivors, there is an increase in sickle cell leukemia, lung, thyroid, breast, skin, and GI tract tumors. A statistically significant risk of cancer has not been demonstrated in populations exposed to doses of less than 100 mSv. The latent period of development of malignancy following radiation exposure is 2–5 years for leukemia, 5 years for thyroid cancer, and 10 or more years for other cancers.

Correct Answer   A 100 mSv

Reference
Laurier, D., Richardson, D. B., Cardis, E., et al. (2017). The international nuclear workers study (in works): a collaborative epidemiological study to improve knowledge about health effects of protracted low-dose exposure. *Radiat Prot Dosimetry*, *173*(1–3), 21–25. PMID: 27885078

3. RATIONALE

The maximum permissible dose (MPD) is the upper limit of the allowed radiation dose that one may receive without the attendant risk of significant side effects. The annual whole-body dose limit for physicians is 50 mSv. The ICRP safety dose recommendations call for a whole-body effective dose limit of 20 mSv/1 year, average dose 5 years. For ocular lens, 20 mSv/yr; skin, 500 mSv/yr; and extremities, 500 mSv/yr. The ICRP system of protection in medical practice stresses the basic principles of justification, optimization dose, and risk limits. It is the responsibility of the hospital and medical personnel to ensure that the radiation equipment is maintained (preventative maintenance) to deliver the lowest dose of radiation and to ensure the safety instructions and all productive measures are adopted by all involved personnel. Hospitals have radiation physicists overseeing the radiation safety, and systems of reporting and immediate measures are in place in situations where the recommended dose limit is exceeded.

Correct Answer   **D** 50 mSv

Reference
Rehani, M. M., Ciraj-Bjelac, O., Vañó, E., et al. (2010). ICRP Publication 117. Radiological protection in fluoroscopically guided procedures performed outside the imaging department. *Ann ICRP*, *40*(6), 1–102. PMID: 22732420

4. RATIONALE

Whenever possible, for diagnostic evaluations, MRI or ultrasound imaging should be considered, as there is no radiation involved with these two modalities. The effective dose of spiral and multislice detector CT scans is 10%–30% higher than with past-generation CT scans. In order to reduce radiation exposure to a CT scan following endovascular aneurysm repair (EVAR), techniques such as automated tube current modulation or attenuation-based kilovoltage selection algorithms can be used. The effective dose of a CT scan of the abdomen and pelvis is in the range of 10–20 mSv, and repeated CT exams following the EVAR effective dose may approach harmful levels. The risk of development of solid organ malignancy from a postoperative CT scan following EVAR is higher in women, young patients, and patients undergoing repeated scans. Dyna CT (three-dimensional rotational angiography) results in a mean dose produced in the range of 3500–4000 u Gym², which is about 8 times a reduction in the radiation as compared to standard multidetector CT.

Correct Answer   **B** 10 mSv

Reference
Smith-Bindman, R., Lipson, J., Marcus, R., et al. (2009). Radiation dose associated with common computed tomography examinations and the associated lifetime attributable risk of cancer. *Arch Intern Med*, *169*(22), 2078–2086. PMID: 20008690

5. RATIONALE

All personnel performing X-ray imaging studies should maintain the maximum distance from the X-ray tube. The image intensifier should be kept as close to the patient and the tube as far away as possible to reduce the dose to the patient's skin. The amount of scattered radiation decreases with the square of the distance to the tube. Exposure equals 1/d2. Therefore, the radiation dose will diminish fourfold if the distance from the operator doubles. The left anterior oblique view exposes the operator extending on the right side of the patient to the greatest amount of radiation, as the tube is closest to the operator. The radiation dose is 3–5 times higher than the right anterior oblique view. Steep gantry angulations also increase radiation exposure. Use of ceiling-mounted plexiglass should be used to decrease exposure from scattered radiation. Raising the fluoroscopic table and lowering the imaging intensifier decreases radiation exposure. A 0.25-mm lead-equivalent apron, lead glasses, and thyroid shields should always be worn. The front of the lead apron should be kept away from the X-ray tube. Protective gloves (at least 0.35-mm lead equivalent) are not often used due to reduced tactical sensitivity. Lead-equivalent surgical caps reduce the exposure to the brain during interventions. Radiation safety training should be a component of every training program in surgery.

Correct Answer   **B** Fourfold

Reference

Haqqani, O. P., Agarwal, P. K., Halin, N. M., & Iafrati, M. D. (2012). Minimizing radiation exposure to the vascular surgeon. *J Vasc Surg*, *55*(3), 799–805. PMID: 22079168

SECTION 4: VASCULAR MEDICINE

MCQs 1–14

Q1. Each of the following antiplatelet medications has been proven to reduce the risk of stroke except:
A. Ticagrelor
B. Aspirin and dipyridamole
C. Clopidogrel
D. Aspirin

Q2. Which statin was the first to be shown to reduce the risk of stroke in patients with previous stroke and no history of coronary artery disease?
A. Atorvastatin
B. Lovastatin
C. Simvastatin
D. Pravastatin

Q3. In the CREST-2 trial the target for lowering LDL is:
A. <130 mg/dL
B. <100 mg/dL
C. <70 mg/dL
D. <50 mg/dL

Q4. A 65-year-old man is scheduled to undergo percutaneous iliac stenting for a common artery occlusion with symptoms of disabling claudication. He is a known former smoker (10 pack-years). He has a history of well-controlled hypertension and dyslipidemia. He denies symptoms of chest pain or shortness of breath. The pre-intervention cardiac assessment should include:
A. Nuclear cardiac stress test
B. CTA coronary arteries
C. 2D echocardiogram
D. Preintervention testing is not necessary

Q5. A 70-year-old woman is scheduled to undergo open repair of a juxtarenal abdominal aortic aneurysm. She quit smoking 1 month ago and has a 50-pack-year history of smoking. Which of the following statements best reflects her risk of developing pulmonary complications?
A. Cessation of smoking 6 months prior to the operation
B. Cessation of smoking 1 year prior to the operation
C. Her risk of pulmonary complications does not increase even if she does not quit smoking prior to the operation
D. Cessation of smoking within 2 months of the operation

Q6. A 50-year-old man with a history of type I diabetes mellitus is scheduled to undergo arteriography of the lower extremities for ischemic gangrene of the right big toe. Serum creatinine is 1.5 mm/dL (eGFR 40 mL). The best strategy for the prevention of contrast-induced nephropathy is:
A. Administration of dopamine
B. Preprocedure hydration with normal saline
C. Preprocedure hydration with normal saline for 12 hours followed by postprocedure hydration with normal saline, reducing the volume of the contrast and use of diluted contrast and using CO_2 angiography whenever feasible
D. Obtain MRA of the lower extremities instead of catheter-based arteriography

DOI: 10.1201/9781003389897-4

Q7. A 62-year-old man had a femoral-tibial bypass for critical limb ischemia 3 days ago. His postoperative course is uncomplicated. His hemoglobin on postoperative day 3 is 7.4 gm/dL. The transfusion trigger in this patient is:
A. Hemoglobin less than 10 gm/dL
B. Hemoglobin less than 9 gm/dL
C. Hemoglobin less than 8 gm/dL
D. Hemoglobin less than 7 gm/dL

Q8. A 66-year-old man on apixaban for atrial fibrillation presents with a ruptured juxtarenal aortic aneurysm not suitable for endovascular repair. The most suitable agent to reverse the action of apixaban is:
A. Fresh-frozen plasma
B. Idarucizumab
C. Recombinant factor XA (Andexxa)
D. Warfarin

Q9. The following are the risk factors for postoperative delirium except:
A. Baseline dementia
B. Poor vision/hearing
C. Presence of infection
D. Age less than 65 years

Q10. The incidence of postoperative atrial fibrillation following open abdominal aortic reconstruction is:
A. <5%
B. 5%–10%
C. 11%–15%
D. >15%

Q11. The most important risk factor for postoperative renal failure following open aortic reconstruction is:
A. Mean blood pressure of 60 mmHg for 2 hours
B. Warm renal ischemia time of 30 minutes
C. Need for blood transfusion
D. Preoperative chronic kidney disease

Q12. The peak incidence of heparin-induced thrombocytopenia following open aortic reconstruction is on postoperative days:
A. 0–4
B. 5–10
C. 11–15
D. 16–20

Q13. A 70-year-old man with a history of atrial fibrillation with a CHADS score of 2 on apixaban is scheduled to undergo open juxtarenal AAA repair. When should apixaban be stopped?
A. Stop apixaban 24 hours before the operation
B. Stop apixaban 48 hours before the operation
C. Stop apixaban 5 days before the operation
D. The patient should undergo hemodialysis to clear the apixaban

Q14. A 76-year-old man presents to the ER with dizziness and presyncope. The patient is in atrial fibrillation with heart rate of 110 per minute. CTA of the neck shows less than 50% stenosis of the bilateral internal carotid arteries with a hypoplastic right vertebral artery and the left vertebral artery has 50% stenosis at its origin. CT scan of the brain shows chronic white matter changes. The optimal management consists of:
A. Vertebral artery transposition into the common carotid artery
B. Urgent cardiology consult
C. ENT consult
D. Discharge patient on antiplatelet medication and beta-blockers

RATIONALE 1–14

1. RATIONALE

Antiplatelet medications are recommended for secondary prevention of noncardioembolic ischemic stroke and TIA. Clopidogrel, extended-release dipyridamole, cilostazol, and ticagrelor have been studied for stroke prevention. The effect of antiplatelet medications is achieved through several mechanisms. Aspirin irreversibly blocks the cyclooxygenase (COX) activity of the prostaglandin H synthase 1 and 2 (COX 1 and COX 2). COX 1 inhibition permanently alters the thromboxane A2–dependent platelet aggregation and vasoconstriction. Dipyridamole and cilostazol are phosphodiesterase inhibitors. Clopidogrel, prasugrel, and ticagrelor inhibit the adenosine-dependent platelet aggregation. Clopidogrel and prasugrel need activation by the cytochrome P-450 enzyme. Aspirin and extended-release dipyridamole are superior to aspirin alone in preventing major vascular events. The optimal medical management for carotid stenosis is antiplatelet medication, statins, targeted blood pressure reduction, and smoking cessation. Guideline-directed treatment of diabetes mellitus, physical activity, medication and diet, and evaluation of sleep apnea are important in reducing the risk of stroke.

Correct Answer **A** Ticagrelor

Reference

Marquardt, L., Geraghty, O. C., Mehta, Z., & Rothwell, P. M. (2010). Low risk of ipsilateral stroke in patients with asymptomatic carotid stenosis on best medical treatment: a prospective, population-based study. *Stroke, 41*(1), e11–17. PMID: 19926843

2. RATIONALE

According to the results of the Stroke Prevention by Aggressive Reduction of Cholesterol Levels (SPARCL) trial, treatment with atorvastatin in patients with carotid stenosis as compared to placebos was associated with a 33% reduction in the risk of any stroke. In 2004 systematic reviews and meta-analysis of randomized trials testing statin drugs concluded that each 10% reduction in LDL was estimated to reduce the risk of all strokes by 15.6%. For patients undergoing interventions such as carotid artery stenting and statin treatment, the incidence of cardiovascular events was significantly lower in patients with statin pretreatment than in those without pretreatment. For patients with symptomatic carotid stenosis, a perspective population-based study from Denmark reported that the early risk of recurrent stroke in patients with symptomatic carotid stenosis is dramatically reduced following urgent aggressive medical therapy, including statins.

Correct Answer **A** Atorvastatin

Reference

Amarenco, P., Bogousslavsky, J., Callahan, A., 3rd, et al. (2006). High-dose atorvastatin after stroke or transient ischemic attack. *N Engl J Med, 355*(6), 549–559. PMID: 16899775

3. RATIONALE

CREST-2 is an ongoing trial to evaluate CEA or CAS compared to intensive medical management for asymptomatic carotid stenosis of 70–99%. Intensive medical management consists of aspirin 325 mg daily, with patients undergoing carotid stenting (CAS) also receiving clopidogrel in addition to aspirin for 30–90 days. The goal of systolic blood pressure is ≤140 mmHg and an

LDL of <70 mg/dL. For patients with hyperlipidemia who are not able to reach the target LDL with statin therapy, treatment with injectable PCK9 inhibitors is a good option, as these medications have shown to reduce cardiovascular events in patients with hyperlipidemia

Correct Answer **C** <70 mg/dL

Reference
Howard, V. J., Meschia, J. F., Lal, B. K., et al. (2017). Carotid revascularization and medical management for asymptomatic carotid stenosis: protocol of the CREST-2 clinical trials. *Int J Stroke*, *12*(7), 770–778. PMID: 28462683

4. RATIONALE

The extent to which the cardiac assessment is to be performed prior to a vascular procedure depends on the overall procedural risks, the patient's comorbidities, and the patient's exercise capacity. A patient who is undergoing a low-risk percutaneous intervention may be sufficiently cleared by a history that is negative for chest pain and shortness of breath, while those who require general anesthesia at a minimum should have a 12-lead electrocardiogram prior to open arterial reconstruction. Patients selected to undergo high-risk open repair such as open abdominal aortic reconstruction, lower extremity bypass, or any patients with a significant history of cardiac disease including unstable angina, known cardiac arrhythmias, severe valvular disease, or congestive heart failure should undergo evaluation by a cardiologist first. Patients with unstable or stable angina involving the left main coronary artery or triple-vessel disease should undergo coronary revascularization prior to major vascular reconstruction. When patients who have reconstructed coronary artery disease need an alternative intervention, existing coronary artery disease should be treated with balloon angioplasty or bare metal stent placement followed by dual antiplatelet therapy for 4–6 weeks.

Correct Answer **D** Preintervention testing is not necessary

Reference
Malek, J., & McElroy, I. (2020). Preoperative risk assessment. In S. S. Hans & M. F. Conrad (Eds.), *Vascular and endovascular complications: a practical approach* (pp. 1–5). Boca Raton, FL: CRC Press.

5. RATIONALE

Pulmonary complications are more common following major open vascular reconstruction performed via a thoracic or thoracoabdominal incision. Active smokers are counseled to stop smoking for at least 2 weeks prior to moderate- and high-risk procedures to decrease the incidence of pulmonary complications. Patients are at highest risk for complications within the first 2 months of quitting smoking, and their risk becomes equal to a nonsmoker after 6 months. For patients with long-standing tobacco use, COPD, and poor baseline respiratory function, preoperative pulmonary function tests and arterial blood gases are recommended. These patients should be started on bronchodilators for at least 2 weeks prior to open arterial reconstruction.

Correct Answer **D** Cessation of smoking within 2 months of the operation

Reference
Malek, J., & McElroy, I. (2020). Preoperative risk assessment. In S. S. Hans & M. F. Conrad (Eds.), *Vascular and endovascular complications: a practical approach* (pp. 1–5). Boca Raton, FL: CRC Press.

6. RATIONALE

For patients at risk for contrast-induced nephropathy prehydration with normal saline for 12 hours, use of diluted contrast (1:1 with normal saline), reducing the volume of the contrast, and continuation of intravenous normal saline for 12 hours following arteriography have a beneficial effect. Whenever possible, CO_2 angiography should be substituted in place of iodinated contrast in patients with CKD, as it does not have allergic potential or risk of renal toxicity. A CO_2 angiography study may be inadequate for visualization of infrapopliteal arteries. Contrast-enhanced MRA with gadolinium in the presence of CKD is associated with nephrogenic systemic fibrosis, and there has been a recent resurgence regarding the application of noncontrast MRA techniques in the evaluation of peripheral artery disease. Newer approaches such as quiescent-interval slice-selective, velocity-sensitive, three-dimensional fast spin echo magnetic resonance angiography is an attractive alternative to CTA or DSA.

Correct Answer   C Preprocedure hydration with normal saline for 12 hours followed by postprocedure hydration with normal saline, reducing the volume of the contrast and use of diluted contrast and use of CO_2 angiography whenever feasible

Reference
Gleeson, T. G., & Bulugahapitiya, S. (2004). Contrast-induced nephropathy. *AJR Am J Roentgenol,* *183*(6), 1673–1689. PMID: 15547209

7. RATIONALE

The decision to transfuse should be based on clinical assessment of the patient's results of laboratory tests and evidence-based guidelines. Pooled results from three trials with 2364 participants showed that a restrictive hemoglobin transfusion trigger of <7 gm/dL resulted in reduced in-hospital mortality, total mortality, rebleeding, acute coronary syndrome, pulmonary edema, and bacterial infections compared with a more liberal strategy.[1]

Another clinical trial showed that a low trigger (Hgb <8.0 gm/dL) was associated with a higher rate of death or major complications and that further trials were recommended.[2]

Correct Answer   D Hemoglobin less than 7 gm/dL

References
1. Salpeter, S. R., Buckley, J. S., & Chatterjee, S. (2014). Impact of more restrictive blood transfusion strategies on clinical outcomes: a meta-analysis and systematic review. *Am J Med,* *127*(2), 124–131. e123. PMID: 24331453
2. Møller, A., Nielsen, H. B., Wetterslev, J., et al. (2019). Low vs high hemoglobin trigger for transfusion in vascular surgery: a randomized clinical feasibility trial. *Blood,* *133*(25), 2639–2650. PMID: 30858230

8. RATIONALE

The procoagulant effects of recombinant factor XA (Andexanet alfa) are anchored through the ability to bind to and sequester factor XA inhibitors. The increase in available factor XA reduces anticoagulant action. In clinical trials the median decline in anti–factor XA activity for apixaban or rivaroxaban was 88% or higher. Andexanet alfa also binds tissue factor inhibitor pathways or peptides that inhibit factor XA. Adverse effects include deep vein thrombosis, arterial thrombosis, pulmonary embolism, and ischemic stroke. Idarucizumab is used for the reversal of dabigatran.

Correct Answer   **C** Recombinant factor XA (Andexxa)

Reference
Siegal, D. M., Curnutte, J. T., Connolly, S. J., et al. (2015). Andexanet alfa for the reversal of factor XA inhibitor activity. *N Engl J Med*, *373*(25), 2413–2424. PMID: 26559317

9. RATIONALE

Delirium occurs in approximately 80% of elderly patients admitted to a critical care unit. Delirium increases the length of stay in a critical care unit and increases the days that a patient is on a ventilator, as well as morbidity and mortality. The risk of delirium is increased in hearing and visually impaired individuals, use of narcotics during the hospital stay, use of restraints, prehospital cognitive impairment, heavy alcohol abuse, and polypharmacy withdrawals. Inadequate pain control may also contribute to delirium. Delirium is characterized by a disorganized thought process, inattention, and altered level of consciousness. Normalization of the patient's environment, usual sleep–wake cycles, presence of family at the bedside, and access to glasses and hearing aids is helpful. Removal of restraining devices and early immobilization are also beneficial. Benzodiazepine and diphenhydramine may contribute to delirium and therefore should be avoided. Dexmedetomidine is a useful drug in the management of delirium.

Correct Answer   **D** Age less than 65 years

Reference
Barr, J., Fraser, G. L., Puntillo, K., et al. (2013). Clinical practice guidelines for the management of pain, agitation, and delirium in adult patients in the intensive care unit. *Crit Care Med*, *41*(1), 263–306. PMID: 23269131

10. RATIONALE

The incidence of atrial fibrillation following open abdominal aortic reconstruction nears 10%. Factors predisposing to atrial fibrillation include advanced age, hypertension, coronary artery disease, valvular heart disease, ischemic cardiomyopathy, prior history of atrial fibrillation, and chronic obstructive pulmonary disease. Treatment is based on controlling the heart rate and reducing the risk of embolic events. In hemodynamically unstable patients, electric cardioversion is the treatment of choice. In patients who are hemodynamically stable, rate control with beta-blockers, calcium channel blockers, and amiodarone is often implemented. If atrial fibrillation persists for longer than 48 hours, anticoagulation with unfractionated heparin should be considered.

Correct Answer   **B** 5%–10%

Reference
Valentine, R. J., Rosen, S. F., Cigarroa, J. E., et al. (2001). The clinical course of new-onset atrial fibrillation after elective aortic operations. *J Am Coll Surg*, *193*(5), 499–504. PMID: 11708506

11. RATIONALE

Acute kidney injury has been shown to occur in as many as one in five patients postoperatively. Patients who have preoperative chronic kidney disease have the highest risk of postoperative renal failure. Other factors include prolonged perioperative hypotension, prolonged renal ischemia, and need for blood transfusion. Use of iodinated contrast and rhabdomyolysis are also contributing factors. Patients who develop postoperative renal failure have been shown to develop other organ dysfunction with longer ICU length of stay and increased mortality. Prevention of acute kidney injury begins preoperatively with appropriate planning to maximize renal protection and continued fluid resuscitation. Adequate replacement of blood products intraoperatively and postoperatively is important in preventing transient hypotension and supporting renal blood flow. Limiting warm renal ischemia time to <40 minutes in open pararenal AAA is an important factor in decreasing the renal metabolic requirements. Intraoperative use of mannitol during aortic cross-clamping, though controversial, improves urine flow rate, attenuates renal cortical blood flow reduction, and scavenges oxygen free radicals. Hemodialysis should be considered for patients with significant acidosis, hyperkalemia, volume overload, and uremic symptoms.

Correct Answer **D** Preoperative chronic kidney disease

Reference
Ellenberger, C., Schweizer, A., Diaper, J., et al. (2006). Incidence, risk factors and prognosis of changes in serum creatinine early after aortic abdominal surgery. *Intensive Care Med, 32*(11), 1808–1816. PMID: 16896848

12. RATIONALE

Heparin-induced thrombocytopenia (HIT) may be encountered after vascular reconstruction due to the exposure to heparin in patients and results of the formation of immunoglobin antibodies against the heparin-platelet factor IV complex. These complexes coat platelets, activate them, and cause them to be removed by macrophages, resulting in thrombocytopenia. There is generally a 30%–50% decline in platelet count 5-10 days after initiation of heparin. Bleeding complications are extremely uncommon in patients with HIT. Thrombotic complications, particularly venous, are the most common. Management of HIT-positive patients begins with immediate discontinuation of unfractionated and low molecular weight heparin on suspicion. If there is a need for anticoagulation, direct thrombin inhibitors are preferable. Anticoagulation is recommended for 1 month for non-thrombotic HIT and for 3-6 months with thrombotic HIT.

Correct Answer **B** 5-10 days

Reference
Arepally, G. M. (2017). Heparin-induced thrombocytopenia. *Blood, 129*(21), 2864–2872. PMID: 28416511

13. RATIONALE

For procedures/surgeries in the high-risk category such as major surgeries lasting longer than 45 minutes, major abdominal/pelvic surgery, cardiothoracic surgery, vascular or urologic surgery, or major orthopedic surgery, a strategy of oral anticoagulation interruption of four to five half-lives preprocedure (5 days off warfarin and 2 days off the DOAC) and resumption 2-3 days postprocedurally. In the case of a treatment dose, UFH or LMWH bridging therapy for warfarin and for DOAC in general would be associated with an acceptable periprocedural bleeding risk. In warfarin-treated patients, resumption of LMWH bridging at the treatment dose after high-bleeding-risk procedures confers a 20-fold higher risk for major bleeds. In patients with atrial fibrillation on warfarin with treatment interrupted for an elective operation or invasive proce-dure, forgoing bridging anticoagulation was non-inferior to perioperative bridging with LMWH for the prevention of arterial thromboembolism and a decreased risk of bleeding.

Correct Answer   **B** Stop apixaban 48 hours before the operation

Reference
Douketis, J. D., Spyropoulos, A. C., Kaatz, S., et al. (2015). Perioperative bridging anticoagulation in patients with atrial fibrillation. *N Engl J Med*, *373*(9), 823–833. PMID: 26095867

14. RATIONALE

The minimal anatomical requirement to justify vertebral artery reconstruction for patients with true hemodynamic symptoms is stenosis greater than 60% in both vertebral arteries if both vertebral arteries are patent and are complete, or the same degree of stenosis in the dominant vertebral artery and if the opposite vertebral artery is hypoplastic and ends in a posteroinferior cerebellar artery or is occluded. Surgical reconstruction is not indicated in an asymptomatic patient with stenotic or occlusive vertebral lesions, as these patients are well compensated by the carotid circulation through the posterior communicating arteries. A single normal vertebral artery is sufficient to adequately perfuse the basilar artery, regardless of the patency status of the contralateral vertebral artery. On the other hand, patients with symptomatic vertebrobasilar ischemia due to emboli are candidates for surgical reconstruction regardless of the condition of the contralateral vertebral artery. The most common site of disease is at the origin of the verte-bral artery and is best displayed by catheter-based arteriography in oblique projection. Patients with suspected vertebral artery compression should undergo dynamic arteriography, which incorporates provocative positioning. Delayed imaging may be able to demonstrate reconstitu-tion of the distal vertebral artery via the cervical collaterals.

Correct Answer   **B** Urgent cardiology consult

Reference
Berguer, R., Flynn, L. M., Kline, R. A., & Caplan, L. (2000). Surgical reconstruction of the extracranial vertebral artery: management and outcome. *J Vasc Surg*, *31*(1 Pt 1), 9–18. PMID: 10642704

SECTION 5: CEREBROVASCULAR DISEASE

MCQs 1–55

Q1. Transcarotid revascularization (TCAR) is considered a better approach to carotid stenting as compared to a transfemoral approach in which of the following circumstances:
- **A.** Patients with type III aortic arch
- **B.** Patients with contralateral recurrent laryngeal palsy
- **C.** Disease in the common carotid artery 4 cm above the clavicle
- **D.** Patients with bilateral common femoral venous thrombosis

Q2. During transcarotid artery revascularization (TCAR), the retrograde flow is confirmed along with the patient's hemodynamic status, with the maintenance of blood pressure between:
- **A.** 100 and 120 mmHg systolic
- **B.** 120 and 140 mmHg systolic
- **C.** 140 and 160 mmHg systolic
- **D.** 160 and 180 mmHg systolic

Q3. A relative contraindication to transfemoral carotid artery (CA) stenting includes all of the following except:
- **A.** Thrombus in the ICA
- **B.** Circumferential plaque calcification
- **C.** Thrombus at the origin of the common carotid artery
- **D.** Type I aortic arch

Q4. During transfemoral CAS there is a change in the neurological status of the patient, and a brisk aspiration of the sheath is performed. The patient's blood pressure, heart rate, and oxygen saturation are satisfactory. Contrast injection (a small amount) shows absent flow in the ICA with deformity of the stent. The next best procedure is:
- **A.** Intravenous nitroglycerin
- **B.** Terminate the procedure and perform a CEA
- **C.** Consider TCAR
- **D.** Aspiration with an export catheter

Q5. During transfemoral carotid angioplasty/stenting, the patient experiences significant bradycardia (heart rate <40/min) with a systolic blood pressure of 100 mmHg. What is the next course of action?
- **A.** Deflate the balloon and administer 1 mg intravenous atropine
- **B.** Temporary pacing
- **C.** Abandon the procedure and perform CEA
- **D.** Continue the procedure with volume resuscitation

Q6. A 70-year-old man presents with chest and back pain. Past history includes coronary artery bypass graft with the left internal mammary artery to the left anterior descending artery bypass and chronic obstructive pulmonary disease. CT scan shows a large penetrating ulcer in the inferior wall of the transverse arch opposite the origin of the left subclavian artery. The most important next step in management is:
- **A.** Repeat CT scan of the chest in 6 months
- **B.** Open repair of the thoracic aorta
- **C.** Endovascular stent graft with repair of the thoracic aorta, with left subclavian artery revascularization if symptoms develop
- **D.** Left common carotid artery to subclavian artery bypass followed by endovascular repair of the thoracic aorta

DOI: 10.1201/9781003389897-5

Q7. A 35-year-old woman presents with worsening right upper extremity ischemia. She has a history of febrile illness in the past year. Her right axillary, brachial, and radial pulses are absent with blood pressure in the right upper extremity of 60 mmHg as compared to 100 mmHg systolic in the left upper extremity. CTA demonstrates brachiocephalic artery occlusion and 50% stenosis of the left common carotid artery. The best management option is:
A. Brachiocephalic artery endarterectomy
B. Axilloaxillary artery bypass
C. Brachiocephalic artery stenting via right brachial artery access
D. Aorto-brachiocephalic (innominate) bypass graft

Q8. Factors affecting both the procedural and long-term outcome for endovascular therapy for supra-aortic trunk vessel occlusive disease include:
A. Length of the lesion
B. Stenosis versus occlusion
C. High burden of ostial calcification
D. Length of the lesion, occlusion of the aortic arch branch as compared to stenosis, and severe ostial calcification

Q9. A 66-year-old woman was referred by her primary care physician for absent left brachial and radial pulses. The right arm blood pressure is 130 systolic and the left arm blood pressure is 74 mmHg. A duplex examination reveals severe stenosis approaching occlusion in the proximal left subclavian artery. She has no symptoms of upper extremity fatigue on exertion or symptoms of vertebrobasilar insufficiency. The best management option for this patient is:
A. Transposition of the left subclavian artery to the left common carotid artery
B. Left carotid–subclavian artery bypass
C. Left subclavian artery stenting
D. Risk factor modification without any intervention

Q10. The incidence of perioperative stroke and death in patients undergoing carotid endarterectomy and simultaneous proximal intervention is:
A. Same as for carotid endarterectomy
B. Two times that of isolated carotid endarterectomy
C. Three times that of isolated carotid endarterectomy
D. Four times that of isolated carotid endarterectomy

Q11. The incidence of stroke following stenting of an aortic arch vessel is:
A. <1%
B. 1%–1.9%
C. 2%–2.9%
D. >3%

Q12. The incidence of brachial artery (access) thrombosis following stenting of an aortic arch lesion is:
A. <1%
B. 2%
C. 3%
D. >3%

Q13. A 62-year-old man sustained a minor stroke (NIH stroke scale 4) in the distribution of the left middle cerebral artery (MCA). Carotid duplex and CTA show greater than 70% stenosis at the origin of the left internal carotid artery with less than 50% stenosis of the right internal carotid artery. MRI of the brain shows a small embolic stroke in the distribution of the left MCA on the diffusion scan. He is at moderate risk for carotid revascularization. What is the next step in the management of this patient?
A. Carotid revascularization should be performed 6 weeks after the stroke
B. Carotid revascularization should only be performed if the patient develops recurrent stroke
C. Early carotid endarterectomy/carotid artery stenting should be considered within 10 days of the stroke
D. Carotid artery stenting has a better outcome than carotid endarterectomy in this setting

Q14. The number of patients requiring shunt placement during carotid endarterectomy (CEA) under cervical block anesthesia (awake) is:
A. Less than 5%
B. Approximately 10%
C. Approximately 15%
D. Approximately 20%

Q15. Patients undergoing CEA under cervical block anesthesia (CBA) as compared to general anesthesia have:
A. A lower incidence of perioperative neurological complications
B. A decreased incidence of neck hematoma
C. More stable hemodynamics during and immediately after CEA
D. Earlier discharge

Q16. A 62-year-old man had just completed a left CEA under general anesthesia with EEG monitoring and is ready to be re-extubated. EEG shows mild ischemic changes on the ipsilateral side along with positive median nerve evoked potential study. He cannot move his right upper extremity. The incision is reopened; the CEA site appears to be satisfactory. On-table carotid arteriogram reveals a normal carotid endarterectomy site but with occlusion of the main trunk of the middle cerebral artery. The next best management option is:
A. Intravenous heparin therapy
B. Initiate tPA infusion into the internal carotid artery and middle cerebral artery
C. Emergent CT scan of the head
D. Neurovascular interventionalist consult for retrieval of the plaque/thrombus with stent-assisted mechanical recanalization for acute MCA occlusion

Q17. The most common nerve injury during carotid endarterectomy is:
A. Vagus
B. Hypoglossal
C. Glossopharyngeal
D. Ramus mandibularis

Q18. Prosthetic patch site infection following carotid endarterectomy is best treated with:
A. Debridement, removal of the patch, autologous reconstruction, and antibiotics
B. Interposition of a synthetic graft, debridement, and antibiotics
C. Ligation of the ICA and antibiotics
D. Antibiotics only

Q19. A 72-year-old man undergoes carotid endarterectomy for 80% stenosis of the right internal carotid artery with contralateral ICA occlusion. Seventy-two hours following the CEA, the patient wakes up with a headache and contralateral motor paralysis. CT scan of the head reveals an intracerebral hemorrhage without midline shift. The next step in the management of this patient is:
A. Continue medical management
B. Insert a ventriculo-jugular shunt
C. Urgent neurosurgical consult for possible craniotomy
D. This complication could have been avoided if carotid artery stenting was performed

Q20. During carotid endarterectomy for high plaque, the distal end of the intimal flap could not be well visualized. The procedure is completed with the application of a patch graft. The next best step to consider should be:
A. Perform on-table carotid/cerebral arteriogram
B. Carotid duplex imaging
C. Transcranial Doppler study
D. No further study is necessary if there is no evidence of neurological deficit

Q21. The most commonly injured nerve during distal (high) exposure of the ICA with division of the posterior belly of the digastric, stylohyoid muscle, and styloid process is:
A. Hypoglossal
B. Vagus
C. Spinal accessory
D. Glossopharyngeal

Q22. A 70-year-old man developed symptoms of focal TIA in the distribution of the right middle cerebral artery with >70% stenosis of the right ICA, with the cephalad end of the plaque at the level of the body of the second cervical vertebra. The plaque is markedly calcified with a suspicion of overlying thrombus. The optimal management is:
A. Carotid artery stenting
B. CEA with high distal exposure
C. Medical management
D. Carotid ligation

Q23. Protamine administration reduces bleeding complications associated with carotid endarterectomy, but it results in:
A. Increased risk of stroke
B. Unincreased risk of stroke
C. Increased incidence of MI
D. Increased incidence of death

Q24. A 60-year-old woman underwent right carotid endarterectomy with bovine pericardial patch under general anesthesia for high-grade stenosis of the right internal carotid artery presenting with symptoms of transient loss of vision in the right eye. Heparin was not reversed at the end of the operation. Six hours later the patient developed tense swelling in the neck without difficulty in breathing. However, the patient has difficulty swallowing her saliva and has a low-pitched, hoarse voice. The next best option is:
A. Immediate CT scan of the neck
B. Reversal of heparin with protamine
C. Emergent re-exploration of the neck in the OR
D. Exploration of the neck at the bedside

Q25. An 80-year-old woman undergoes carotid endarterectomy for high-grade symptomatic carotid stenosis. Postoperatively myocardial infarction (MI) is diagnosed with new ST-segment changes and elevated troponin level. Which statement reflects the long-term survival in this patient?
A. The patient has the same long-term survival as compared to those who did not sustain postoperative MI after carotid endarterectomy

B. The patient is more likely to have decreased survival during the first 5 years postoperatively
C. The patient is more likely to develop cardiac arrhythmias in the follow-up
D. The patient is more likely to need coronary revascularization

Q26. The Eversion Carotid Endarterectomy Versus Standard Trial (EVEREST) demonstrated that:
A. Eversion carotid endarterectomy had no difference in restenosis rates when compared with primary closure carotid endarterectomy
B. Eversion carotid endarterectomy and patch angioplasty had significantly lower restenosis rates as compared to primary closure carotid endarterectomy
C. Eversion carotid endarterectomy had significantly higher restenosis rates when compared with patch angioplasty closure after conventional carotid endarterectomy
D. Eversion carotid endarterectomy had a significantly lower restenosis rate as compared with primary closure after carotid endarterectomy

Q27. In comparing eversion carotid endarterectomy with standard carotid endarterectomy with patch angioplasty:
A. Eversion carotid endarterectomy has a higher rate of stroke and perioperative mortality as compared with carotid endarterectomy and patch angioplasty
B. The rate of perioperative stoke and perioperative mortality is similar in patients undergoing eversion carotid endarterectomy or carotid endarterectomy with patch angioplasty
C. The incidence of perioperative stroke and perioperative mortality is lower in patients undergoing eversion carotid endarterectomy as compared to standard carotid endarterectomy with patch grafting
D. None of the above

Q28. The advantages of eversion carotid endarterectomy versus standard carotid endarterectomy include:
  A. Shortening of the redundant ICA
  B. Easier detection of distal intimal flaps
  C. Faster closure and all autologous reconstruction
  D. Shortening of the redundant ICA, faster closure, all autologous reconstruction, and easier detection of distal intimal flaps

Q29. During the performance of eversion carotid endarterectomy, the distal endpoint of the plaque could not be well visualized. The best option is:
  A. Interposition graft between the distal CCA to ICA
  B. Convert to standard carotid endarterectomy with patch graft
  C. Intraoperative carotid stenting
  D. Arteriotomy in the transected ICA is extended cephalad to reach the endpoint. The transected ICA is brought anterior to the hypoglossal nerve and is sutured at the carotid bulb, and a patch graft is sutured anteriorly

Q30. The reported incidence of carotid restenosis following carotid endarterectomy and carotid stenting is:
  A. <4%
  B. 4%–10%
  C. 10%–20%
  D. >20%

Q31. Which statement best reflects the complications of repeat carotid endarterectomy for symptomatic atherosclerotic restenosis of the ICA?
  A. Incidence of perioperative stroke is higher than with primary carotid endarterectomy
  B. Incidence of cranial nerve palsy is the same as with primary carotid endarterectomy
  C. Incidence of neck hematomas is higher than with primary carotid endarterectomy
  D. Incidence of perioperative stroke is the same as in primary carotid endarterectomy, but the incidence of cranial nerve palsy is greater in patients undergoing repeat carotid endarterectomy as compared to primary carotid endarterectomy

Q32. A 72-year-old man presents to the hospital with aphasia, right supranuclear facial palsy, flaccid paralysis of the right upper extremity, grade 0 strength, and grade 3 motor strength in the right lower extremity (NIH scale 18). Clinical examination and imaging studies showed 70% stenosis of the left ICA with a moderate-sized infarct in the left middle cerebral artery (MCA) distribution without edema or midline shift. He had a left carotid endarterectomy performed 8 years ago. The best management option is:
  A. Urgent carotid stenting
  B. Urgent left CEA
  C. PT, OT, speech therapy, and medical management
  D. PT, OT, speech therapy, medical management, and reevaluation of neurological status. If the neurological deficit improves (NIH stroke scale less than 15), consider left carotid intervention (CAS or CEA) in 10–14 days after medical optimization

Q33. A patient with a recent mild stroke in the distribution of the middle cerebral artery (NIH stroke scale 6) presents with weakness of the right upper extremity (motor strength 3/5) with 70% stenosis of the left ICA. MRI shows a small area of perfusion defects in the left middle cerebral artery distribution. The patient is scheduled for a left carotid endarterectomy 5 days following the stroke. During carotid clamping, the decision to place an indwelling shunt should be:
  A. Performed in all patients with recent stroke
  B. Selective depending on EEG changes under general anesthesia and ischemic symptoms with carotid cross-clamping under cervical block anesthesia

C. Eversion carotid endarterectomy should be considered, as it can be performed faster without the necessity of a shunt in most cases

D. Carotid endarterectomy should be postponed for 6 weeks, as the need for a shunt will diminish as the collateral circulation develops

Q34.

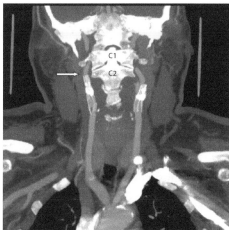

Two years after carotid artery stenting, a patient develops stent fracture and stent failure, with stenosis developing above the level of the stent at the junction of the first and second cervical vertebral bodies. Control of the distal internal carotid artery during carotid interposition graft operation is best achieved by:

A. Conventional control of the distal ICA

B. Distal control is not necessary

C. Distal ICA controlled with balloon occlusion

D. Clamp the internal carotid artery, including the stent, with a soft Fogarty jaw vascular clamp

Q35. The most satisfactory conduit for a carotid interposition graft in a patient undergoing radical neck dissection for oral cancer with involvement of the carotid artery is:

A. Superficial femoral artery

B. Tapered PTFE graft

C. Bovine xenograft

D. External carotid artery

Q36.

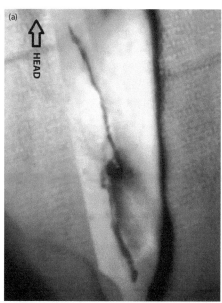

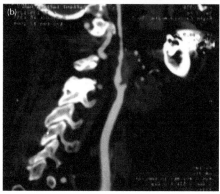

Following carotid interposition grafting with a prosthetic graft, a patient has increased drainage from the sinus in the neck. CTA of the neck shows a soft tissue mass surrounding the interposition graft. The best management option is:

A. Antibiotics; removal of the prosthetic graft; and replacement with a superficial femoral artery/superficial femoral vein, autologous great saphenous vein, and possible myocutaneous flap

B. Debridement, antibiotics, and antibiotics-soaked prosthetic graft

C. Placement of covered stent graft and long-term antibiotics

D. Debridement, antibiotics, removal of interposition graft, and ligation of the proximal internal carotid artery

Q37. Symptomatic radiation-induced carotid stenosis is often:
A. Bilateral and the plaque extends cephalad for a considerable distance
B. Always unilateral
C. Carotid endarterectomy is contraindicated
D. Carotid endarterectomy is associated with a lower incidence of cranial nerve complications and a lower incidence of wound complications as compared to CAS

Q38. Onset of seizures following carotid endarterectomy usually occurs:
A. Immediately following carotid endarterectomy
B. Always preceded by a headache
C. More common if carotid endarterectomy is performed for asymptomatic high-grade carotid stenosis
D. 12 hours to 10 days after carotid endarterectomy

Q39. The most common presentation of a carotid body tumor is:
A. Cranial nerve deficit
B. Asymptomatic neck mass
C. Dysphagia
D. Hoarseness

Q40. The Shamblin classification of carotid bypass tumor is based on:
A. Pathological type of paraganglioma
B. Symptomatology at the time of presentation
C. Biochemical evaluation of the functional nature of the tumor
D. Size of the tumor, difficulty of resection, and risk of neurovascular complications

Q41. Which statement best describes the baroreceptor failure following resection of a carotid body tumor?
A. Occurs after resection of a unilateral carotid body tumor
B. Occurs if local anesthetic is not infiltrated at the carotid bifurcation during removal of the carotid body tumor
C. Bradycardia and hypotension are common manifestations
D. Occurs 24–72 hours after bilateral carotid body tumor resection manifesting as headaches, anxiety with tachycardia, and hypertension

Q42. A malignant carotid body tumor is treated with en bloc resection and carotid artery bifurcation followed by:
A. Chemotherapy
B. Radiation therapy
C. Chemotherapy and radiation
D. Surveillance

Q43. The following statement best reflects the postoperative complications of resection of unilateral Shamblin II and III carotid body tumors:
A. Baroreceptor failure is common
B. Incidence of stroke is higher than cranial nerve palsy
C. Incidence of cranial nerve palsy is higher than stroke
D. Preoperative embolization decreases the incidence of postoperative stroke

Q44. The most common cause of an extracranial carotid aneurysm is:
A. Mycotic
B. Atherosclerosis
C. Connective tissue disorders
D. Cystic medial necrosis

Q45. The most commonly used imaging study for planning resection of an extracranial carotid aneurysm is:
A. Duplex ultrasound
B. CTA
C. MRA
D. Transcranial Doppler

Q46. The optimal method of treatment for a 2-cm-diameter internal carotid artery aneurysm 1.5 cm from its origin with associated redundancy of the internal carotid artery is:
A. Resection of the aneurysm with end-to-end anastomosis
B. Resection of the aneurysm with interposition of a synthetic graft
C. Covered carotid stent
D. Coil embolization of the aneurysmal sac

Q47. The most common complication following repair of an extracranial carotid aneurysm is:
A. Thrombosis at the site of anastomosis
B. Cranial nerve palsy
C. Perioperative stroke
D. Neck hematoma

Q48. Primary extracranial vertebral artery aneurysms most commonly are:
- A. Congenital in origin
- B. Atherosclerotic
- C. Mycotic
- D. A connective tissue disorder

Q49. All of the following statements about carotid kinks are true except:
- A. Is defined as an angle of less than or equal to 90 degrees in the two segments of the carotid artery
- B. Atherosclerosis is a strong predictive factor for developing kinks
- C. Carotid kinks are more frequently bilateral than unilateral
- D. Carotid kinks affect women more than men

Q50. The risk of stroke in patients who experience vertebrobasilar TIA with associated vertebral artery disease over 5 years is:
- A. <10%
- B. 10%–21%
- C. 22%–35%
- D. >35%

Q51.

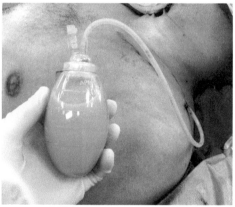

Two days following vertebral artery transposition into the common carotid artery a patient develops 170 cc of milky drainage in the neck in 24 hours' time. Initial management consists of:
- A. Thoracic duct embolization
- B. Immediate re-exploration of the neck to identify the site of the leak and its ligature
- C. Local compression, dietary manipulation, and octreotide
- D. Total parental mutation with minimal calories from fat

Q52. The incidence of perioperative stroke following open repair of a carotid aneurysm is:
- A. <2%
- B. 2%–4%
- C. 5%–9%
- D. 10%–12%

Q53. Spontaneous extracranial internal carotid artery dissection accounts for how many percentages of all initial strokes?
- A. Less than 2%
- B. 2.5%–3%
- C. 3.1%–3.5%
- D. 3.6%–4%

Q54. The most common presenting symptom of cervical and vertebral artery dissection is:
- A. Unilateral headache, neck, and facial pain
- B. Stroke
- C. Horner syndrome
- D. Pulsatile tinnitus

Q55. The optimal management of ischemic stroke and TIA caused by cervical artery dissection is:
- A. Thrombolytic therapy
- B. Carotid/vertebral artery stenting
- C. Anticoagulation/antithrombotic therapy
- D. Open surgical repair

RATIONALE 1–55

1. RATIONALE

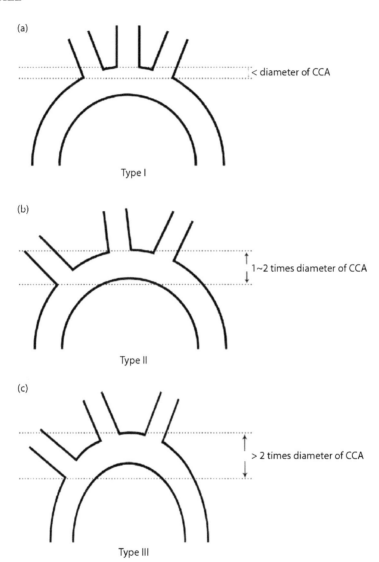

The aortic arch can be divided into three types according to the ratio between the diameter of the common carotid artery (CCA) to the distance between the horizontal line through the superior-most aspect of the aortic arch and the horizontal line through the orifice of the innominate artery.

- Type I: Less than 1 time the diameter of the CCA
- Type II: Between 1 and 2 times the diameter of the CCA
- Type III: More than 2 times the diameter of the CCA

In patients with steep aortic arches (type II and type III) and excessive proximal calcifications at the origin of the major arch arteries, TCAR is preferable. This technique of carotid stenting requires 5 cm of normal CCA proximal to the common carotid bifurcation in the neck as measured from the clavicle. This measurement can be obtained from the preprocedure carotid duplex study. In addition, this segment of the CCA should be relatively disease-free at the access site. Approximately 2 cm of the CCA are circumferentially exposed in the lower neck using a transverse or a short vertical incision. Nerve injury and injury to the lymphatics are carefully avoided. The proximal CCA is encircled with a Rummel tourniquet or silastic vessel loop. An arteriogram is performed confirming satisfactory anatomy to proceed with placement of the sheath and stenting. An 8 French femoral venous sheath supplied in the en route system is placed in the contralateral femoral vein under ultrasound guidance and secured with a suture. A retrograde forward flow system is established and confirmed. A 0.014″ wire is advanced fluoroscopically into the distal ICA, and the stent is positioned and deployed and orthogonal images are obtained.

Correct Answer   A Patients with type III aortic arch

Reference
Kwolek, C. J., Jaff, M. R., Leal, J. I., et al. (2015). Results of the ROADSTER multicenter trial of transcarotid stenting with dynamic flow reversal. *J Vasc Surg*, *62*(5), 1227–1234. PMID: 26506270

2. RATIONALE

During the establishment of retrograde flow during TCAR, the systolic blood pressure should be maintained between 140 and 160 mmHg systolic. In patients undergoing TCAR under regional block, should there be any evidence that the patient cannot tolerate retrograde flow, the procedure should be terminated and standard CEA or transfemoral carotid artery stenting with cerebral protection should be performed instead.

Correct Answer   C 140–160 mmHg systolic

Reference
Malas, M. B., Leal, J., Kashyap, V., Cambria, R. P., Kwolek, C. J., & Criado, E. (2017). Technical aspects of transcarotid artery revascularization using the ENROUTE transcarotid neuroprotection and stent system. *J Vasc Surg Cases*, *65*(3), 916–920. PMID: 28236931

3. RATIONALE

Marked calcification may lead to inadequate expansion or deformity of the stent. Even late stent fractures have been reported. Excessive internal carotid artery tortuosity makes protective filter placement contraindicated. Thrombus in the origin of the ICA with near occlusion (string sign) is also a relative contraindication to CAS. Patients at high risk for transfemoral CAS include those with type II and type III aortic arches. TCAR does eliminate some of the aforementioned risks, but patient selection requires a complete understanding of the potential complications and steps taken to eliminate the risks of perioperative stroke. As the great vessels come off more proximally from the ascending aorta (type II) and aortic arch (type III), this often results in additional manipulation of catheters in a potentially diseased aortic arch with the risk of embolization to the brain.

Correct Answer   D Type I aortic arch

Reference
Molnar, R. G., & Malhotra, N. G. (2018). Technical aspects of carotid artery stenting. In S. S. Hans (Ed.), *Extracranial carotid and vertebral artery disease: contemporary management* (pp. 187–196). Switzerland: Springer International Publishing.

4. RATIONALE

In this unfortunate situation, the export catheter should be advanced up to the level of the embolic protection filter and aspirated. Large-size thrombotic and embolic debris can be more easily aspirated with a 6 French sheath. The sheath can be slowly advanced to the stent up to the filter, and repeated aspirations will usually remove the debris. Any spasm resulting from manipulation of the ICA can be relieved with intraarterial injection of nitroglycerin. If thrombus is suspected, 1–2 mg of alteplase can be injected locally.

Correct Answer   D Aspiration with an export catheter

Reference

Molnar, R. G., & Malhotra, N. G. (2018). Technical aspects of carotid artery stenting. In S. S. Hans (Ed.), *Extracranial carotid and vertebral artery disease: contemporary management* (pp. 187–196). Switzerland: Springer International Publishing.

5. RATIONALE

During carotid angioplasty/stenting of the carotid bulb, activation of the baroreceptors resulting in bradycardia or even cardiac pause can take place. This can be prevented by administering 1 mg atropine prior to stenting and angioplasty. Should the heart rate decrease due to angioplasty, it is important to deflate the angioplasty balloon immediately and recheck the heart rate. Asking the patient to cough can also increase the heart rate. Temporary pacing is necessary if there is persistent bradycardia with associated hypotension.

Correct Answer   A Deflate the balloon and administer 1 mg intravenous atropine

Reference

Molnar, R. G., & Zuhali, B. (2018). Carotid angioplasty and stenting. In S. S. Hans, A. D. Shepard, P. G. Bove, H. R. Weaver, & G. W. Long (Eds.), *Endovascular and open vascular reconstructions: a practical approach* (pp. 3–8). Boca Raton, FL: CRC Press.

6. RATIONALE

In patients with a symptomatic thoracic aortic penetrating ulcer, endovascular repair of the thoracic aorta is performed. Prior to such repair, a left carotid to subclavian artery bypass is performed with a prosthetic graft, with a subclavian artery anastomosis performed first followed by carotid anastomosis. Typically, a 6- to 8-mm-diameter Dacron graft or a PTFE graft is selected. Carotid to subclavian artery bypass has low morbidity and mortality with a 5-year patency of 75%–90%.

Correct Answer   D Left common carotid artery to subclavian artery bypass followed by endovascular repair of the thoracic aorta

Reference

Weaver, M. R. (2018). Reconstruction for occlusive lesions of aortic arch branches. In S. S. Hans (Ed.), *Extracranial carotid and vertebral artery disease* (pp. 197–214). Cham, Switzerland: Springer.

7. RATIONALE

A preoperative cardiopulmonary evaluation with a low threshold for obtaining a coronary angiography prior to proceeding with open reconstruction using a median sternotomy, left brachiocephalic vein is mobilized, and the ascending aorta is dissected free. Distally, the right subclavian artery and common carotid artery are mobilized in their proximal portions, protecting the recurrent laryngeal nerve. Following systemic heparinization, the anesthesiology team is requested to keep the blood pressure around 100 mmHg systolic. A side biting clamp such as Lemole–Strong is applied to the ascending aorta. The excluded aorta is aspirated with a needle to ensure that there is no clamp leak. The clamp is applied at a disease-free site, and an aortotomy incision is made in the excluded ascending aorta. A 10- or 12-mm knitted Dacron graft is sutured to the ascending aorta. The patient is temporarily placed in Trendelenburg position to protect against air trapped at the anastomosis embolizing. A distal anastomosis is typically performed to the brachiocephalic bifurcation. The mortality rate ranges from 2.7% to 8% with stroke from a rate of 2.7% to 11%. Graft patency is excellent at 5 years and is reported to be 94%–98% and at 10 years 88%–96%.

Correct Answer **D** Aorto-brachiocephalic (innominate) bypass graft

Reference

Berguer, R., Morasch, M. D., & Kline, R. A. (1998). Transthoracic repair of innominate and common carotid artery disease: immediate and long-term outcome for 100 consecutive surgical reconstructions. *J Vasc Surg*, *27*(1), 34–41; discussion 42. PMID: 9474080

8. RATIONALE

Endovascular techniques are considered to be the first-line therapy for the treatment of short-segment occlusive lesions of the supra-aortic trunk vessel without circumferential calcification. Important procedural considerations include access, therapeutic intervention, and use of distal thromboembolic protection devices. Access options include antegrade approach to the vessel via the femoral artery or retrograde approach via the carotid or brachial arteries. Aortic arch vessels are displayed in the LAO projection. Arteriography in the right anterior oblique projection defines the bifurcation of the right brachiocephalic artery more accurately. For retrograde brachial access, open exposure is preferrable because of the necessity of using larger sheaths (6 Fr or larger) in order to decrease the incidence of access site complications. When the transfemoral approach is used, distal embolic protection has been used both routinely and selectively in some series. Some investigators have reported supra-aortic branch stenting without the use of any cerebral protection devices.

Correct Answer **D** Length of the lesion and occlusion of the aortic arch branch as compared to stenosis and severe ostial calcification

Reference

Paukovits, T. M., Lukács, L., Bérczi, V., et al. (2010). Percutaneous endovascular treatment of innominate artery lesions: a single-centre experience on 77 lesions. *Eur J Vasc Endovasc Surg*, *40*(1), 35–43. PMID: 20435490

9. RATIONALE

Most patients with asymptomatic proximal subclavian artery occlusive disease do not require intervention because of the presence of a rich collateral network around the shoulder joint (branches of the axillary artery). Blood pressure monitoring should only be performed in the unaffected upper extremity. Even patients with diminished antegrade flow to the vertebral artery or the presence of retrograde vertebral artery flow usually do not have symptoms of so-called "vertebral steal." This is usually an interesting angiographic finding and is clinically insignificant in most cases, unless the contralateral vertebral artery has severe disease.

Asymptomatic subclavian artery stenosis is associated with an increased risk of morbidity and mortality related to the underlying atherosclerotic disease burden in other vascular beds.

Correct Answer   **D** Risk factor modification without any intervention

Reference
Clark, C. E., Taylor, R. S., Shore, A. C., et al. (2012). Association of a difference in systolic blood pressure between arms with vascular disease and mortality: a systematic review and meta-analysis. *Lancet, 379*(9819), 905–914. PMID: 22293369

10. RATIONALE

A review of the vascular quality initiative data obtained in 404 patients who underwent carotid endarterectomy combined with ipsilateral proximal intervention showed a combined stroke and death rate that was twice that of isolated carotid endarterectomy. After risk adjustment, predictors of stroke and death were diabetes mellitus, symptomatic statis, and carotid endarterectomy combined with ipsilateral proximal endovascular intervention. Symptomatic patients should preferably not have the combined procedures, and consideration should be given to the open surgical bypass cerebral protection and staged procedures.

Correct Answer   **B** Two times that of isolated carotid endarterectomy

Reference
Wang, L. J., Ergul, E. A., Conrad, M. F., et al. (2019). Addition of proximal intervention to carotid endarterectomy increases risk of stroke and death. *J Vasc Surg, 69*(4), 1102–1110. PMID: 30553728

11. RATIONALE

The incidence of stroke following endovascular treatment of the branches of the aortic arch is <3%. Periprocedural stroke is usually caused by embolization, thrombosis, or dissection. The routine use of preoperative dual antiplatelet therapy and intraprocedural anticoagulation reduces the risk of micro-emboli by stabilizing the plaque prior to intervention. Several of the largest studies have reported stroke rates of 0%–2.6% without the use of neuroprotection. Technical aspects of stenting are important, as inaccurate placement of a stent risks covering the ostium of the carotid or ostium of the vertebral artery, resulting in thrombosis of the artery. Baseline imaging of the intracerebral circulation should be performed before intervention. A neurointerventionalist consult is often necessary if there is intracerebral artery occlusion of the MCA or its main division during the procedure. The results of neurorescue are mixed. Patients with periprocedural strokes have a threefold increase in 4-year mortality.

Correct Answer   **C** 2%–2.9%

Reference
Zhang, X., Ma, H., Li, L., et al. (2019). A meta-analysis of transfemoral endovascular treatment of common carotid artery lesions. *World Neurosurg, 123*, 89–94. PMID: 30453085

12. RATIONALE

The incidence of thrombosis of the brachial artery is around 2%. The small vessel diameter, large diameter sheath (6 Fr or greater), and relatively easy compressibility compared to the femoral artery render the brachial artery more prone to thrombosis. In a series of 732 patients who underwent the procedure for brachial artery access in the vascular quality initiative data, there was a 9% complication rate as compared to 3% for femoral artery access. The complication rate after brachial artery cut down (4.1%) was significantly lower than ultrasound-guided percutaneous access (11.8%).[1] However, another study reported that the percutaneous brachial artery approach leads to similar rates of complication as compared to femoral access. Management of brachial artery thrombosis is surgical with a brachial artery thrombectomy using a transverse arteriotomy. A large series of brachial artery access with cardiac catheterization procedures performed at the Cleveland Clinic revealed that the cause of brachial artery thrombosis was most often due to posterior intimal disruption from percutaneous puncture.[2] Therefore, segmental resection after mobilization of the brachial artery with an oblique end-to-end anastomosis to prevent recurrent thrombosis is the preferred approach.

Correct Answer   B 2%

References
1. Kret, M. R., Dalman, R. L., Kalish, J., & Mell, M. (2016). Arterial cutdown reduces complications after brachial access for peripheral vascular intervention. *J Vasc Surg*, *64*(1), 149-154. PMID: 27021376
2. Kitzmiller, J. W., Hertzer, N. R., & Beven, E. G. (1982). Routine surgical management of brachial artery occlusion after cardiac catheterization. *Arch Surg*, *117*(8), 1066-1071. PMID: 7103726

13. RATIONALE

It has been well established in the last three decades that early carotid endarterectomy (within 2 weeks of a stroke) should be performed in patients with mild-to-moderate stroke. A meta-analysis of 47 studies reporting periprocedural stroke/death after CEA/CAS related to the time between the development of neurological symptoms and intervention was performed. Among 47 studies, 30 were on carotid endarterectomy and 7 on CAS; 5 involved both procedures. The results demonstrated that CEA within 15 days from the onset of stroke (transient ischemic attack) can be performed with periprocedural stroke risk of less than 3.5% as compared to 4.8% with carotid artery stenting.[1] In clinical practice, it is better to wait at least 48-72 hours following a stroke to assess the cardiopulmonary risk and if any edema around the infarct improves before carotid intervention. Carotid revascularization is not recommended in patients in whom the neurological deficit is severe (NIH stroke scale greater than 15).[2]

Correct Answer   C Early carotid endarterectomy/carotid artery stenting should be considered within 10 days of the stroke

References
1. De Rango, P., Brown, M. M., Chaturvedi, S., et al. (2015). Summary of evidence on early carotid intervention for recently symptomatic stenosis based on meta-analysis of current risks. *Stroke*, *46*(12), 3423-3436. PMID: 26470773
2. Hans, S. S., Acho, R. J., & Catanescu, I. (2018). Timing of carotid endarterectomy after recent minor to moderate stroke. *Surgery*, *164*(4), 820-824. PMID: 30072249

14. RATIONALE

Patients undergoing carotid endarterectomy under general anesthesia with EEG monitoring are reported to require a shunt in 12%-18% and under regional anesthesia (CBA) in about 10% of patients.[1] Normal cerebral blood flow is about 50 mL/100 g/min, and cerebral ischemia resulting in an unresponsive state occurs if the cerebral blood flow is less than 20 mL/100 g/min. If the cerebral ischemia is not prolonged, brain function may return on restoration of cerebral perfusion. Ischemic EEG changes during carotid cross-clamping under general anesthesia overestimate the need for the shunt. Since cerebral embolization is the most common cause of perioperative stroke, meticulous operative technique with careful mobilization of carotid bifurcation should be carried out.[2]

Correct Answer   B Approximately 10%

References
1. Hans, S. S., & Jareunpoon, O. (2007). Prospective evaluation of electroencephalography, carotid artery stump pressure, and neurologic changes during 314 consecutive carotid endarterectomies performed in awake patients. *J Vasc Surg*, *45*(3), 511–515. PMID: 17275248
2. Calligaro, K. D., & Dougherty, M. J. (2005). Correlation of carotid artery stump pressure and neurologic changes during 474 carotid endarterectomies performed in awake patients. *J Vasc Surg*, *42*(4), 684–689. PMID: 16242555

15. RATIONALE

In a controlled trial 3526 patients (multicentered randomized study) undergoing carotid endarterectomy were randomly assigned to surgery under general (*n* = 1753) or local (*n* = 1773) anesthesia between 1997 and 2007. The primary outcome was the proportion of patients with stroke, MI, and 30-day mortality. The primary outcome was 4.8% under general anesthesia and 4.5% under local anesthesia, showing no difference between general anesthesia and local anesthesia for CEA.[1] Gassner et al. reported from a retrospective study lesser hemodynamic lability in patients undergoing CEA under cervical block anesthesia as compared to those undergoing CEA under general anesthesia.[2]

Correct Answer   C More stable hemodynamics during and immediately after CEA

References
1. Lewis, S. C., Warlow, C. P., Bodenham, A. R., et al. (2008). General anaesthesia versus local anaesthesia for carotid surgery (GALA): a multicentre, randomised controlled trial. *Lancet*, *372*(9656), 2132–2142. PMID: 19041130
2. Gassner, M., Bauman, Z., Parish, S., et al. (2014). Hemodynamic changes in patients undergoing carotid endarterectomy under cervical block and general anesthesia. *Ann Vasc Surg*, *28*(7), 1680–1685. PMID: 24704052

16. RATIONALE

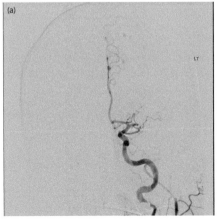
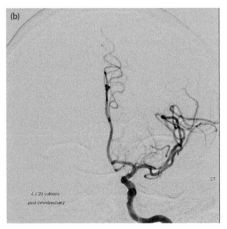

(a) MCA occlusion by the plaque.   (b) Completing filling of MCA following neurointervention.

Perioperative stroke is the most serious complication of carotid endarterectomy, and its incidences ranges from 1% to 5%. The incidence is lowest in patients undergoing CEA for asymptomatic stenosis and higher in patients undergoing CEA for recent strokes. The most common cause is plaque embolization either during the operation or in the immediate postoperative period. Another important cause of postoperative stroke following normal neurological function following completion of carotid endarterectomy is due to thrombosis at the endarterectomy site, most commonly due to a retained distal intimal flap. Cerebral ischemia due to nonuse of the shunt or malfunction of the shunt with inadequate cerebral collateral flow may also result in stroke, depending on the duration of cerebral ischemia. If the patient develops a neurological deficit in the recovery room or a few hours later, emergent non-contrast CT scan of the head should be performed. As ischemic infarct does not become distinctly visible on the CT scan of the head for a few hours, it may manifest as decreased parenchymal attenuation with effacement of sulci initially. A hyperattenuated middle cerebral artery sign may be present. Intracranial plaque retrieval by a neurovascular interventionalist should be performed within the 6- to 8-hour window so that a satisfactory neurological outcome is obtained.

Correct Answer   **D** Neurovascular interventionalist consult for retrieval of the plaque/thrombus with stent-assisted mechanical recanalization for acute MCA occlusion

Reference

Roth, C., Papanagiotou, P., Behnke, S., et al. (2010). Stent-assisted mechanical recanalization for treatment of acute intracerebral artery occlusions. *Stroke, 41*(11), 2559–2567. PMID: 20947848

17. RATIONALE

Most nerve injuries associated with carotid endarterectomy affect the hypoglossal or vagus nerves, and a vast majority of nerve injuries are transient. Data from the *European Carotid Surgery Trial* (ECST) were gathered on the largest series of patients undergoing CEA in which neurological assessment was performed before and after surgery. The study revealed that a 4% risk of moderate cranial nerve injury persisted beyond hospital discharge. A meta-analysis of 26 articles published between 1972 and 2015 corresponding to 20,860 CEAs revealed the vagus nerve is the most frequent nerve injured (3.99%) followed by the hypoglossal nerve (3.79%). Some variations in reporting may reflect temporary weakness being permanent nerve injury, thus accounting for a higher incidence of hypoglossal nerve palsy. Cranial nerve injury is more common in patients undergoing repeat carotid endarterectomy and CEA for high plaque.

Correct Answer   **B** Hypoglossal

Reference

Kakisis, J. D., Antonopoulos, C. N., Mantas, G., et al. (2017). Cranial nerve injury after carotid endarterectomy: incidence, risk factors, and time trends. *Eur J Vasc Endovasc Surg, 53*(3), 320–335. PMID: 28117240

18. RATIONALE

Patch graft closure with CEA is almost universally performed. The most common patches used are bovine pericardial patch, Dacron PTFE, and autologous vein patch. Carotid vein patch blowout has been reported in the past. At present, the autologous vein patch is not as commonly used. Approximately 0.25%–0.5% of all synthetic patches appear to get infected following CEA. Patch graft infection may appear early or late and has a bimodal distribution depending on the virulence of the microorganism. Postoperative hematoma is associated with late development of infection. Most patients with patch graft infections present with neck swelling, pseudoaneurysm, or a draining sinus at the time of the incision. CT angiography of the neck is necessary for complete evaluation. Complete excision of the infected tissue and arterial reconstruction with autologous interposition vein graft should be considered. In patients with a history of neck radiation with poorly vascularized tissues such as the sternocleidomastoid muscle (if present) or pectoralis major, a myocutaneous flap should be performed. An interposition vein graft tends to develop myointimal hyperplasia at follow-up. The site of myointimal hyperplasia is usually at the site of the valves. Carotid stenting is an option for carotid restenosis due to myointimal hyperplasia. Long-term results of carotid stenting for carotid interposition graft stenosis are not well defined.

Correct Answer   **A** Debridement, removal of patch, autologous reconstruction, and antibiotics

Reference
Knight, B. C., & Tait, W. F. (2009). Dacron patch infection following carotid endarterectomy: a systematic review of the literature. *Eur J Vasc Endovasc Surg, 37*(2), 140–148. PMID: 19041268

19. RATIONALE

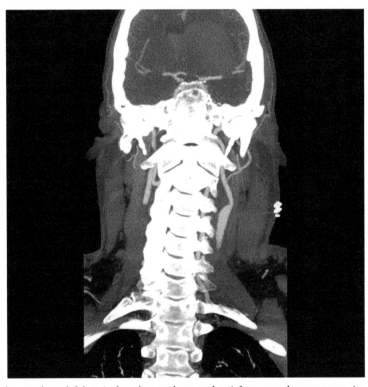

Postoperative CTA showing large left hemisphere hemorrhage and satisfactory endarterectomy site.

In a small number of patients, opening a high-grade stenosis in the CCA/ICA can result in a significant increase in regional cerebral blood flow with loss of autoregulation resulting in hyperperfusion and intracerebral hemorrhage. In its milder form, hyperperfusion syndrome manifests as headaches or seizures, which are the result of cerebral edema. Following CEA/CAS, intracerebral hemorrhage occurs in less than 1% of patients with a mortality of approximately 50%, with associated significant morbidity in most survivors. There is a higher risk of postoperative intracerebral hemorrhage among patients undergoing CAS as compared to patients undergoing CEA. Intracerebral hemorrhage occurs in the first 24 hours following CAS and 2–7 days following CEA. Systemic hypertension, if not controlled, is an important risk factor for intracerebral hemorrhage. Intracerebral hemorrhage, if localized to the frontal lobe, can be treated urgently by a neurosurgeon with craniotomy. However, a large intracerebral hemorrhage in the parietal lobe with midline shift requires reversal of anticoagulation, modest blood pressure reduction, and in some cases intracranial pressure monitoring. Treatment options are limited. Ipsilateral CEA should preferably be delayed for at least 3 months after contralateral CEA for asymptomatic stenosis in order to reduce the risk of hyperperfusion syndrome.

Correct Answer   C Urgent neurosurgical consult for possible craniotomy

Reference

Wang, G. J., Beck, A. W., DeMartino, R. R., et al. (2017). Insight into the cerebral hyperperfusion syndrome following carotid endarterectomy from the national vascular quality initiative. *J Vasc Surg, 65*(2), 381–389.e382. PMID: 27707618

20. RATIONALE

In patients undergoing CEA for high plaque mobilization of the internal carotid artery, division of the sternocleidomastoid branch of the occipital artery and often the occipital artery itself is required. This maneuver helps to mobilize the hypoglossal nerve cephalad. The posterior belly of the digestive muscle is retracted cephalad, or it may have to be divided to gain distal exposure of the internal carotid artery. For the hypoglossal nerve to be mobilized, the ansa hypoglossi may need to be divided. The hypoglossal nerve is gently looped with a silastic vessel loop and retracted cephalad.[1] Following endarterectomy, the distal intima is inspected. If there is any question about the smooth tapering of the intima and hence its complete removal, completion operative arteriogram via a microcatheter in the CCA or via catheter in the superior thyroid artery is performed, and carotid stenting may be necessary (rarely). If there is any concern that the distal intima is not adequately removed to its distal feathery end with difficulty in visualizing the endpoint of endarterectomy, intraoperative carotid stenting is performed via a 6 or 7 Fr sheath inserted into the common carotid artery just above the clavicle with a micro puncture technique and a 0.014 microwire advanced cranially.[2]

Correct Answer   A Perform on-table carotid/cerebral arteriogram

References

1. Vang, S., & Hans, S. S. (2019). Carotid endarterectomy in patients with high plaque. *Surgery, 166*(4), 601–606. PMID: 31405580
2. Ross, C. B., & Ranval, T. J. (2000). Intraoperative use of stents for the management of unacceptable distal internal carotid artery end points during carotid endarterectomy: short-term and midterm results. *J Vasc Surg, 32*(3), 420–427; 427–428. PMID: 10957648

21. RATIONALE

During routine carotid endarterectomy the most common nerves to be injured are either the hypoglossal or vagus. In patients undergoing CEA for high plaque, the division of the stylohyoid muscle and styloid process may result in injury to the glossopharyngeal nerve, which manifests as difficulty in swallowing with weakened or missing gag reflex and risk of aspiration. The patient may need a temporary feeding tube. In addition, the patient has impaired gustation and reduced sensation over the posterior third of the tongue, palate, and pharynx.

Correct Answer   **D** Glossopharyngeal

Reference

Rosenbloom, M., Friedman, S. G., Lamparello, P. J., Riles, T. S., & Imparato, A. M. (1987). Glossopharyngeal nerve injury complicating carotid endarterectomy. *J Vasc Surg*, *5*(3), 469–471. PMID: 3509601

22. RATIONALE

Carotid artery stenting (TCAR or transfemoral) for severely calcified plaque is not a satisfactory option, as the stent may not expand or become deformed. Medical management and carotid ligation are not satisfactory options either. The best medical management includes cessation of smoking, antiplatelet medications, and cholesterol-lowering drugs are very important in the management of cerebrovascular occlusive disease. Obtaining distal exposure of the internal carotid artery requires that the cephalad end of the incision be extended towards and behind the ear lobule with retraction of the posterior belly of the digastric muscle. The sternocleidomastoid branch of the occipital artery is divided and, in some cases, the occipital artery itself is divided and the hypoglossal nerve is carefully retracted cephalad with a silastic vessel loop. In certain situations, the stylohyoid muscle and stylohyoid process need to be divided. A caudal retraction with a double silastic vessel loop around the common carotid artery and external carotid artery is often helpful in bringing the carotid bifurcation inferiorly. Following arteriotomy and removal of the plaque, two stay sutures are placed at the origin of the internal carotid artery on either side (3:00 and 9:00), and traction is placed outward and downwards. Intraluminal control of the internal carotid artery is obtained by the passage of a 4- or 4.5-mm arterial dilator (Teleflex Medical, Morrisville, NC), and cephalad dissection is done around the stem of the dilator. Another option would be to place a distal Pruitt balloon occlusion catheter (LeMaitre Vascular, Burlington, ME). If the plaque is at the level of the superior body of the second cervical vertebra, nasotracheal intubation and mandibular subluxation by an ENT surgeon or oral/maxillofacial surgeon should be considered to gain satisfactory exposure.

Correct Answer   **B** CEA with high distal exposure

Reference

Vang, S., & Hans, S. S. (2019). Carotid endarterectomy in patients with high plaque. *Surgery*, *166*(4), 601–606. PMID: 31405580

23. RATIONALE

Stone et al. reviewed 4587 carotid endarterectomies performed at a vascular study group of northern New England and observed that protamine reduced serious bleeding requiring reoperation during carotid endarterectomy without increasing the risk of MI, stroke, or death. In their series multivariant logistic regression confirmed that protamine administration was an independent predictor of diminished reoperation for bleeding.[1] In a meta-analysis of seven studies reporting on 3817 patients receiving protamine after CEA and 6070 patients not receiving protamine, heparin reversal reduced the risk of wound hematoma without increasing the risk of stroke.[2]

Correct Answer   B Does not increase the risk of stroke

References
1. Stone, D. H., Nolan, B. W., Schanzer, A., et al. (2010). Protamine reduces bleeding complications associated with carotid endarterectomy without increasing the risk of stroke. *J Vasc Surg*, *51*(3), 559–564, 564.e551. PMID: 20045609
2. Kakisis, J. D., Antonopoulos, C. N., Moulakakis, K. G., et al. (2016). Protamine reduces bleeding complications without increasing the risk of stroke after carotid endarterectomy: a meta-analysis. *Eur J Vasc Endovasc Surg*, *52*(3), 296–307. PMID: 27389942

24. RATIONALE

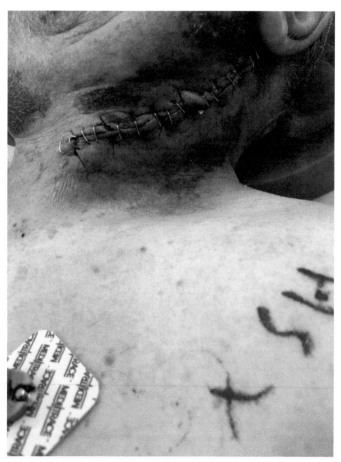

Post-CEA neck hematoma.

Bleeding after carotid endarterectomy is an important complication to avoid, as large cervical hematomas may result in airway compromise and death. Postoperative bleeding is reported to occur in <3% of cases, and in most patients, hematomas are small, non-expansile, and resolve in a few days. If a significant cervical hematoma is identified, as was in the aforementioned patient, the patient should be immediately taken back to the OR for wound exploration and hematoma evacuation. In patients with small non-expanding hematomas, anticoagulation should be reversed and patients should continue to be monitored very closely. Some surgeons prefer to place a drain prior to closing the incision to monitor bleeding, although the benefit of placing a drain is not well established. Endotracheal intubation may be challenging as a result of hematoma in the neck causing tracheal deviation. The suture line should be opened under local anesthesia, and removal of deeper sutures will help in evacuation of hematoma and endotracheal intubation may be performed if necessary.

Correct Answer   **C** Emergent re-exploration of the neck in the OR

Reference
Greenstein, A. J., Chassin, M. R., Wang, J., et al. (2007). Association between minor and major surgical complications after carotid endarterectomy: results of the New York Carotid Artery Surgery study. *J Vasc Surg*, *46*(6), 1138–1144; discussion 1145–1136. PMID: 18154989

25. RATIONALE

The Carotid Revascularization Endarterectomy Versus Stenting Trial (CREST) found that patients who had an MI with EKG changes in the postoperative period with biomarker elevation were significantly more likely to die in the follow-up period even after adjusting for other risk factors for mortality. Carotid endarterectomy is considered an intermediate-risk procedure. Patients who also have at least 4.0 METS (metabolic equivalents), which is consistent with moderate activity, do not require preoperative cardiac testing. Walking on a level ground at about 6 kilometers an hour or carrying groceries up a flight of stairs expands about 4 METS of activity. Generally, greater than 7 METS of activity tolerance is considered excellent and less than 4 is considered poor for surgical risk stratification. In patients without such functional capacity or with recent onset of symptoms, cardiac evaluation, including a stress test, is recommended.[1] Preoperative optimal medical therapy (beta-blockers, statins, aspirin) should be continued throughout the perioperative period. The rate of myocardial infarction after carotid endarterectomy is under 1% in a contemporary series of 8315 patients undergoing CEA and CAS from 2003 to 2011. During the first 5 years, multivariable modeling showed postoperative stroke and postoperative MI remained independent predictors of decreased survival.[2]

Correct Answer   **D** The patient is more likely to need coronary revascularization

References
1. Fleisher, L. A., Fleischmann, K. E., Auerbach, A. D., et al. (2014). 2014 ACC/AHA guideline on perioperative cardiovascular evaluation and management of patients undergoing noncardiac surgery: a report of the American College of Cardiology/American Heart Association Task Force on Practice Guidelines. *Circulation*, *130*(24), e278–e333. PMID: 25085961
2. Simons, J. P., Goodney, P. P., Baril, D. T., et al. (2013). The effect of postoperative stroke and myocardial infarction on long-term survival after carotid revascularization. *J Vasc Surg*, *57*(6), 1581–1588. PMID: 23402875s

26. RATIONALE

Results of the EVEREST (Eversion Carotid Endarterectomy Versus Standard Trial) validated the short- and long-term safety and efficacy of eversion carotid endarterectomy. This prospective multicenter randomized trial compared rates of carotid occlusion, restenosis rate, major stroke, and death among standard carotid endarterectomy ($n = 675$) and eversion carotid endarterectomy ($n = 678$). Long-term results showed a significantly lower restenosis rate in the eversion group (2.7% vs. 5.6%, $p = 0.01$) at a mean follow-up of 33 months. A single-institution series demonstrated there is no significant difference between the eversion and standard carotid endarterectomy in early (<30 days) and late postoperative complications. Eversion carotid endarterectomy is associated with a higher incidence of return to the operating room for bleeding (1.4% for conventional carotid endarterectomy versus 8% for eversion carotid endarterectomy, $p = 0.002$).

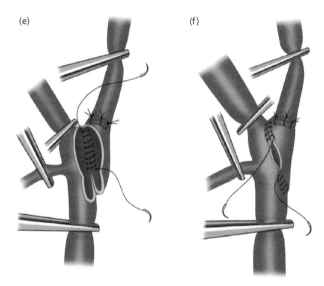

(e)   (f)

Schematics of anastomosis of eversion endarterectomy with a separate incision in the internal carotid artery for removal of a residual flap.

Correct Answer   B Eversion carotid endarterectomy and patch angioplasty had a significantly lower restenosis rate as compared to primary closure carotid endarterectomy

Reference
Schneider, J. R., Helenowski, I. B., Jackson, C. R., et al. (2015). A comparison of results with eversion versus conventional carotid endarterectomy from the Vascular Quality Initiative and the Mid-America Vascular Study Group. *J Vasc Surg, 61*(5), 1216–1222. PMID: 25925539

27. RATIONALE

A Cochrane review of the literature of 2465 patients from five controlled clinical trials showed that incidence of perioperative stroke and perioperative mortality was similar in patients undergoing eversion carotid endarterectomy as compared to standard carotid endarterectomy with patch grafting. There were no significant differences in the rate of perioperative stroke and death and stroke and death during follow-up between eversion and conventional CEA. Eversion CEA was associated with a lower rate of restenosis.

Correct Answer   B The pate of perioperative stroke and perioperative mortality is similar in patients undergoing eversion carotid endarterectomy or carotid endarterectomy with patch angioplasty

Reference
Cao, P. G., de Rango, P., Zannetti, S., et al. (2001). Eversion versus conventional carotid endarterectomy for preventing stroke. *Cochrane Database Syst Rev, 2000*(1), Cd001921. PMID: 11279740

28. RATIONALE

Conventional carotid endarterectomy, even with patch grafting, is associated with appreciable rates of residual or recurrent stenosis. Management of the endpoint may be challenging, especially in patients with a high plaque. Eversion carotid endarterectomy with reimplantation is preferred if the internal carotid artery is tortuous, <4 mm in diameter, and in women. In these situations, eversion carotid endarterectomy can shorten a redundant ICA and provide better visualization of the endpoint and easier detection of distal intimal flaps and faster closure by simple anastomosis of the ICA to the carotid bulb.

Correct Answer   D Shortening of the redundant ICA, faster closure, all autologous reconstruction, and easier detection of distal intimal flaps

Reference
Kieny, R., Hirsch, D., Seiller, C., et al. (1993). Does carotid eversion endarterectomy and reimplantation reduce the risk of restenosis? *Ann Vasc Surg, 7*(5), 407–413. PMID: 8268085

29. RATIONALE

Eversion carotid endarterectomy is performed by circumferential elevation of the plaque with a Penfield plaque and removal of the intima and media from the transected ICA while the plaque is held by the assistant. The adventitia and outer layer of the media are everted, and the aforementioned atheromatous plaque is held in tension until the endpoint is reached and there is no residual intimal flap. If the endpoint cannot be obtained, then a longitudinal arteriotomy incision in the ICA is performed, extending cephalad until the endpoint is ascertained and, if needed, tacking of the distal intima is performed. The transected ICA at its origin is then sutured to the carotid bulb at the posterior wall extending from the 3 to 9 o'clock position (suture line) and a patch graft applied anteriorly.

Correct Answer   D Arteriotomy in the transected ICA is extended cephalad to reach the endpoint. The transected ICA is brought anterior to the hypoglossal nerve and is sutured at the carotid bulb, and a patch graft is sutured anteriorly

Reference
Lim, J. C. (2018). Eversion carotid endarterectomy. In S. Hans (Ed.), *Extracranial carotid artery and vertebral artery disease: contemporary management* (pp. 151–157). Cham, Switzerland: Springer.

30. RATIONALE

Duplex ultrasound surveillance of patients following carotid endarterectomy and carotid artery stenting has increased the incidence of recurrent disease. Carotid artery restenosis following carotid endarterectomy and CAS averages 4%–6% nationally. Recurrent carotid disease after carotid endarterectomy can be categorized into three different entities:

A. Residual disease

B. Early recurrent stenosis (within 24 months) due to myointimal hyperplasia

C. Late recurrent stenosis (due to atherosclerotic plaque formation)

Recurrent carotid stenosis following carotid artery stenting may be found in the stented segment of the artery proximal to the stent, distal to the stent, or as a combination of both. The frequency of severe post-stent recurrence varies significantly, ranging from 2% to 14% in the CAVATAS study. In-stent restenosis is likely due to intimal and medial injury resulting in an inflammatory response followed by a proliferative cellular response. Intraluminal remodeling results in hyperplastic restenosis.

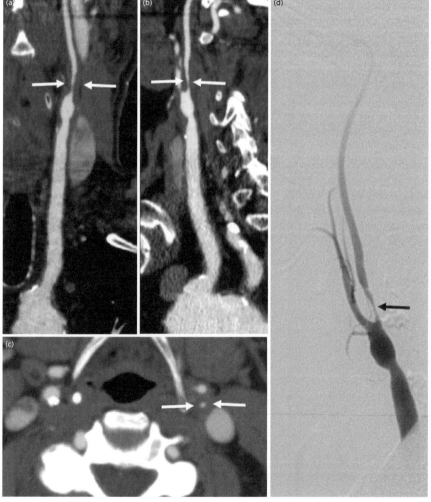

Myointimal hyperplasia following carotid endarterectomy. Curved planar reformats (a, b) and axial (c) CT angiogram demonstrate circumferential luminal narrowing within the proximal left internal carotid artery. (d) Conventional angiogram confirms the luminal narrowing compatible with restenosis.

Correct Answer   B 4%–10%

References
1. Lal, B. K., Hobson, R. W., 2nd, Goldstein, J., et al. (2003). In-stent recurrent stenosis after carotid artery stenting: life table analysis and clinical relevance. *J Vasc Surg, 38*(6), 1162–1168; discussion 1169. PMID: 14681601
2. Endovascular versus surgical treatment in patients with carotid stenosis in the Carotid and Vertebral Artery Transluminal Angioplasty Study (CAVATAS): a randomised trial. (2001). *Lancet, 357*(9270), 1729–1737. PMID: 11403808

31. RATIONALE

Tu et al. reported results of a meta-analysis of patients undergoing repeat carotid endarterectomy versus carotid artery stenting for patients with carotid restenosis after endarterectomy. The incidence of myocardial infarction and cranial nerve palsy was increased in the repeat carotid endarterectomy group, though cranial nerve palsy is often reversible. Carotid artery stenting for recurrent carotid stenosis is an acceptable alternative and may be preferable to a repeat carotid endarterectomy in certain situations. However, there is a higher incidence of carotid in-stent restenosis than those treated with repeat carotid endarterectomy over long-term follow-up. The approach to the management of recurrent carotid stenosis should be based on morphology, symptomology, and location of the lesion; associated medical comorbidities; and anticipated life expectancy.

Correct Answer   D Incidence of perioperative stroke is the same as in primary carotid endarterectomy, but incidence of cranial nerve palsy is higher in patients undergoing repeat carotid endarterectomy as compared to primary carotid endarterectomy

Reference
Tu, J., Wang, S., Huo, Z., et al. (2015). Repeated carotid endarterectomy versus carotid artery stenting for patients with carotid restenosis after carotid endarterectomy: systematic review and meta-analysis. *Surgery, 157*(6), 1166–1173. PMID: 25840718

32. RATIONALE

The timing of carotid endarterectomy after recent stroke in the territory of the ipsilateral MCA has been studied, and for patients with minor to moderate stroke (NIH stroke scale less than 15), early carotid endarterectomy (within 14 days of symptoms) is preferable, as there is no increase in the incidence of complications as compared to delayed CEA (6 weeks after the onset of symptoms). In patients with severe stroke (NIH stroke greater than 15), carotid intervention is not recommended. Delay in carotid endarterectomy in patients with NIH stroke scale of less than 15 may subject the patient to the risk of recurrent stroke.

Correct Answer   D PT, OT, speech therapy, medical management, and reevaluation of neurological status. If the neurological deficit improves (NIH stroke scale less than 15), consider left carotid intervention (CAS or CEA) in 10–14 days after medical optimization

Reference
Hans, S. S., Acho, R. J., & Catanescu, I. (2018). Timing of carotid endarterectomy after recent minor to moderate stroke. *Surgery, 164*(4), 820–824. PMID: 30072249

33. RATIONALE

Empirically, surgeons have recommended the use of a shunt in all patients undergoing carotid endarterectomy for recent stroke to maintain the blood flow in the areas around the ischemic infarct during carotid cross-clamping. A cerebral blood flow reduction below certain values leads to functional biochemical and structural changes leading to irreversible neuronal death. The ischemic penumbra is defined as a functionally impaired yet still viable brain tissue surrounding the ischemic core. The penumbra includes ischemic areas that recover spontaneously (benign oligemia) and areas that progress to irreversible changes unless effective treatment is undertaken. The rate of progression to infarction depends on the degree of collateral circulation, duration of ischemia, and repeat ischemic insults.

Shunt requirement during carotid endarterectomy for patients with recent acute stroke is similar to other indications for carotid endarterectomy. Patients undergoing carotid endarterectomy for recent stroke have a similar incidence of postoperative neurological deficits, mortality, MI, and cranial nerve palsy as compared to other indications of carotid endarterectomy, but had a higher incidence of postoperative seizures.

Correct Answer   B Selective use of a shunt depending on EEG changes under general anesthesia and ischemic symptoms with carotid cross-clamping under cervical block anesthesia

Reference

Hans, S. S., & Catanescu, I. (2015). Selective shunting for carotid endarterectomy in patients with recent stroke. *J Vasc Surg*, *61*(4), 915–919. PMID: 25601503

34. RATIONALE

In order to obtain distal control of the ICA in a patient where the lesion extends to the junction of C1 and C2, intraluminal control with balloon occlusion is the safest and most practical technique. A short 6 Fr sheath is placed in the proximal common carotid artery above the clavicle and a 0.014″ wire is advanced into the ICA towards the base of the skull and a #3 Fogarty balloon catheter is advanced over the wire under fluoroscopy and balloon inflation is performed. The common carotid artery is clamped proximal to the sheath, and a double silastic loop is tightened around the external carotid artery after the patient has been fully heparinized. Prior to arteriotomy in the common carotid artery and internal carotid artery, the Fogarty balloon is inflated with diluted contrast and is confirmed under fluoroscopy. The removal of the stent and carotid operation can then proceed in the usual manner.

Correct Answer   C Distal ICA controlled with balloon occlusion

Reference

Hans, S. S. (2018). Carotid interposition grafting. In S. S. Hans (Ed.), *Extracranial carotid artery and vertebral artery disease: contemporary management* (pp. 167–170). Cham, Switzerland: Springer.

35. RATIONALE

The superficial femoral artery should be examined by duplex imaging, and the ankle-brachial index should be obtained. The superficial femoral artery as a conduit is preferable to a prosthetic graft in patients undergoing resection of head and neck cancer invading the carotid artery in patients with radiation failure. The superficial femoral artery can be resected in many patients without the need for revascularization of the lower extremity. If the lower extremity shows evidence of ischemia, then an above-knee femoral-popliteal bypass graft should be considered. By using immediate reconstruction with autologous arterial grafting, carotid artery resection without the additional need of myocutaneous flaps to provide tissue coverage can be carried out without the risk associated with the use of prosthetic grafts.

Correct Answer   A Superficial femoral artery

Reference
Jacobs, J. R., Korkmaz, H., Marks, S. C., et al. (2001). One stage carotid artery resection: reconstruction in radiated head and neck carcinoma. *Am J Otolaryngol, 22*(3), 167–171. PMID: 11351284

36. RATIONALE

In a patient with an infected distal CCA/ICA with a synthetic graft or carotid stent, the stent and infected artery must be removed and autologous reconstruction performed with either the superficial femoral artery or great saphenous vein. Tissue coverage of carotid reconstruction will depend on the quality of the surrounding tissue. If the sternocleidomastoid muscle has been removed or the carotid artery has poorly vascularized surrounding tissues, then autologous reconstruction with a myocutaneous flap based on the pectoralis major flap is a desirable option. If the surrounding tissues are well vascularized following debridement and autologous reconstruction can be carried out, standard closure can be completed without the necessity of a myocutaneous flap.

Correct Answer   A Antibiotics, removal of the prosthetic graft, and replacement with a superficial femoral artery/superficial femoral vein, autologous great saphenous vein, and possible myocutaneous flap

Reference
Fatima, J., Federico, V. P., Scali, S. T., et al. (2019). Management of patch infections after carotid endarterectomy and utility of femoral vein interposition bypass graft. *J Vasc Surg, 69*(6), 1815–1823. e1811. PMID: 30591294

37. RATIONALE

Radiation-induced carotid stenosis is often bilateral, and the plaque is invariably long and extends for a considerable distance cephalad. Carotid stenting (transfemoral or TCAR) is preferable in patients with a history of head and neck cancer treated with prior radiation and radical neck dissection with or without tracheostomy. Carotid endarterectomy in patients with a history of neck radiation is associated with slightly increased incidence of cranial nerve palsy, cervical hematoma, and wound complications. Patients undergoing carotid artery stenting are at a higher risk of restenosis, mostly asymptomatic, and can be managed without repeat intervention in a majority of patients. The exact mechanism of radiation-induced carotid stenosis is not well established. The process is inflammatory, and plaque characteristics are similar to those present in atherosclerotic disease.

Correct Answer   A Bilateral and plaque extends cephalad for a considerable distance

Reference
Fokkema, M., den Hartog, A. G., Bots, M. L., et al. (2012). Stenting versus surgery in patients with carotid stenosis after previous cervical radiation therapy: systematic review and meta-analysis. *Stroke, 43*(3), 793–801. PMID: 22207504

38. RATIONALE

The onset of seizure is between 12 hours and 10 days following carotid endarterectomy, probably as a result of hyperperfusion. Reperfusion is a more apt description of the hemodynamic mechanism for the development of seizures. No changes in the middle cerebral artery or mean flow velocities were detected by transcranial Doppler. The white matter edema (vasogenic) correlates with breakthrough of an autoregulatory mechanism, which has been demonstrated in patients with hyperperfusion syndrome on CT scan and T2-weighted MR imaging. Most patients have a history of labile hypertension and associated severe carotid and vertebral disease. Akinetic mutism and confusion as a manifestation of non-convulsive status epilepticus has been reported following carotid endarterectomy for severe carotid stenosis. This can be easily confused with aphasia as a symptom of stroke following carotid endarterectomy. Urgent neurological consult, especially with a neurologist with an interest in seizure disorders, should be obtained.

Correct Answer   D 12 hours to 10 days after carotid endarterectomy

Reference

Naylor, A. R., Evans, J., Thompson, M. M., et al. (2003). Seizures after carotid endarterectomy: hyperperfusion, dysautoregulation or hypertensive encephalopathy? *Eur J Vasc Endovasc Surg*, *26*(1), 39–44. PMID: 12819646

39. RATIONALE

The most common presentation of a carotid body tumor is an asymptomatic neck mass. Larger tumors can manifest as fullness, pain, dysphagia, odynophagia, and hoarseness due to pressure on the surrounding structures. Tumors of 3 cm or larger size can be appreciated as a neck mass. The mass may be displaced laterally but not vertically (Fontaine sign). These tumors can be diagnosed by carotid duplex and CT angiography. A rare functional carotid body tumor may produce neuro-endocranial secretions resulting in catecholamine-related symptoms such as palpitations, headaches, hypertension, tachycardia, and flushing.

Correct Answer   B Asymptomatic neck mass

Reference

Kakkos, S. K., Reddy, D. J., Shepard, A. D., et al. (2009). Contemporary presentation and evolution of management of neck paragangliomas. *J Vasc Surg*, *49*(6), 1365–1373.e1362. PMID: 19497493

40. RATIONALE

The Shamblin classification divides carotid body tumors into type I – tumors are small lesions at the carotid bifurcation and can be removed without difficulty – and type II – tumors are larger and significantly splay the carotid bifurcation but do not circumferentially encase the carotid arteries. Type III tumors are large, encapsulate the internal carotid artery and/or external carotid artery, and may be adherent to adjacent cranial nerves.

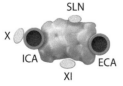

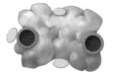
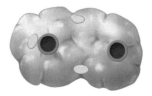

Shamblin Type I   Type II   Type III

Shamblin classification of carotid body tumors.

Correct Answer **D** Size of the tumor, difficulty of resection, and risk of neurovascular complications

Reference
Davila, V., Chang, J., Stone, W., et al. (2016). Current surgical management of carotid body tumors. *J Vasc Surg Cases*, *64*(6), 1703–1710. PMID: 27871494

41. RATIONALE

Baroreceptor failure is a very rare but serious complication following bilateral carotid body tumor resection. It should be suspected with the development of tachycardia and hypertension 24–72 hours postoperatively. Prompt identification of such a syndrome is imperative, as complications may include stroke and hypertensive encephalopathy. This condition does not occur after unilateral carotid body tumor resection, indicating the contralateral preservation of the baroreceptor is adequate to maintain normal physiological balance. Treatment is largely empiric. During hypertensive crisis, medications with a quick onset of action and a short half-life such as nitroprusside, phentolamine, and labetalol are preferred. For long-term treatment, clonidine is the drug of choice.

Correct Answer **D** Occurs 24–72 hours after bilateral carotid body tumor resection manifesting as headaches, anxiety with tachycardia, and hypertension

Reference
Ketch, T., Biaggioni, I., Robertson, R., & Robertson, D. (2002). Four faces of baroreflex failure: hypertensive crisis, volatile hypertension, orthostatic tachycardia, and malignant vagotonia. *Circulation*, *105*(21), 2518–2523. PMID: 12034659

42. RATIONALE

Malignant carotid body tumors are rare and carry a poor prognosis compared with benign carotid body tumors. Malignant tumors have a more advanced Shamblin classification and larger tumor size. These tumors are often adherent to the internal carotid artery and external carotid artery and surrounding nerves. Postoperative radiation therapy is recommended. The role of chemotherapy is limited. Besides loco-regional spread, distant metastasis may develop at a late follow-up.

Correct Answer **B** Radiation therapy

Reference
Gu, G., Wang, Y., Liu, B., et al. (2020). Distinct features of malignant carotid body tumors and surgical techniques for challengeable lesions: a case series of 11 patients. *Eur Arch Otorhinolaryngol*, *277*(3), 853–861. PMID: 31807890

43. RATIONALE

A standard approach beginning with exposure of the common carotid artery in the lower neck and progressing the dissection cephalad with early identification of the vagus nerve is used. Cranial nerve injuries are the most frequent complication of this operation, and the risk increases with tumor size. The dissection plane is carried out in the subadventitial plane with the use of bipolar cautery. This avascular plane between the tumor and the media is the so-called white line. The majority of blood flow to the carotid body tumor is from the external carotid artery, and these tumors are highly vascular. The external carotid artery can be ligated, if necessary, with a decrease in vascularity of the tumor, and this will facilitate dissection of the tumor from the internal carotid artery. An internal-to-external carotid dissection with freeing of the tumor from the internal carotid artery with Mayo dissection scissors is conducted, and the external carotid artery is the last one to be dissected. This approach lessens the chance of injury to the internal carotid artery. A cranial-to-caudal dissection has also been described based on the course of the ascending pharyngeal artery, which can be the main source of the blood supply to the tumor. As the dissection begins at a more cephalad level, the tumor is devascularized earlier and there is less blood loss. In addition, the nerves are dissected first and are preserved with less chance of cranial nerve injury. The role of preoperative embolization of the tumor blood supply is controversial but should be considered in tumors larger than 5 cm in diameter. When embolization is performed, surgical resection is recommended within 24–48 hours to avoid a post-embolization inflammatory response in surrounding tissues. Recently, coil embolization of the branches of the external carotid artery was supplanted by direct injection of the Onyx liquid embolic system (Medtronic, Minneapolis, MN) into the tumor with a marked decrease in its vascularity.

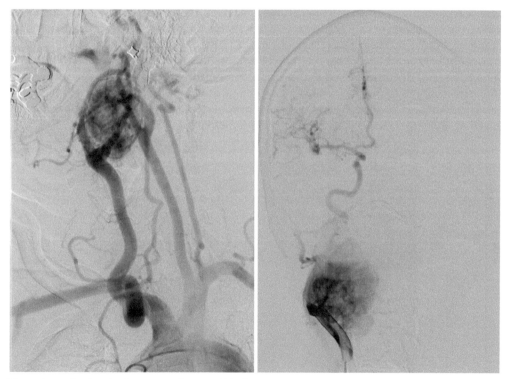

Carotid arteriography showing hypervascular carotid body tumor.

Correct Answer   C Incidence of cranial nerve palsy is higher than stroke

Reference
van der Bogt, K. E., Vrancken Peeters, M. P., van Baalen, J. M., & Hamming, J. F. (2008). Resection of carotid body tumors: results of an evolving surgical technique. *Ann Surg, 247*(5), 877–884. PMID: 18438127

44. RATIONALE

The incidence of carotid aneurysm is low (0.1%–3.7%). Atherosclerotic disease of the carotid artery is the most common cause of extracranial carotid artery aneurysm. True aneurysms can be either fusiform or saccular. Fusiform aneurysms tend to be bilateral, degenerative, and located near the carotid bifurcation. Saccular aneurysms are unilateral and occur in the ICA. Pseudoaneurysms typically occur in the disrupted vessel along the suture line of the patch angioplasty. Less common causes of carotid artery pseudoaneurysms include carotid dissection and blunt and penetrating traumatic injuries involving the common/internal carotid artery.

Correct Answer   **B** Atherosclerosis

Reference
Srivastava, S. D., Eagleton, M. J., O'Hara, P., et al. (2010). Surgical repair of carotid artery aneurysms: a 10-year, single-center experience. *Ann Vasc Surg, 24*(1), 100–105. PMID: 20122464

45. RATIONALE

Both CTA and MRA are helpful in determining the extent of the aneurysm and its location in surgical planning. CTA is helpful in providing clear information about the extent of the aneurysm and its relation to bony structures such as the styloid process, angle of the mandible, and vertebral bodies. Catheter-based carotid/cerebral arteriography has also been used to delineate the carotid aneurysm, but there is a small risk of cerebral embolization with neurological complications, and CTA can provide all the necessary information required for treatment planning. Balloon occlusion testing has used carotid/cerebral artery arteriography in cases of high carotid artery aneurysms (near the base of the skull) for consideration of internal carotid artery ligation in order to assess the cross-filling from the contralateral side.

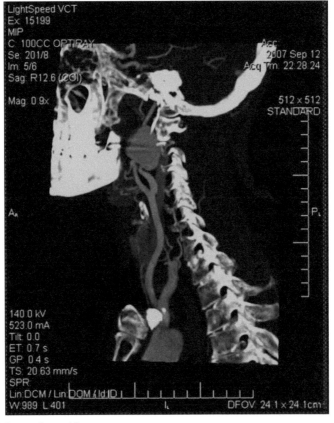

CTA showing large right internal carotid aneurysm.

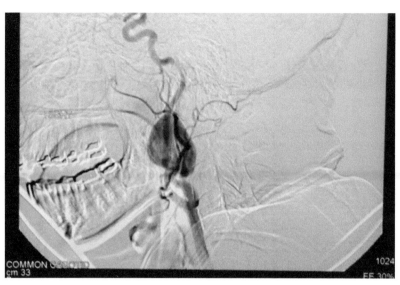

Carotid arteriogram showing right internal carotid aneurysm.

Correct Answer B CTA

Reference
Srivastava, S. D., Eagleton, M. J., O'Hara, P., et al. (2010). Surgical repair of carotid artery aneurysms: a
10-year, single-center experience. *Ann Vasc Surg, 24*(1), 100–105. PMID: 20122464

46. **RATIONALE**

The goal of treatment is to remove the aneurysm and restore vessel continuity. Aneurysm resection can be challenging depending on its size, surrounding inflammation, and the location.
Smaller aneurysms with associated redundancy of the internal carotid artery may be resected
with direct end-to-end anastomosis of the mobilized internal carotid artery in a continuous or
interrupted fashion, spatulating both ends of the internal carotid artery with preservation of
the luminal diameter. It is preferable to bring the anastomosed internal carotid artery in front
of the hypoglossal nerve. Interposition grafting with a synthetic or vein graft conduit has been
described. The choice of conduit depends on the vessel diameter and operative field. In mycotic
aneurysms, autologous arterial or venous conduits are the preferred options. Patency of a synthetic graft is only slightly inferior to a vein interposition graft. With its easy availability, a prosthetic graft in a challenging or high-risk patient is justified. Tapered grafts may be more suitable
when transitioning from a large-diameter common carotid artery to a smaller-diameter internal
carotid artery. For aneurysms with a cephalad location, nasotracheal intubation with or without
mandibular subluxation, with distal exposure and mobilization of the internal carotid artery by
dividing the posterior belly of the digastric and stylohyoid muscles may be required. In mycotic
aneurysms, use of an autologous vein or superficial femoral artery as a conduit for interposition grafting is preferred. Ligation of the internal carotid artery is usually not recommended
unless the aneurysm is in an inaccessible location and the patient has demonstrated satisfactory intracerebral collateral blood flow during preoperative cerebral arteriography with balloon
occlusion and confirmed with intraoperative assessment of satisfactory backpressure with no
evidence of ischemia on EEG monitoring. Endovascular treatment with a covered stent or coil
embolization for carotid pseudoaneurysm has been described in patients with a hostile neck
with or without an inaccessible location of such aneurysms.

74 Section 5: Cerebrovascular Disease

Correct Answer **A** Resection of the aneurysm with end-to-end anastomosis

Reference
Srivastava, S. D., Eagleton, M. J., O'Hara, P., et al. (2010). Surgical repair of carotid artery aneurysms: a 10-year, single-center experience. *Ann Vasc Surg, 24*(1), 100–105. PMID: 20122464

47. RATIONALE

The most common complication of the repair of an extracranial carotid aneurysm is cranial nerve palsy. The incidence of temporary cranial nerve palsy has been reported to be as high as 20%. Permanent cranial nerve palsy has been reported to be in 6.3% of patients. The postoperative stroke rate is reported to be 1.6%. Thrombosis at the site of anastomosis is uncommon and is usually due to technical factors. The 5-year survival is 90%, and 10-year survival of 77% has been reported with a stroke-free survival rate of 80%–87%. The stroke rate of untreated carotid aneurysms has been reported at greater than 50%.

Correct Answer **B** Cranial nerve palsy

Reference
Attigah, N., Külkens, S., Zausig, N., et al. (2009). Surgical therapy of extracranial carotid artery aneurysms: long-term results over a 24-year period. *Eur J Vasc Endovasc Surg, 37*(2), 127–133. PMID: 19046645

48. RATIONALE

Most extracranial vertebral artery aneurysms are pseudoaneurysms, usually associated with trauma or dissection. Primary cervical vertebral artery aneurysms are even rarer and are most often the result of a connective tissue disorder including Ehlers–Danlos syndrome, Marfan disease, and neurofibromatosis. The natural history of vertebral artery aneurysms is not well defined. Open repair in the form of resection and vertebral artery bypass with the great saphenous vein, external carotid artery autograft, and vertebral artery transposition into the common carotid artery has been described. Endovascular occlusion is not recommended because of the risk of posterior circulation stroke. In a few instances hybrid techniques with bypass combined with occlusion of the aneurysm with balloons and detachable coils have been described. In patients with Ehlers–Danlos syndrome, the repair is extremely difficult due to tissue degradation. Anastomosis should be performed with interrupted monofilament sutures using mini-pledgets. Despite careful technique, the repair may break down, requiring vertebral artery ligation.

Correct Answer **D** Connective tissue disorder

Reference
Morasch, M. D., Phade, S. V., Naughton, P., et al. (2013). Primary extracranial vertebral artery aneurysms. *Ann Vasc Surg, 27*(4), 418–423. PMID: 23540677

49. RATIONALE

The internal carotid artery is normally coiled, and straightening occurs when the fetal heart and great vessel descend into the mediastinum. If the descent is incomplete, coiling will occur. Conversely, kinking occurs when a tortuous carotid artery develops an acute angulation with subintimal deposits, loss of elasticity, and elongation, and occasionally aneurysmal degeneration will occur. Based on angiographic studies coils occur in 10%–16% of the general population and are equally common in men and women. Hypertension is present in 80%–85% of patients with carotid kinks. Most carotid kinks are asymptomatic, but a patient may present with dizziness. Patients with carotid kinks have a higher incidence of abdominal aortic aneurysm as compared to the general population. Patients with symptomatic carotid kinks should be considered for resection of a kinked or coiled internal carotid artery with end-to-end anastomosis in a spatulated manner. The redundant internal carotid artery may be resected and reimplanted into a more proximal site in the common carotid artery.

Correct Answer   **D** Carotid kinks affect women more than men

Reference
Ballotta, E., Thiene, G., & Baracchini, C. (2005). Surgical vs medical treatment for isolated internal carotid artery elongation with coiling or kinking in symptomatic patients: a prospective randomized clinical study. *J Vasc Surg*, *42*(5), 838–846; discussion 846. PMID: 16275432

50. RATIONALE

Atherosclerosis is the most common disease affecting the vertebral artery. Approximately 25% of all ischemic strokes occur in the vertebrobasilar territory. One half of patients will present initially with stroke, and 26% of patients present with transient ischemic symptoms rapidly followed by stroke. The mortality associated with posterior circulation stroke is 20%–30%, which is higher than that for the anterior circulation stroke. Ischemia affecting the temporo-occipital area of cerebral hemispheres, segments of the brainstem, and cerebellum characteristically produce bilateral symptoms. The classic symptoms of vertebrobasilar ischemia are dizziness, vertigo, drop attacks, diplopia, perioral numbness, tinnitus, dysphasia, dysarthria, and ataxia. Ischemic manifestations can be due to hemodynamic changes and embolic phenomena. Symptoms occur as a result of transient "end organ" (brainstem, cerebellum, occipital lobes) hypoperfusion and rarely result in infarction. For hemodynamic symptoms to occur, occlusive lesions must be present in both of the paired vertebral arteries. In addition, collateral cerebral flow via the circle of Willis must be incomplete. Up to one-third of vertebrobasilar ischemic episodes are caused by embolization from plaques as mural lesions of the subclavian, vertebral, and/or basilar arteries. Actual infarction in the vertebrobasilar distribution is most often the result of an embolic event.

Correct Answer   **C** 22%–35%

Reference
Caplan, L. R., Wityk, R. J., Glass, T. A., et al. (2004). New England Medical Center Posterior Circulation registry. *Ann Neurol*, *56*(3), 389–398. PMID: 15349866

51. RATIONALE

This will be considered a low-output chyle leak. Changing the enteral diet to a diet in which only medium-chain triglycerides are present can markedly decrease the amount of drainage. Adding the somatostatin analog octreotide is also helpful. Octreotide causes smooth muscle vasoconstriction in the splenic and lymphatic vessels to decrease lymph production and flow. Surgical management is reserved for patients who fail conservative management and is more often necessary in high-output chyle fistulas. Total parental nutrition with the patient kept nothing by mouth is recommended if more aggressive measures become necessary. Thoracic duct embolization may be necessary if the patient has a chylothorax.

Correct Answer **C** Local compression, dietary manipulation, and octreotide

Reference
Nandy, K., Jayaprakash, D., Rai, S., et al. (2022). Management of chyle leak after head and neck surgery; our meritorious experience in 52 cases and review of literature. *Indian J Otolaryngol Head Neck Surg, 74*(Suppl 3), 5978–5983. PMID: 36742724

52. **RATIONALE**

Surgical repair of an extracranial carotid artery aneurysm is associated with a perioperative stroke rate of 6%–9% and a mortality rate of 1%–2%. The most common complication of carotid aneurysm repair is cranial nerve palsy and ranges from 3% to 17%. Zhow et al. reported 42 cases of carotid aneurysms divided into two groups. Group 1 (1984–1994) had 22 patients and group 2 (1995–2004) had 20 patients. In group 1, all patients underwent open repair; while in group 2, 14 patients underwent endovascular repair, 5 interposition grafting following resection, and 1 carotid ligation. Most aneurysms in their series were degenerative (atherosclerotic), but 36% were pseudoaneurysms. The 30-day mortality/stroke rate was 14% in group 1 and 5% in group 2 ($P < 0.04$).

Correct Answer **C** 5%–9%

Reference
Zhou, W., Lin, P. H., Bush, R. L., et al. (2006). Carotid artery aneurysm: evolution of management over two decades. *J Vasc Surg, 43*(3), 493–496; discussion 497. PMID: 16520161

53. **RATIONALE**

Spontaneous extracranial internal carotid artery dissection has an incidence of 2.6–2.9 per 100,000 people annually, with a median age of 45 years, with a male-to-female ratio of 57:53. Carotid artery dissection can also occur when there is major or minor trauma that causes the neck to hyperextend laterally, rotate, or have abnormal lateral displacement. The most common location is 2–3 cm above the carotid bifurcation in the extracranial segment of the internal carotid artery and accounts for 2.5% of all initial strokes. Patients are more likely to have hypertension but are less likely to have hyperlipidemia. It is postulated that genetic factors have a role in the pathophysiology of carotid artery dissection. Inherited connective tissue conditions such as Ehlers–Danlos syndrome, Marfan syndrome, osteogenesis imperfecta, and FMD increase the risk of carotid artery dissection by 16- to 18-fold. Family history of arterial dissection has been shown to be another risk factor for recurrent arterial dissection. Recurrent ischemic events seem to be rare and usually occur during the first 4 weeks after dissection. At 1 year, the rate of ischemic recurrences has been estimated to be 0.4%–13.3%. Factors associated with an increased risk of recurrent ischemic events are multiple dissections and a history of hypertension. The prognosis of recurrent carotid artery dissection is usually benign.

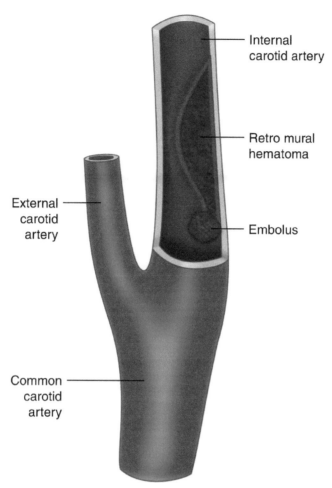

Internal
carotid artery

Retro mural
hematoma

External
carotid
artery

Embolus

Common
carotid
artery

Carotid artery dissection.

Correct Answer **B** 2.5%–3%

Reference
Schievink, W. I., Mokri, B., & O'Fallon, W. M. (1994). Recurrent spontaneous cervical-artery dissection. *N Engl J Med, 330*(6), 393–397. PMID: 8284004

54. RATIONALE

The classic triad of carotid and vertebral artery dissection includes unilateral pain of the head and neck or face, partial Horner syndrome (ptosis, miosis), and cerebral or retinal ischemia. However, less than one-third of patients will present with all three components. The pathogenesis of a cervical artery dissection (carotid or vertebral) involves a hematoma that develops within the layers of the wall of the carotid or vertebral artery due to an intimal tear, direct bleeding into the arterial wall from a ruptured vasa vasorum or an intramural hematoma expanding towards the intima or adventitial layers resulting in stenosis, or aneurysmal dilation of the carotid/vertebral artery.

Correct Answer   **A** Unilateral headache, neck, and facial pain

Reference
Schievink, W. I., Mokri, B., & O'Fallon, W. M. (1994). Recurrent spontaneous cervical-artery dissection. *N Engl J Med*, *330*(6), 393–397. PMID: 8284004

55. RATIONALE

Antithrombotic therapy with either anticoagulation or antiplatelet drugs has been used for ischemic stroke and TIA caused by cervical artery dissection. Anticoagulation may prevent occlusion of a stenotic vessel and minimize distal embolization. Extension of intramural hematoma in the presence of an anticoagulant medication is rare; however, the evidence suggests no advantage of anticoagulation over antiplatelet medications. In a randomized trial assigned to either antiplatelet or anticoagulant treatment for 3 months in patients with extracranial carotid or vertebral artery dissection, a meta-analysis did not show any significant differences between the two treatment groups. Similarly, one meta-analysis of nonrandomized studies with over 1300 patients who had acute carotid dissection also found no differences in outcome or complication rates when anticoagulation was used in place of antiplatelet therapy.

Correct Answer   **C** Anticoagulation/antithrombotic therapy

Reference
Markus, H. S., Hayter, E., Levi, C., Feldman, A., Venables, G., & Norris, J. (2015). Antiplatelet treatment compared with anticoagulation treatment for cervical artery dissection (CADISS): a randomised trial. *Lancet Neurol*, *14*(4), 361–367. PMID: 25684164

SECTION 6: VASCULAR SURGICAL CRITICAL CARE

MCQs 1–15

Q1. A 75-year-old man with a history of chronic obstructive pulmonary disease develops ARDS on the fourth postoperative day following open abdominal aortic aneurysm repair and is placed on ventilatory support with a PEEP of 10 mmHg. The ideal tidal volume for this patient is:
A. 4–6 mL/kg
B. 7–10 mL/kg
C. 11–15 mL/kg
D. 15–20 mL/kg

Q2. Sixteen hours after open repair of a ruptured abdominal aortic aneurysm in a 74-year-old man with a prior history of coronary artery bypass graft, urine output is low, <25 cc/hr for 4 hours. He received 10 liters of crystalloids in the operating room and 8 units of packed red blood cells and 4 units of frozen plasma. What is the best measure to evaluate fluid responsiveness?
A. Central venous pressure (CVP)
B. Aggressive crystalloid bolus
C. Insertion of pulmonary artery catheter
D. Bedside cardiac ultrasonography

Q3. Eight days following femoral-tibial bypass for critical limb ischemia, an 80-year-old woman has inferior wall myocardial infarction and respiratory complications necessitating mechanical ventilation. She develops fever and is diagnosed with a ventilator-associated pneumonia caused by *Klebsiella pneumoniae*. The proper duration for antibiotics is:
A. Until the chest X-ray is clear
B. Until the WBC count is normal and fever has resolved

C. 7–8 days
D. 15 days

Q4. A 68-year-old woman is currently sedated and intubated following open repair of a ruptured abdominal aortic aneurysm. She has received propofol and fentanyl for sedation and analgesia. In regard to her pulmonary management, what intervention is most likely to lead to prompt liberation from the ventilator?
A. Measurement of rapid shallow breathing index
B. Early tracheostomy
C. Assisted controlled ventilation
D. Daily sedation holiday

Q5. A 74-year-old woman with a history of diabetes mellitus underwent left femoral-peroneal in situ bypass for an ischemic ulcer of the left big toe with cellulitis. She is being treated with intravenous antibiotics. Five days later she develops diarrhea with a white blood cell count of 36,000/mm³. The most appropriate therapy for suspected *Clostridioides difficile* infection in this patient would be:
A. 400 mg of oral rifaximin three times daily
B. 500 mg of oral metronidazole four times a day
C. 200 mg of oral fidaxomicin two times a day
D. 1 gm of intravenous vancomycin every 12 hours

Q6. Microcirculatory perfusion improves by using:
A. RBCs stored for 4 weeks
B. RBCs stored for 5 weeks
C. RBCs stored for 6 weeks
D. Fresh non-leukoreduced RBC transfusion

DOI: 10.1201/9781003389897-6

Q7. Following open repair of a ruptured AAA, an 81-year-old man requires ventilatory assistance. He has dilutional coagulopathy. Gastrointestinal (GI) bleeding prophylaxis should result in:
A. No important reduction in GI bleeding
B. An important reduction in GI bleeding
C. An important reduction in GI bleeding but may result in an increased incidence of pneumonia
D. An important reduction in GI bleeding without any increased incidence of pneumonia

Q8. An 85-year-old man had open repair of a ruptured AAA. He is in ICU 3 weeks following repair on mechanical ventilation, renal replacement therapy, and pneumonia. He develops invasive candidiasis. The optimal management consists of:
A. Nystatin
B. Voriconazole
C. Micafungin
D. Liposomal amphotericin B

Q9. A 68-year-old man had anterior resection for rectosigmoid cancer 5 days ago. He developed massive swelling of the leg. Duplex venous study showed acute deep vein thrombosis involving the entire deep venous system of the left lower extremity. He was started on unfractionated heparin with elevation of the left lower extremity. The following morning, the patient became unresponsive with a heart rate of 132 beats/minute. He's afebrile. His blood pressure is 76/38 mmHg. Oxygen saturation is 90% with FiO_2 100%, WBC count 13,000/mm³, HCT 36%, and serum creatinine 0.9 mg/dL. The patient was started on a norepinephrine drip to maintain systolic blood pressure above 80 mm. A CT pulmonary actogram showed a large thrombus in the main trunk extending to both pulmonary arteries. What is the next step in management?
A. Argatroban
B. Alteplase
C. Enoxaparin
D. Rivaroxaban

Q10. Following repair of a ruptured AAA, a 78-year-old man is hypothermic. He has received 14 units of packed cells, 6 units of fresh-frozen plasma, 5 units of platelets, and is on ventilatory support. Which of the following is the most effective method of active rewarming for this patient?
A. Aluminum-lined head covers
B. Increase room temperature
C. Heating/cotton blankets and forced air warming
D. Ventilator circuit heating

Q11. A 76-year-old man undergoes open repair of a ruptured AAA. On the fourth postoperative day, the patient is in severe metabolic acidosis without response to sodium bicarbonate supplements intravenously. His blood pressure is 80 mm systolic. He is intubated and is on assist control ventilation mode with FiO_2 of 80% and PO_2 of 70%. Serum lactate is 4 mmol/L and WBC count is 16,000/mm³ with a shift to the left. The next step in the management of this patient is:
A. CT of the abdomen and pelvis
B. Stool for *Clostridium difficile* toxin
C. Laparotomy
D. Measurement of intraabdominal pressure for possible compartment syndrome

Q12. A 76-year-old man with diabetes mellitus, non-alcoholic cirrhosis, and chronic kidney disease undergoes a femoral–anterior tibial bypass for critical limb ischemia. On postoperative day 2, he developed a sudden onset of atrial fibrillation with a rapid ventricular response. Despite rate control and diuresis, he remains in atrial fibrillation 6 days later. Which of the following risk factors is useful in determining the initiation of anticoagulation?
A. Diabetes mellitus
B. Chronic kidney disease
C. Liver cirrhosis
D. Persistent atrial fibrillation

Q13. A 75-year-old, 110-kg man intubated after open repair of a large juxtarenal AAA using a left retroperitoneal approach becomes combative on the third postoperative day, striking at the staff and trying to pull out the lines and endotracheal tube. In addition to pain management, which of the following is the best management strategy?

A. Haloperidol 10 mg intravenously every 6 hours

B. Lorazepam 5 mg intravenously every 6 hours

C. Dexmedetomidine 0.7 μg/kg/hr intravenous infusion

D. Propofol (Diprivan) 10 mg/mL targeted controlled infusion

Q14. A 63-year-old man with a long-standing history of cigarette smoking presents for preoperative evaluation for a femoral-popliteal bypass for ischemic rest pain, which is scheduled for 4 weeks. With respect to smoking cessation and its effect on the postoperative course:

A. There is no outcome difference between smokers and non-smokers who undergo elective surgery

B. Perioperative smoking cessation reduces the incidence of surgical site infection

C. A remote smoking history does not increase the risk of long-term healing complications

D. Smoking cessation less than 2 months before surgery results in an increase in postoperative complications

Q15. An 82-year-old man is 6 days postoperative following open repair of a ruptured AAA with a horseshoe kidney. His BMI is less than 30, and he is critically ill with multiple organ failure. The recommended caloric requirements for this patient are:

A. 20 kcal/kg/day

B. 25 kcal/kg/day

C. 30 kcal/kg/day

D. 12 kcal/kg/day

RATIONALE 1–15

1. RATIONALE

Pulmonary complications have been reported in up to 80% of postoperative patients undergoing open vascular reconstruction. Risk factors for pulmonary complications include advanced age, male gender, current or former smoking history, history of chronic obstructive pulmonary disease, acuity of the procedure, more complex operation, obesity, and higher American Society of Anesthesiologists classification. Acute respiratory failure may manifest as hypoxemia due to difficulty with oxygenation or difficulty with ventilation leading to hypercapnia. Management includes identification and correction of the underlying cause resulting in the persistence of respiratory failure and significant underlying systemic inflammatory response. The patient may develop acute respiratory distress syndrome (ARDS), which is defined as acute onset (within 1 week) of bilateral lung opacity with exclusion of cardiogenic pulmonary edema. A P/F ratio (PO_2/FiO_2) of 300–200 is mild, 200–100 is moderate, and <100 is severe ARDS with PEEP equal to or greater than 5 cm of water. Management of ARDS revolves around protective lung ventilation with a decreased tidal volume (4–6 mL/kg) and limitation of plateau pressure (<35 cm water).

Correct Answer   **A** 4–6 mL/kg

Reference

Johnson, R. G., Arozullah, A. M., Neumayer, L., Henderson, W. G., Hosokawa, P., & Khuri, S. F. (2007). Multivariable predictors of postoperative respiratory failure after general and vascular surgery: results from the patient safety in surgery study. *J Am Coll Surg*, *204*(6), 1188–1198. PMID: 17544077

2. RATIONALE

Preload responsiveness may be difficult to determine accurately in a critical care setting after a major intraabdominal surgery. Several modalities are available, and there is a preponderance of evidence for the use of bedside ultrasonography (BCU). In spontaneously breathing patients, a stroke volume increase of more than 12% during passive leg raising is highly suggestive of fluid responsiveness. A cutoff value of 15% change in inferior vena cava (IVC) diameter between inspiration and expiration and positive pressure ventilation accurately separates patients who will respond to fluid administration in contrast to those who will not. Passive leg raising and IVC collapsibility measures are unable to predict fluid responsiveness in patients with intraabdominal hypertension. Recent data has suggested that central venous pressure does not correlate with fluid resuscitation. Overly aggressive crystalloid-based resuscitation may result in untoward outcomes.

Correct Answer   **D** Bedside cardiac ultrasonography

Reference

Levitov, A., Frankel, H. L., Blaivas, M., et al. (2016). Guidelines for the appropriate use of bedside general and cardiac ultrasonography in the evaluation of critically Ill patients-Part II: cardiac ultrasonography. *Crit Care Med*, *44*(6), 1206–1227. PMID: 27182849

3. RATIONALE

Recommendations from the Infectious Diseases Society of America and the American Thoracic Society supported by well-controlled randomized trials showed that a short course of 7–8 days is as safe and effective as 14–15 days of antibiotics. The chest X-ray findings may be abnormal due to other causes such as atelectasis or pleural effusion. Normalization of pulmonary infiltrates caused by pneumonia often lags behind the resolution of pneumonia. Continuation of antibiotics for a prolonged period is not necessary and may result in side effects.

Correct Answer   **C** 7–8 days

Reference

Zilahi, G., McMahon, M. A., Povoa, P., & Martin-Loeches, I. (2016). Duration of antibiotic therapy in the intensive care unit. *J Thorac Dis*, *8*(12), 3774–3780. PMID: 28149576

4. RATIONALE

The optimal time to liberate a patient from the ventilator is often difficult to determine and should be addressed on a frequent basis to decrease the time for ventilator assistance. The benefits are the decreased length of ICU length of stay as well as decrease in morbidity and mortality. There is often an overuse of sedation in managing patients on ventilatory support. Patients should preferably receive intermittent sedation as needed. Regardless of the time on the ventilator, the use of spontaneous breathing trials in conjunction with a protocol of daily sedation holidays has the greatest effect in decreasing the days that patient is on ventilatory support. Regardless of the medications used or mode of ventilation, protocols that discontinue sedation and allow for early extubation lead to improved outcomes. Early tracheostomy after laparotomy for aneurysm repair should not be performed. The weaning parameters for extubation include adequate tidal volume, appropriate vital capacity, appropriate negative inspiratory force, and rapid shallow breathing index (<105) to help predict successful extubation.

Correct Answer   **D** Daily sedation holiday

Reference

Juern, J. S. (2012). Removing the critically ill patient from mechanical ventilation. *Surg Clin North Am*, *92*(6), 1475–1483. PMID: 23153880

5. RATIONALE

According to the guidelines published by the Infectious Diseases Society of America, either oral fidaxomicin or oral vancomycin is the drug of choice for *Clostridioides difficile* colitis. Metronidazole should be used only in mild-to-moderate disease in younger patients who have no or only low risk factors for the recurrence of *C. difficile* colitis. Elderly and immunocompromised patients are at greater risk for recurrence. Fecal microbiota transplantation should be offered to patients with frequent recurrences of *C. difficile* infection.

Correct Answer   **C** 200 mg of oral fidaxomicin two times a day

Reference

McDonald, L. C., Gerding, D. N., Johnson, S., et al. (2018). Clinical practice guidelines for clostridium difficile infection in adults and children: 2017 update by the Infectious Diseases Society of America (IDSA) and Society for Healthcare Epidemiology of America (SHEA). *Clin Infect Dis*, *66*(7), e1–e48. PMID: 29462280

6. RATIONALE

The effects of storage (time) and leukocyte content probably interact since a longer storage duration is thought to cause a greater accumulation of leukocyte-derived cytokines and red blood cell (RBC) injury. A randomized assignment of two groups of mixed surgical patients Group A (fresh stored less than 1 week) and Group B (stored more than 3 weeks) were transfused. Both groups had an increase in hemoglobin concentration. From a randomized assignment into two groups, with group A receiving fresh and group B receiving aged RBC transfusion, in both groups RBC transfusion caused an increase in hemoglobin concentration. RBC transfusions increased the functional capillary density in group A (fresh RBC), while functional capillary density (FCD) remained unaffected in group B (aged RBCs). Fresh non-leukoreduced RBC transfusions, but not RBCs stored for more than 3 weeks, were effective in improving microcirculatory perfusion by elevating the number of perfused microvessels in mixed surgical patients.

Correct Answer D Fresh non-leukoreduced RBC transfusion

Reference

Ayhan, B., Yuruk, K., Koene, S., et al. (2013). The effects of non-leukoreduced red blood cell transfusions on microcirculation in mixed surgical patients. *Transfus Apher Sci, 49*(2), 212–222. PMID: 23402838

7. RATIONALE

The results from a meta-analysis of 72 published trials comprising 12,660 patients that compared GI bleeding prophylaxis with proton pump inhibitors (PPIs), histamine-2 receptor antagonists (H2RAs), and sucralfate showed that for patients at highest risk (>8%) or high risk (4%–8%) for bleeding, both PPIs and H2RAs probably reduce clinically important GI bleeding compared with placebo or no prophylaxis. Both will increase the risk of pneumonia as compared with no prophylaxis. It is likely that neither affects mortality and morbidity as a result of *Clostridium difficile* infection, length of ICU stay, or duration of mechanical ventilation.

Correct Answer C An important reduction in GI bleeding but may result in an increased incidence of pneumonia

Reference

Wang, Y., Ye, Z., & Ge, L. (2020). Efficacy and safety of gastrointestinal bleeding prophylaxis in critically ill patients: systematic review and network meta-analysis. *BMJ, 368,* l6744. PMID: 31907166

8. RATIONALE

Invasive candidiasis is present in seriously ill patients. A double-blind, randomized, multinational, non-inferiority trial to compare micafungin (100 mg/day) with liposomal amphotericin B as the first-line treatment of candidemia and invasive candidiasis included 267 patients randomly assigned to receive liposomal amphotericin B and 264 randomly assigned to received micafungin. Treatment success was observed in 89.6% patients treated with micafungin and 89.5% treated with liposomal amphotericin B. Efficacy was independent of the *Candida* species and the primary site of infection as well as neutropenic status, APACHE II score, and whether a catheter was removed or replaced during the study. There were fewer treatment-related adverse events, including those that were serious or led to treatment discontinuation, with micafungin than there were with liposomal amphotericin B, concluding that micafungin was as effective and caused fewer adverse events than liposomal amphotericin B as the first-line treatment of candidemia and invasive candidiasis.

Correct Answer   **C** Micafungin

Reference
Kuse, E. R., Chetchotisakd, P., da Cunha, C. A., et al. (2007). Micafungin versus liposomal amphotericin B for candidaemia and invasive candidosis: a phase III randomised double-blind trial. *Lancet, 369*(9572), 1519–1527. PMID: 17482982

9. RATIONALE

Pulmonary embolism (PE) is a life-threatening complication of acute deep venous thrombosis. The appearance of a clot on CTA of the chest is suggestive that this patient has developed saddle embolus resulting in complete cardiovascular collapse and sudden onset of hypoxia, severe hypotension, and right heart strain. In a patient with PE but without any changes in hemodynamic status, the treatment of choice is heparin. In patients with hypotension, systemic thrombolytic therapy is recommended. Thrombolytic therapy can reduce mortality or recurrent embolism by 55% compared with heparin alone. The disadvantages include an obligatory 2-hour infusion with contraindications to systemic thrombolysis in 50% of patients and major bleeding complications in 20% of patients. Catheter-assisted pulmonary embolectomy allows significantly reduced doses of thrombolytic directly into the pulmonary artery using tenecteplase and tissue plasminogen activator (tPA). Catheter-based thrombectomy with use of the Angiojet rheolytic thrombectomy catheter (Medrad Interventional, Warrendale, PA) has a reported mortality in patients with massive PE ranging from 12% to 25%. Ultrasound-assisted therapies using the EKOS device (EKOS Endovascular System, Boston Scientific, Boston, MA) using a much smaller amount of tPA included in the ULTIMA (ultrasound-assisted, catheter-directed thrombolysis for acute and intermediate risk pulmonary embolism) study. The study conclusion was that ultrasound-assisted, catheter-directed thrombolysis using fixed-dose recombinant tPA (rtPA) is superior to heparin alone in improving right ventricle function in patients with submassive PE, without any increase in bleeding complications.

Correct Answer   **B** Alteplase

Reference
Kucher, N., Boekstegers, P., Müller, O. J., et al. (2014). Randomized, controlled trial of ultrasound-assisted catheter-directed thrombolysis for acute intermediate-risk pulmonary embolism. *Circulation, 129*(4), 479–486. PMID: 24226805

10. RATIONALE

Hypothermia is detrimental in patients with massive blood loss from a ruptured AAA because it may result in coagulopathy. Active internal warming is the most effective route of rewarming and can be performed with continuous arteriovenous rewarming and cardiopulmonary bypass, but these cannot be performed in this patient. Heating blankets and forced air warming are most effective, providing about 20 kcal/hr room warming, and the use of aluminum-lined head covers is another passive rewarming technique.

Correct Answer   **C** Heating/cotton blankets and forced air warming

Reference
Warttig, S., Alderson, P., Campbell, G., & Smith, A. F. (2014). Interventions for treating inadvertent postoperative hypothermia. *Cochrane Database Syst Rev,* (11), CD009892. PMID: 25411963

11. RATIONALE

Persistent acidosis with elevated lactate levels suggests intestinal ischemia, most likely colon infarction. Clinically significant colon ischemia occurs in 1%–2% of patients following abdominal aortic aneurysm (AAA) repair and is more common after repair of a ruptured AAA, resulting in 50%–75% mortality. The mortality can be as high as 90% if bowel resection is required. The presence of early postoperative diarrhea, melena, and hematochezia mandates fiberoptic sigmoidoscopy. Persistent metabolic acidosis following repair of ruptured AAA is an ominous finding, and the patient should undergo emergent laparotomy.

Correct Answer   C Laparotomy

Reference
Chaikof, E. L., Dalman, R. L., Eskandari, M. K., et al. (2018). The Society for Vascular Surgery practice guidelines on the care of patients with an abdominal aortic aneurysm. *J Vasc Surg,* 67(1), 2–77. e72. PMID: 29268916

12. RATIONALE

Initial management of atrial fibrillation with a rapid ventricular response is directed to obtain ventricular rate control, correct electrolytes (potassium and magnesium), and of the necessity for cardioversion. Thromboembolic risk is increased when atrial fibrillation is sustained longer than 48 hours. The risk of hemorrhage may outweigh the risk of a thromboembolic event in patients with postoperative atrial fibrillation of less than 48 hours' duration. Factors supporting anticoagulation are (a) CHADS/CHA2 DS2-VASC score of greater than 2, (b) age >75, (c) congestive heart failure, (d) hypertension, and (e) diabetes mellites, which all have a score of 1 point each. Stroke/TIA and thromboembolism have a score of 2 points. Based on the score, the approximate annual stroke risks are as follows: Score <1 (low), score 2–3 (intermediate), score 4–6 (high), with a stroke risk of 4% with score <1; stroke risk of 5%–6% with an intermediate score (2–3), and 18% stroke risk with a high score (4–6).

Correct Answer   A Diabetes mellitus

Reference
Hsu, J., Maddox, T., Kennedy, K., et al. (2016). Oral anticoagulant therapy prescription in patients with atrial fibrillation across the spectrum of stroke risk: insights from the NCDR PINNACLE registry. *JAMA Cardiol,* 1(1), 55–92. PMID: 27437655

13. RATIONALE

This patient with hyperactive delirium represents with an insidious hospital-acquired complication resulting in increased mortality and prolonged length of stay in the hospital and in the intensive care unit. Risk factors include preexisting dementia, uncontrolled pain, sleep deprivation, sepsis, and advanced age. Out of the proposed medications in the question, dexmedetomidine infusion is the best option, but it may cause bradycardia. Benzodiazepines are contraindicated for postoperative delusions. Haloperidol may result in torsade de pointes.

Correct Answer   **C** Dexmedetomidine 0.7 µg/kg/hr intravenous infusion

Reference
Barr, J., Fraser, G. L., Puntillo, K., et al. (2013). Clinical practice guidelines for the management of pain, agitation, and delirium in adult patients in the intensive care unit. *Critical Care Medicine, 41*(1), 263–306. PMID: 23269131

14. RATIONALE

Smoking has a negative effect on postoperative morbidity. Postoperative healing complications are increased in smokers as well as in former smokers compared with those patients who do not or have not ever smoked. There is a decrease in surgical site infection when a smoker stops smoking at least 4 weeks before surgery, but other healing problems are not reduced. Patients should try to stop smoking as early as possible. Health professionals should advise smokers to quit at least any time before surgery. The adverse effect of smoking on surgical site infections is due to (a) vasoconstriction, (b) impaired inflammatory response such as oxidative burst, and (c) delay of a proliferative healing phase with altered collagen metabolism.

Correct Answer   **B** Perioperative smoking cessation reduces the incidence of surgical site infection

Reference
Myers, K., Hajek, P., Hinds, C., & McRobbie, H. (2011). Stopping smoking shortly before surgery and postoperative complications: a systematic review and meta-analysis. *Arch Intern Med, 171*(11), 983–989. PMID: 21403009

15. RATIONALE

Most critically ill patients in the intensive care unit with sepsis, massive trauma, burns, or multiple organ system failure should receive 30 kcal/kg/day of nutritional support in 24 hours with a BMI of 30 or less. Patients who are sedated and are on mechanical ventilation will have a lower energy expenditure, and their requirement is only 20 kcal/kg/day. In patients with a BMI greater than 30, caloric intake should exceed 60%–70% of targeted energy requirements, or 11–14 kcal/kg actual body weight per day.

Correct Answer   **C** 30 kcal/kg/day

Reference
Barton, R. G. (2019). Nutrition support. In J. E. Parillo & R. P. Dellinger (Eds.), *Critical care medicine: principals of diagnosis and management in the adult* (5th ed., pp. 1273–1286). Philadelphia, PA: Elsevier Saunders.

SECTION 7: THORACIC OUTLET SYNDROME

MCQs 1–8

Q1. In patients with neurogenic thoracic outlet syndrome with an associated cervical rib, optimal decompression of the thoracic outlet consists of:
- **A.** Removal of the cervical rib and scalenectomy
- **B.** Removal of the first rib only
- **C.** Removal of the first rib, scalenectomy, and removal of cervical rib
- **D.** Removal of the cervical rib with staged removal of the first rib

Q2. A 32-year-old man undergoes left first rib resection for neurogenic thoracic outlet syndrome and presents to the outpatient clinic with a winged scapula on the left side. The nerve injury responsible for this appearance is:
- **A.** Thoracodorsal nerve
- **B.** Intercostal brachial nerve
- **C.** Long thoracic nerve
- **D.** Lower cord of brachial plexus

Q3. A 30-year-old man undergoes right first rib resection via a supraclavicular and infraclavicular incision for venous thoracic outlet syndrome and presents with recurrent swelling of the right upper extremity 6 months later. Venous duplex study shows long segmental occlusion of the subclavian and axillary vein. The best treatment option is:
- **A.** Stenting
- **B.** Open thrombectomy
- **C.** Compression sleeve
- **D.** Anticoagulation

Q4. Arterial thoracic outlet syndrome represents what percentage of patients of thoracic outlet syndrome?
- **A.** <1%
- **B.** 1%–3%
- **C.** 4%–5%
- **D.** 6%–8%

Q5. The incidence of recurrent neurogenic thoracic outlet syndrome after thoracic outlet decompression using a supraclavicular approach is approximately:
- **A.** 2%
- **B.** 3%–4%
- **C.** 5%
- **D.** >5%

Q6. The incidence of brachial plexus injury in surgery for thoracic outlet syndrome can be increased by the following factors:
- **A.** Anatomic variations and pathological findings
- **B.** Intraoperative bleeding
- **C.** Preoperative repetitive hyperextension neck trauma
- **D.** Anatomic variations, intraoperative bleeding, and preoperative repetitive hyperextension neck trauma

Q7. The number of patients with neurogenic thoracic outlet syndrome who exhibit physical findings that are isolated to the subcoracoid space is:
- **A.** Up to 10%
- **B.** Up to 20%
- **C.** Up to 25%
- **D.** Up to 30%

DOI: 10.1201/9781003389897-7

Q8. As compared to the supraclavicular approach, the advantage of the transaxillary first rib resection is:

A. Incision in the hidden axillary space and sufficient exposure for resection of the first rib

B. Incision in the hidden axillary space and sufficient exposure for the resection of both the first rib and cervical rib

C. Ability to form complete brachial plexus neurolysis

D. Ability to perform subclavian vein reconstruction in patients with venous thoracic outlet syndrome

RATIONALE 1–8

1. RATIONALE

The thoracic outlet region is composed of three anatomic spaces: The scalene triangle, the costoclavicular space, and the pectoralis minor space. The neurovascular bundle, which consists of the subclavian artery, subclavian vein, and brachial plexus, courses from the scalene triangle to the costoclavicular space and through the pectoralis minor space. Neurogenic thoracic outlet syndrome results from brachial plexus compression, which leads to neurological symptoms involving the upper extremity. Abnormal anatomy of the thoracic outlet region, as well as injuries and repetitive physical activities, can predispose a patient to the development of thoracic outlet syndrome. Because of the lack of objective criteria for neurogenic thoracic outlet syndrome, it is difficult to diagnose this condition. The presence of a cervical rib and a positive response to scalene muscle block are reliable indicators for surgery. The decompression can be performed by a supraclavicular or transaxillary approach, depending on the experience of the surgeon and the manifestation of thoracic outlet syndrome. Most surgeons prefer the supraclavicular approach in the presence of a cervical rib, but excellent results have also been reported using transaxillary approach even in the presence of the cervical rib. In patients with a cervical rib requiring thoracic outlet decompression, scalenectomy, and removal of the first rib as well as the cervical rib are necessary in order to obtain relief of symptoms.

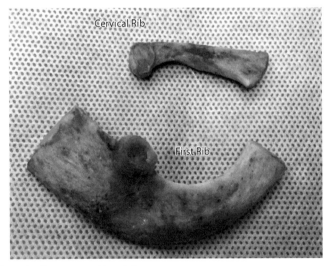

First rib with cervical rib, typically connected by a joint.

Correct Answer **C** Removal of the first rib, scalenectomy, and removal of cervical rib

Reference
Illig, K. A., Donahue, D., Duncan, A., et al. (2016). Reporting standards of the Society for Vascular Surgery for thoracic outlet syndrome: executive summary. *J Vasc Surg*, *64*(3), 797–802. PMID: 27565596

2. RATIONALE

Long thoracic nerve injury during decompression of the thoracic outlet may result in paralysis, pain, weakness, and limitation of shoulder elevation. The scapula tends to protrude at an awkward angle from the body. The patient may benefit from physical and massage therapy in addition to muscle relaxants and antiinflammatory drugs. Decompression of the thoracic outlet can be performed by either a supraclavicular or transaxillary approach. During the supraclavicular exposure, the phrenic nerve is identified in front of the scalenus anticus, and scalenectomy at its attachment to the first rib is performed, preferably using Mayo scissors, and the scalenus anticus origin is divided from the C6 transverse process. The brachial plexus will become apparent after division of the scalenus anticus. It should be brought forward with gentle retraction to expose the scalenus medius. Before dividing the scalenus medius, the long thoracic nerve must be identified. This nerve exists at the anterolateral border of the scalenus medius and courses inferolaterally. The posterior neck of the first rib is exposed with a periosteal elevator. The lateral musculofascial attachments to the first rib are then released anteriorly from its posterior neck to the scalene tubercle. The pleural apex is bluntly dissected from the inferior surface of the first rib. With the brachial plexus roots well protected from the neck of the first rib, which is divided sharply with a bone cutter, the anterior portion of the first rib is then exposed underneath the clavicle and similarly divided just medial to the level of the scalene tubercle, with protection of the subclavian vein, artery, and nerve roots. When the cervical rib is present, it should be resected after the middle scalenectomy is completed. It is exposed at its posterior origin and the neck of the rib is divided, protecting the origin of the nerve root (C8 and T1). The proximal end of the first rib is detached from its attachment of the first rib and removed as a specimen. When the cervical rib is present, it is resected after the middle scalenectomy is completed. It is exposed at its posterior origin and the neck of the rib is divided, protecting C8 and T1 from injury as the proximal end of the cervical attachment of the rib is detached from its first rib.

Correct Answer   C Long thoracic nerve

Reference
Karam, J., & Thompson, R. (2017). Neurogenic thoracic outlet syndrome. In S. S. Hans, A. D. Shepard, H. R. Weaver, P. G. Bove, & G. W. Long (Eds.), *Endovascular and open vascular reconstructions: a practical approach* (pp. 377–382). Boca Raton, FL: CRC Press.

3. RATIONALE
Effort-induced axillary-subclavian vein thrombosis, also known as Paget–Schroetter syndrome, is an underrecognized cause of upper extremity deep venous thrombosis. This represents venous manifestation of thoracic outlet syndrome, where the underlying cause is the compression of and repetitive injury to the subclavian vein between the first rib and clavicle. In patients with an acute-to-subacute presentation, restoring the patency of the subclavian vein is of paramount importance and is most rapidly achieved by pharmocomechanical thrombolysis. After thrombolysis, patients are maintained on systemic anticoagulation to prevent early recurrent thrombosis. Surgical management of venous thoracic outlet syndrome can be performed by the transaxillary approach and infraclavicular approach. A paraclavicular approach for venous thoracic outlet syndrome allows for complete decompression of the thoracic outlet and possible reconstruction of the subclavian vein during the same operation. Following the standard supraclavicular decompression, complete medial resection of the first rib and external venolysis of the subclavian vein after thoracic outlet decompression are performed. The decision to perform patch angioplasty or bypass grafting is made using the venogram. Visualization of the vein and digital palpation, cryopreserved femoral vein grafts, patch angioplasty, or bypass should be considered, and the patient is anticoagulated with intravenous heparin and continuous

infusion of Dextran. A patient presenting with swelling 6 months after thoracic outlet decompression with long segment chronic occlusion of the subclavian/axillary vein should be managed with compression therapy. In some cases where a long bypass graft is constructed, a temporary (12 weeks) conjunctive radiocephalic fistula may also be constructed for those at risk to improve venous flow.

Correct Answer   **C** Compression sleeve

Reference
Karam, J., & Thompson, R. (2017). Vascular thoracic outlet syndrome. In S. S. Hans, A. D. Shepard, H. R. Weaver, P. G. Bove, & G. W. Long (Eds.), *Endovascular and open vascular reconstructions: a practical approach* (pp. 371–376). Boca Raton, FL: CRC Press.

4. RATIONALE

Patients with arterial thoracic outlet syndrome have fixed arterial lesions such as stenosis, occlusion, or aneurysmal dilatation of the subclavian artery as it passes over the first rib, which is the least frequent form of thoracic outlet syndrome, representing 1%–3% of all thoracic outlet syndrome cases. This is usually due to compression by an osseous abnormality such as a cervical rib (70%), whereas anomalous first ribs and a tight ligamentous band or other bony abnormalities account for the rest of the structural anomalies causing compression of the subclavian artery. Clinical manifestations include arterial ischemia caused by embolic or thrombotic occlusions. Patients presenting with acute arm ischemia are treated initially with thrombolysis or surgical thrombectomy depending on the level of the occlusion and type of presentation. After distal circulation is restored, patients are prepared for thoracic outlet decompression within a few days of the initial procedure. The operative procedure is similar to the one used for neurogenic thoracic outlet syndrome. The decision to repair the subclavian artery with a bypass graft versus patch angioplasty depends on the extent of the aneurysm or embolizing lesion along its course. A paraclavicular approach using a cryopreserved femoral vein graft from the subclavian artery to axillary artery may be necessary.

Correct Answer   **B** 1%–3%

Reference
Karam, J., & Thompson, R. (2017). Vascular thoracic outlet syndrome. In S. S. Hans, A. D. Shepard, H. R. Weaver, P. G. Bove, & G. W. Long (Eds.), *Endovascular and open vascular reconstructions: a practical approach* (pp. 371–376). Boca Raton, FL: CRC Press.

5. RATIONALE

Residual neurological symptoms of numbness and tingling in the hand or fingers are common early after thoracic outlet decompression arising as a result of previous neurological damage, intraoperative mobilization of the brachial plexus, and postoperative inflammation and perineural wound healing. Spontaneous resolution of such symptoms usually occurs within several days to weeks but may persist for several months. Some patients with long-standing neurogenic thoracic outlet syndrome can often display residual symptoms that may not be completely eliminated by thoracic outlet decompression. In some patients, peri-incisional skin hypersensitivity after the operation may be quite significant, and when combined with hypersensitivity symptoms extending to the upper limb, consideration should be given to the diagnosis of complex regional pain syndrome (CRPS). Early recognition of CRPS and specific forms of physical therapy, stellate ganglion blocks, may be useful in symptomatic relief of recurrent symptoms that are often accompanied by an increase in arm activity and from secondary injury.

Correct Answer   C 5%

Reference
Rochlin, D. H., Likes, K. C., Gilson, M. M., et al. (2012). Management of unresolved, recurrent, and/or contralateral neurogenic symptoms in patients following first rib resection and scalenectomy. *J Vasc Surg, 56*(4), 1061–1067; discussion 1068. PMID: 22770848

6. RATIONALE

Nerve injury after decompression of thoracic outlet syndrome often manifests as persistent nerve dysfunction over time. In most of these situations, nerve injury rarely presents as an obvious injury identified in the operating room or as a significant deficit immediately after the operation, but more often is evident as persistent nerve dysfunction over time. In patients where the affected nerve was observed to be anatomically intact at the time of surgery, full functional recovery can be anticipated after several weeks to months. Minimizing handling of the nerves, dissecting perineural tissue under direct vision, and minimal nerve retraction of individual nerve roots should be taken under consideration. The presence of a cervical rib or ligamentous band may displace the brachial plexus much more forward, and scalene muscle abnormalities (a scalene minimus muscle) and fibroelastic band may obscure the lower nerve root. Division of the anterior scalene muscle from the first rib should be done with a finger placed between the muscle and the underlying brachial plexus and subclavian artery using scissors rather than electrocautery. Prior to resection of the scalene medius, the brachial plexus should also be mobilized in such a way that all five nerve roots are visible and gently retracted medially. Full visualization of the T1 nerve root should also be obtained, where it passes underneath the first rib to join the C8 nerve root before dividing at the posterior neck of the first rib. Although the C8 nerve root typically joins within 1–2 cm of the first rib, one anomaly that can increase the risk of injury is a long T1 nerve root, which may run for 3–4 cm underneath the first rib before passing across the bone to join the C8 nerve root. In this setting an unrecognized long T1 nerve root may be injured by the instrument used to divide the rib, reinforcing the need to divide the rib under direct vision and protect the C8–T1 junction and lower trunk of the brachial plexus before dividing the posterior portion of the first rib.

Correct Answer   D Anatomic variations, intraoperative bleeding, and preoperative repetitive hyperextension neck trauma

Reference
Duwayri, Y. M., & Thompson, R. W. (2014). Supraclavicular approach for surgical management of thoracic outlet syndrome. In Elliott L. Chaikof and Richard P. Cambria (Eds.), *Atlas of vascular surgery and endovascular therapy* (pp. 172–192). Philadelphia, PA: Elsevier Saunders.

7. RATIONALE

Brachial plexus compression by the pectoralis minor muscle has become increasingly appreciated as a factor contributing to neurogenic thoracic outlet syndrome. It has been reported that up to 10% of patients with neurogenic thoracic outlet syndrome exhibit physical findings that are isolated to the subcoracoid space, and 85%–90% have findings that co-localize to both the scalene triangle and the subcoracoid space. Even in patients with findings predominately localized to the scalene triangle, residual nerve compression at the site of the pectoralis minor muscle may be a source of persistent or recurrent neurogenic thoracic outlet syndrome. Simple division of the pectoralis minor tendon below the coracoid process may provide substantial relief of brachial plexus compression with minimal addition to the operative procedure.

Correct Answer   **A** Up to 10%

Reference
Vemuri, C., Wittenberg, A. M., Caputo, F. J., et al. (2013). Early effectiveness of isolated pectoralis minor tenotomy in selected patients with neurogenic thoracic outlet syndrome. *J Vasc Surg, 57*(5), 1345–1352. PMID: 23375605

8. RATIONALE

The primary advantage of the supraclavicular approach is excellent exposure of all the relevant anatomy, allowing more complete decompression with first rib resection, complete scalenectomy, and thorough brachial plexus neurolysis. This approach is thereby applicable to all three forms of thoracic outlet syndrome with a transaxillary approach; first rib resection as well as cervical rib resection can be carried out with a hidden incision. Following decompression, an upright chest X-ray is performed in the recovery room and a few days after decompression to detect any air or pleural fluid collection. Postoperative analgesia is initially provided by patient-controlled intravenous opiates. Continuous-infusion local anesthesia may also be used for several days, administered through small-caliber perfusion catheters placed at the time of surgery. A closed-suction drain placed at the time of the operation is removed when daily output is less than 50 cc, usually 5–7 days after supraclavicular decompression. Full activity is permitted after 2–3 months.

Correct Answer   **B** Incision in the hidden axillary space and sufficient exposure for the resection of both the first rib and cervical rib

Reference
Rinehardt, E. K., Scarborough, J. E., & Bennett, K. M. (2017). Current practice of thoracic outlet decompression surgery in the United States. *J Vasc Surg, 66*(3), 858–865. PMID: 28579292

SECTION 8: AORTOILIAC DISEASE

MCQs 1–105

Q1. During open repair of an abdominal aortic aneurysm (AAA) without involvement of the common and external iliac arteries, distal anastomosis to the femoral artery should be avoided in order to prevent:
- **A.** Increased incidence of surgical site infection and late development of anastomotic aneurysm
- **B.** Increased incidence of retrograde ejaculation
- **C.** Increased incidence of graft limb occlusion
- **D.** Increased incidence of sigmoid colon ischemia

Q2. A 70-year-old man with a 7-cm juxtarenal abdominal aortic aneurysm with moderately severe COPD has a left retroaortic renal vein on CTA imaging. The preferred method of repair is:
- **A.** Transperitoneal midline approach
- **B.** Transperitoneal transverse incision approach
- **C.** Left retroperitoneal approach with the left kidney remaining in its anatomical position
- **D.** Left retroperitoneal approach with the plane of dissection behind the left kidney

Q3. The incidence of incisional hernia following 6 years of open midline repair of an abdominal aortic aneurysm is:
- **A.** <5%
- **B.** <10%
- **C.** 10%–15%
- **D.** 16%–20%

Q4. Significant colon ischemia following open repair of an unruptured AAA occurs in:

- **A.** <1% of patients
- **B.** 1%–2% of patients
- **C.** 2%–4% of patients
- **D.** Colon ischemia occurs in patients with a history of left colectomy with an incidence of 5%

Q5. Graft infection following repair of an uncomplicated AAA occurs in:
- **A.** <1% of patients
- **B.** 1%–2% of patients
- **C.** >2% of patients
- **D.** Graft infection occurs only following repair of a ruptured AAA

Q6. During repair of a large juxtarenal AAA with a 3.4-cm right common iliac artery aneurysm via the transperitoneal approach, proximal clamping of the aorta is facilitated by:
- **A.** Ligation of the left renal vein medial to the gonadal and adrenal vein
- **B.** Division of the left renal vein and its reanastomosis after completion of proximal anastomosis
- **C.** Supraceliac control
- **D.** Balloon occlusion of the suprarenal aorta

Q7. During open repair of a suprarenal aortic aneurysm, the best exposure can be achieved using a:
- **A.** Midline celiotomy with inframesocolic approach
- **B.** Thoracoabdominal incision through the 7th intercostal space
- **C.** Midline celiotomy with medial visceral rotation
- **D.** Left flank retroperitoneal approach through the left 10th intercostal space

Q8. In a patient with a proximal AAA extending to the level of the SMA, proximal control of the aorta is best obtained by:
A. Clamp placement at the supraceliac level
B. Clamp placement above the SMA but below the celiac
C. Intraluminal control by advancing and inflating an aortic balloon occlusion catheter
D. Supraceliac balloon occlusion using left brachial access

Q9. During open repair of a para-visceral AAA, renal ischemia time >30 minutes is anticipated. The best management strategy to reduce the risk of AKI consists of:
A. Mannitol infusion prior to aortic cross clamp
B. Infusion of sodium bicarbonate during the period of proximal aortic clamping
C. Perfusion of the renal arteries with a solution of cold Ringer's lactate, heparin, mannitol, and methylprednisolone during aortic occlusion
D. Maintaining the patient's temperature at 32–34°C

Q10. During open repair of a para-visceral AAA, the left renal artery can be reconstructed:
A. Leaving it on an anterior tongue of the aorta including the right renal, SMA, and celiac artery
B. Bypassing with a sidearm graft previously sewn on the aortic prosthesis
C. Reimplanting it directly onto the aortic prosthesis
D. All of the above are acceptable techniques depending on the local anatomy

Q11. Repair of a thoracoabdominal aortic aneurysm repair (TAAA) should be considered when the aneurysm reaches the maximum transverse/AP diameter of:
A. 5.0 cm
B. 5.5 cm
C. 6.0 cm
D. 7.0 cm

Q12. The best strategy for reducing the risk of spinal cord ischemia during repair of a TAAA is:

A. Epidural cooling
B. Distal aortic perfusion using a temporary axillary femoral shunt
C. Distal aortic perfusion with intraoperative motor evoked potential monitoring
D. Quick clamp and sew technique without distal aortic perfusion

Q13. During repair of a TAAA, the left atrial femoral bypass is initiated. Mean distal perfusion pressures should be maintained at:
A. 35–39 mmHg
B. 40–50 mmHg
C. 51–59 mmHg
D. 60–70 mmHg

Q14. Operative mortality for open TAAA repair is 8%–16%. Open repair of such an aneurysm is contraindicated in patients with CKD with a GFR less than:
A. 30 cc
B. 40 cc
C. 50 cc
D. 60 cc

Q15. The most common predictors of spinal cord ischemia after TAAA repair are:
A. Repair of type IV thoracoabdominal aortic aneurysm
B. Advanced age
C. Type I–III thoracoabdominal aortic aneurysm
D. Type I–III thoracoabdominal aortic aneurysm and urgency of operation

Q16. The incidence of mesenteric ischemia following open repair of a thoracoabdominal aneurysm is:
A. <1%
B. 1%–2%
C. 2%–3%
D. >3%

Q17. An inflammatory abdominal aortic aneurysm has a thickened aortic wall with dense adhesions to the:
A. Jejunum
B. Duodenum and ureter
C. Sigmoid colon
D. Left renal veins

Q18. During transperitoneal repair of an inflammatory abdominal aortic aneurysm, the surgical approach is as follows:
   A. The third portion of the duodenum should be separated from the aneurysmal wall in order to obtain adequate exposure
   B. The third and proximal fourth portions of the duodenum should be left attached to the aneurysmal wall
   C. The ligament of Treitz should not be mobilized
   D. Mandatory ligation and division of left renal vein and inferior mesenteric vein

Q19. During repair of an inflammatory abdominal aortic aneurysm, there is an injury to the right common iliac vein, which is repaired by lateral venorrhaphy. On the second postoperative day the patient develops mild discomfort in the right thigh without any significant swelling of the right lower extremity. The patient should now undergo:
   A. Venogram of the right lower extremity
   B. EMG of the right lower extremity
   C. Close observation with serial hematocrit levels
   D. Duplex venous study of the right lower extremity

Q20. A completion arteriogram following deployment of a stent graft for repair of an infrarenal abdominal aortic aneurysm with a suprarenal fixation device shows a normal flow to the right kidney but partial coverage of the left renal artery origin. Optimal management consists of:
   A. Follow-up CTA of the abdomen and pelvis in 1 week
   B. Bare-metal stent in the left renal artery using femoral access
   C. Self-expanding stent in the left renal artery via brachial access
   D. Bare-metal balloon-expandable stent using left brachial access in the left renal artery

Q21. A completion arteriogram following EVAR reveals 80% coverage of the right hypogastric artery with known severe stenosis of the contralateral hypogastric artery. Optimal management consists of:
   A. No treatment necessary
   B. Left brachial access with deployment of a bare-metal stent into the right hypogastric artery
   C. Left brachial access with both balloon angioplasty and stenting of the left hypogastric artery
   D. Ipsilateral wire access into the right hypogastric artery via the right femoral artery with distal limb extension and internal iliac artery stenting that extends into the external iliac artery to permit retrograde perfusion via the snorkel technique

Q22. A type IA endoleak is seen following EVAR in an 80-year-old woman with aortic neck angulation of 45 degrees. There is no resolution following repeat aortic balloon neck angioplasty. The next best option is:
   A. Snorkeling
   B. Consider a large bare-metal stent (Palmaz) or endostapling
   C. Coil embolization of the endoleak site
   D. No treatment at this time, but follow-up CTA scan of the abdomen and pelvis in 4 weeks

Q23. A 67-year-old man presents with right lower extremity ischemia 6 weeks following EVAR with absent right femoral pulse. ABI on the right is 0.4 and on the left is 1.0. CTA of the abdomen and pelvis shows right graft limb occlusion with reconstitution of the proximal external iliac artery and filling of branches of the right hypogastric artery. Optimal management consists of:
   A. Crossover femoral-femoral graft
   B. Thrombolysis and relining the endograft and extension of the graft to the right external iliac artery with coil embolization of the hypogastric artery
   C. Anticoagulation
   D. Right axillofemoral graft

Q24. One year following EVAR a 75-year-old man developed a type II endoleak from a patent inferior mesenteric artery with sac enlargement by 5 mm. The next best management option should be:
A. Translumbar sac embolization
B. No intervention at present; follow-up CTA of the abdomen and pelvis in 6 months
C. Sac embolization using femoral access with passage of a catheter within the iliac limb of the endograft and native iliac artery
D. Coil embolization of the inferior mesenteric artery via the superior mesenteric artery using a microcatheter

Q25. The incidence of ischemic stroke following chimney parallel grafting (ch. EVAR) is:
A. <2%
B. 2%–2.9%
C. 3%–3.5%
D. >3.5%

Q26. Branch stent endoleaks following FEVAR and branched endografts requiring intervention for renal arteries occur in:
A. <1%
B. 1%–2%
C. 2%–3%
D. >3%

Q27. Results of a U.S. multicenter prospective study evaluating the Zenith fenestrated endovascular graft for treatment of a juxtarenal abdominal aortic aneurysm showed secondary interventions for renal artery stenosis/occlusion in:
A. 30% of patients
B. 22% of patients
C. 12% of patients
D. 6% of patients

Q28. Use of intraoperative C-arm cone-beam computed tomography (CBCT) in fenestrated/branched aortic endografting showed:
A. Fewer operative minutes
B. Lower fluoroscopy time

C. Lower contrast dose
D. No difference in detection of early complications

Q29. The prevalence of iliac artery aneurysms from the most common to least common is ranked as:
A. Hypogastric artery, common iliac artery, external iliac artery
B. Common iliac artery, hypogastric artery, external iliac artery
C. External iliac artery, hypogastric artery, common iliac artery
D. Common iliac artery, external iliac artery, hypogastric artery

Q30. Which of the following is an anatomical requirement for the use of an iliac branch device?
A. Aortic to iliac bifurcation length <5 cm
B. Hypogastric artery landing zone length <10 mm
C. Iliac bifurcation inner diameter >16 mm
D. Hypogastric artery landing zone diameter 12 mm

Q31. The incidence of abdominal compartment syndrome following open repair of a ruptured AAA is:
A. 10%
B. 15%
C. 20%
D. >20%

Q32. Spinal cord ischemia (SCI) following repair of a ruptured AAA occurs in:
A. <1% of patients
B. 1%–2% of patients
C. >2% of patients
D. Spinal cord ischemia occurs only following repair of a thoracic aortic aneurysm

Q33. A 72-year-old woman with profound hypotension secondary to a ruptured juxtarenal AAA should be taken to the hybrid OR, and proximal control should be obtained by:
A. Thoracic aortic balloon occlusion using femoral artery access in the OR
B. Thoracic aortic balloon occlusion using left brachial artery access in the OR

C. Laparotomy and supraceliac control

D. Retrograde passage of a large balloon Foley catheter advanced from an opening in the aortic neck during laparotomy

Q34. During open repair of a ruptured AAA, there is injury to the left renal vein lateral to the gonadal vein and adrenal vein with a 30% loss of circumference. Mean blood pressure is 70 mmHg. Optimal management consists of:

A. Lateral venorrhaphy

B. Ligation of the left renal vein

C. Splenic vein to left renal vein bypass

D. Vascular clamps on either side of the left renal vein and repair after proximal aortic anastomosis is completed

Q35. The incidence of pancreatitis and duodenal obstruction is highest following:

A. Open repair of unruptured AAA

B. Aortobifemoral grafting

C. Open repair of ruptured AAA

D. Open repair of type IV thoracoabdominal aneurysm

Q36. Following completion of distal anastomosis during open repair for ruptured AAA, the patient has diffuse oozing from exposed surfaces. Lab data: hemoglobin 9.2 gm, hematocrit 26, platelets 84,000, INR 1.8, fibrin split products normal. The most common cause of this abnormality is:

A. Disseminated intravascular coagulopathy

B. Secondary fibrinolysis due to visceral ischemia from supraceliac clamping

C. Dilutional coagulopathy

D. Primary fibrinolysis

Q37. A 64-year-old man presents to the emergency room with a leaking AAA. CT scan shows a horseshoe kidney with small retroperitoneal hematoma. The most important criterion in deciding the method of repair (open or endovascular) is:

A. Experience of the surgeon

B. Open repair is mandatory in all patients with a horseshoe kidney

C. Endovascular repair should be preferred

D. Should be decided by the anatomy of the aneurysm and arterial supply to the horseshoe kidney

Q38. A 78-year-old man presents to the emergency room with a leaking AAA with antecedent endovascular aneurysm repair. The optional management is:

A. Mandatory open repair

B. Repair of ruptured AAA in a patient with a prior endograft is uniformly fatal so only palliative care should be recommended

C. Mandatory endovascular repair

D. Choice of endovascular versus open repair depends on the findings of the CTA of the abdomen and pelvis and clinical condition of the patient

Q39. Endovascular repair of a ruptured AAA in a high-risk patient with prior EVAR with a large type IA endoleak required intentional coverage of one renal artery. The following best reflects the outcome in this situation:

A. Single renal artery coverage does not increase the odds of permanent dialysis/30-day mortality

B. Single renal artery coverage increases the risk of dialysis but does not increase the 30-day mortality

C. Single renal artery coverage increases the odds of permanent dialysis/30-day mortality primarily due to the need for permanent dialysis

D. Single renal artery coverage results in prohibitive mortality and should not be performed

Q40. The incidence of late open conversion following EVAR is:

A. <1%

B. 1%–5%

C. 0%–10%

D. 11%–12%

Q41. The best strategy to facilitate complete removal of suprarenal stents during total explant of an aortic endograft is:
  A. Release of barbs from the main body with a wire cutter circumferentially
  B. Use of a 20-cc syringe as a sheath to encircle and collapse the suprarenal segment
  C. Iced saline on nitinol elements to help collapse the metal
  D. Release of barbs with a wire cutter and iced saline in a syringe to collapse the suprarenal segment

Q42. The following statement best reflects the incidences of late conversion and delayed rupture risks following EVAR:
  A. Overall incidence of late conversion is 1% and delayed risk of rupture is 0.5% per year
  B. Overall incidence of late conversion is 1.9% and delayed risk of rupture is 1% per year
  C. Overall incidence of late conversion is 5% and delayed risk of rupture is 2% per year
  D. Overall incidence of late conversion is 7% and delayed risk of rupture is 4% per year

Q43. A 76-year-old man is to undergo repair of an aortoenteric fistula following open AAA repair 10 years previously. The patient is hemodynamically stable. The best conduit for aortic reconstruction following removal of a remotely placed prosthetic graft is:
  A. Rifampin socked Dacron graft
  B. Cryopreserved arterial allograft
  C. Reconstruction using deep veins (femoral and popliteal)
  D. Axillobifemoral graft

Q44. For repair of a secondary aortoenteric fistula, the best method for proximal control of the aorta is:
  A. Suprarenal via midline laparotomy
  B. Supraceliac via midline laparotomy
  C. Balloon occlusion of distal descending thoracic aorta using femoral artery access
  D. Proximal clamp between superior mesenteric artery and celiac artery

Q45. Following repair of a secondary aorto-enteric fistula with a direct in-line aortic reconstruction, antibiotic therapy should be administered for:
  A. 2 weeks
  B. 6 weeks
  C. 3 months
  D. 6 months/possibly lifelong

Q46. During transperitoneal repair of a juxtarenal AAA, a proximal aortic clamp is applied below the right renal artery and above the left renal artery. Following completion of a proximal aortic anastomosis with release of the clamp, there is bleeding secondary to a tear in the aorta at the origin of the left renal artery, which is controlled by passage of a 30-cc balloon Foley catheter to the left limb of the Dacron graft and inflating at the supraceliac limb. Management of an aortic tear involving the left renal artery should be performed by:
  A. Primary repair
  B. Patch graft at the site of laceration using a PTFE patch
  C. End-to-side bypass graft from the suprarenal aorta to the left renal artery with an end-to-end anastomosis
  D. Bypass graft to the left renal artery with origin from the main body or the left limb of the prosthetic graft (end-to-side) to the left renal artery with end-to-end anastomosis distally

Q47. A 72-year-old man with a 6.5-cm transverse/AP infrarenal AAA has a left kidney anatomically located in the pelvis with its arterial supply from the origin of each common iliac artery (two renal arteries). The optimal management is:
  A. Open repair of AAA with renal auto-transplantation
  B. Temporary axillofemoral bypass graft to maintain retrograde perfusion to the kidney during repair
  C. Endovascular aneurysm repair with fenestration at the site of two renal arteries to the pelvic kidney
  D. Reimplantation of renal arteries supplying the pelvic kidney incorporating in the aortobiiliac graft reconstruction

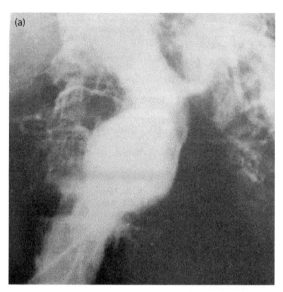

(a)

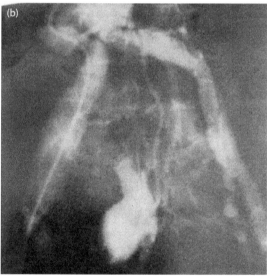

(b)

Q48. A 74-year-old man has a 7.5-cm transverse diameter infrarenal AAA with a
15-mm neck and normal common iliac
arteries. The patient has a large inferior
mesenteric artery with an arc of Riolan
on preoperative aortography. There is
associated occlusion of the celiac artery
and 50% stenosis of the superior mesenteric artery. The best management
option is:
  A. Standard EVAR
  B. Open repair with inferior mesenteric
  artery reimplantation

C. EVAR with a custom-made fenestration at
the site of the origin of the large inferior
mesenteric artery
D. Superior mesenteric artery stenting followed by EVAR

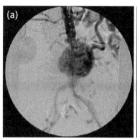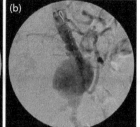

Q49. During transperitoneal repair of a
juxtarenal AAA, a double inferior vena
cava was encountered. A preoperative
CT scan was not obtained because of a
history of anaphylaxis to contrast agent.
Management options include:
  A. Ligation of the left-sided inferior vena
  cava
  B. Mobilization of the left-sided inferior
  vena cava near the aortic neck
  C. Division of the left-sided inferior vena
  cava with end-to-end anastomosis after
  completion of aortic anastomosis
  D. Left retroperitoneal approach should
  have been selected for repair of AAA

Q50. Which of the following statements best
applies to a patient with compensated
liver cirrhosis (MELD score <10)
undergoing open AAA repair:
  A. Open repair of AAA in patients with
  liver cirrhosis should not be considered
  because of a high risk of complications
  B. Incidence of perioperative complications
  in patients with compensated cirrhosis
  of the liver is similar to those without
  cirrhosis but there is greater blood loss,
  increased operative time, and increased
  length of stay
  C. Always administer preoperative fresh-
  frozen plasma even in patients with
  normal INR
  D. Open repair without heparin administration during aortic cross-clamping should
  be routine in patients with liver cirrhosis

Q51. A 79-year-old man undergoes open repair of an inflammatory AAA (6.2 cm), right common iliac artery aneurysm (3.5 cm), right hypogastric aneurysm (2.5 cm), left common iliac aneurysm (2.5 cm), and a small thrombosed left hypogastric aneurysm. During repair, major venous bleeding from a left common iliac vein injury necessitated repair with ligation of the left common iliac artery above its bifurcation in order to gain exposure. Reconstruction was performed with aorto-right external iliac bypass and a left common femoral bypass graft. In the recovery room, the patient was found to be paraplegic. The most likely cause of spinal cord ischemia is:

A. Abnormal origin of the greater radicular artery (artery of Adamkiewicz)
B. Intraoperative hypotension
C. Prolonged aortic clamping
D. Interruption of hypogastric arterial flow

Q52. A 53-year-old man underwent open repair of a ruptured AAA with aortobifemoral graft reconstruction. One year later he presents with an infected graft (methicillin-sensitive *Staphylococcus aureus*). Graft incision and cryopreserved allograft reconstruction were performed. One week later the patient presented with rupture of the cryopreserved graft and underwent ligation of the infrarenal aorta with bilateral axillofemoral grafting, with distal anastomosis performed to the proximal superficial femoral artery using lateral tunnels. The patient had multiple occlusions of an axillofemoral graft in the subsequent 2 years and is free from infection. The patient is an acceptable risk for major vascular reconstruction. The next best management option is:

A. In-line rifampin-soaked Dacron aortobifemoral graft
B. Deep vein autograft (femoral and popliteal veins)

C. Aortofemoral reconstruction using a left flank retroperitoneal approach with bilateral groin incisions with a prosthetic graft as a conduit
D. Thoracic aorta to femoral artery bypass

Q53. A 79-year-old man with multiple comorbidities presents with a 7-cm AAA with a neck measuring 4 mm in length and 20 mm in diameter with <30° angulation without any significant thrombus and <25% circumferential calcification. Endovascular repair in this patient is best performed:

A. Using a fenestrated endograft
B. EVAR with Heli-FX endo-anchors
C. Standard endovascular repair with Palmaz stent at the aortic neck
D. Chimney or snorkel technique for obtaining a proximal seal

Q54. The incidence of sac enlargement in a patient with a type II endoleak following EVAR is:

A. <5%
B. 6%–8%
C. 9%–10%
D. 11%–12%

Q55. Results of the IMPROVED trial comparing EVAR to open repair for ruptured AAA, demonstrated an all-cause mortality at 1 year of:

A. 60% for open repair, 50% for EVAR
B. 50% for open repair, 60% for EVAR
C. 45% for open repair, 41% for EVAR
D. 50% for open repair, 45% for EVAR

Q56. Type III endoleak following EVAR occurs in:

A. <2% of patients
B. 2%–3% of patients
C. 3.1%–4% of patients
D. Type III endoleaks do not occur with third-generation endografts

Q57. An existing aortic endograft in a patient with ruptured AAA:

A. Provides acute survival benefit
B. Provides 1-year survival benefit
C. Provides both acute and 1-year survival benefit
D. Provides neither acute nor 1-year survival benefit

Q58. An 80-year-old man presented with a large left iliac anastomotic aneurysm (6.5 cm) with left hydronephrosis. Twenty years after open repair of AAA with an aorto-biiliac graft, the left hypogastric artery is occluded. The best management option is:

A. Ureteral stent followed by endovascular repair using a covered stent

B. Endovascular repair using a covered stent by left femoral and brachial access with coil embolization of the hypogastric artery if patent

C. Open repair

D. Coil embolization or use of glue (Onyx)

Q59. A large (6-cm) hypogastric artery aneurysm is diagnosed 15 years following open repair of AAA with an aortobiiliac graft. Endovascular repair is selected, which should be performed using:

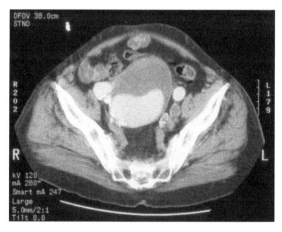

A. Contralateral femoral artery access with deployment of the iliac-extension limb of the stent graft

B. Brachial access and deployment of the coil in the two main trunks of the hypogastric artery with covered stent placement extending to the proximal external iliac artery

C. Ipsilateral femoral access and deployment of a covered stent across the origin of the hypogastric artery

D. Ipsilateral femoral access with placement of coils in the outflow branches of the hypogastric artery and a covered stent across the outflow of the hypogastric artery

Q60. The incidence of paraplegia following TEVAR is:

A. 5% or less

B. 10% or less

C. 10%–15%

D. 16%–20%

Q61. When comparing TEVAR to open repair for a ruptured descending thoracic aortic aneurysm, the following statement best reflects perioperative 30-day mortality:

A. TEVAR has a mortality of 30%, and open repair 30%

B. TEVAR has a mortality of 30%, and open repair 43%

C. TEVAR has a mortality of 19%, and open repair 33%

D. TEVAR has a mortality of 10%, and open repair 30%

Q62. The incidence of retrograde type A aortic dissection as a complication of TEVAR occurs in:

A. 1% of patients

B. 1%–2% of patients

C. 2.5% of patients

D. 3%–4% of patients

Q63. Posterior circulation stroke as a complication of TEVAR occurs in:

A. 2% of patients

B. 3%–3.5% of patients

C. 3.6%–4% of patients

D. >4% of patients

Q64. Transfemoral access for TEVAR is feasible in:

A. 90% of patients

B. 80% of patients

C. 70% of patients

D. 60% of patients

Q65. Type IA or type IB endoleak in patients undergoing TEVAR occurs in:

A. <1%

B. 1%–2%

C. 2.1%–3%

D. 3.1%–3.5%

Q66. Perioperative stroke as a complication of TEVAR occurs in:
A. <3% of cases
B. 3%–5% of cases
C. 5.1%–6% of cases
D. >6% of cases

Q67. The incidence of clinically manifest foregut ischemia following TEVAR occurs in:
A. 0%–6% of patients
B. 0%–12% of patients
C. 12.1%–15% of patients
D. 15.1%–20% of patients

Q68. In order to prevent maldeployment of the endograft in the false lumen of acute type B aortic dissection, the best strategy is:
A. Careful preoperative CTA evaluation
B. Intravascular ultrasound
C. Imaging catheter placed via the right brachial artery or a long 14 Fr sheath from the femoral artery through which angiography is performed via the sidearm at the level of each branch vessel
D. Careful evaluation of preoperative CTA, use of intravascular ultrasound, and intraoperative angiography at the level of each branch vessel

Q69. The incidence of graft infection after TEVAR is reported as:
A. <1%
B. 1%–1.5%
C. 1.6%–2%
D. 2%–2.5%

Q70. The incidence of graft migration following TEVAR is reported to be:
A. <4%
B. 4%–6%
C. 7%
D. 10%

Q71. An aberrant right subclavian artery aneurysm should be repaired:
A. Only if the patient is symptomatic
B. If the aneurysm measures 2.5–3 cm in diameter
C. If the aneurysm is >3 cm to <4 cm in diameter
D. If the aneurysm is 4 cm or greater in the AP/transverse diameter

Q72. An aneurysm resulting from chronic thoracic aortic dissection (type B) should be treated by:
A. TEVAR
B. TEVAR with fenestration
C. Open repair
D. Fenestration alone

Q73. For open repair of an isolated distal descending thoracic aortic aneurysm, the best approach is:
A. Posterolateral thoracotomy via 8th intercostal space
B. Anterolateral thoracotomy via 8th intercostal space
C. Posterolateral thoracotomy via 4th intercostal space
D. Anterolateral thoracotomy

Q74. The most common complication after open descending thoracic aortic aneurysm repair is:
A. Cardiac arrhythmias
B. Respiratory failure
C. Chylothorax
D. Renal failure

Q75. The most common reason for repair of a subclavian artery aneurysm is:
A. To prevent thromboembolic complications
B. Brachial plexopathy
C. Subclavian vein compression
D. To prevent rupture

Q76. The most common nerve injured during open repair of a subclavian artery aneurysm in its second portion is:
A. Vagus
B. Recurrent laryngeal
C. Phrenic
D. Lower cord of brachial plexus

Q77. The incidence of axillary and brachial artery aneurysms among peripheral artery aneurysms is:
A. <1%
B. 1%–3%
C. 3.1%–4%
D. 4.1%–5%

Q78. Repair of an axillary and brachial artery aneurysm is recommended for an aneurysm size of:
A. 0.5–1 cm
B. 1.1–1.5 cm
C. 1.6–1.9 cm
D. >2 cm

Q79. A repeat aortobifemoral graft for aortoiliac occlusive disease is associated with a mortality of:
A. <5%
B. 5%–7%
C. 7.1%–8%
D. >8% but <10%

Q80. During a repeat aortobifemoral bypass, exposure can most easily be achieved using a:
A. Midline celiotomy with an inframesocolic approach
B. Midline celiotomy with medial visceral rotation
C. Left flank retroperitoneal approach
D. Transverse celiotomy through an infra-umbilical incision

Q81. The complication rate after aortofemoral bypass grafting can be as high as:
A. 5%
B. 10%
C. 15%
D. 20%

Q82. The following statement best describes primary patency of an aortofemoral bypass at 5 and 10 years:
A. Primary patency 80%–85% at 5 years and 65%–70% at 10 years
B. Primary patency 85%–92% at 5 years and 80%–85% at 10 years
C. Primary patency 92%–99% at 5 years and 80%–85% at 10 years
D. Primary patency 75%–80% at 5 years and 60%–65% at 10 years

Q83. The average time from index aortofemoral reconstruction to symptomatic infection is:
A. 3.5–5 years
B. 5.1–5.5 years
C. 6.5–7 years
D. 7.5–8 years

Q84. Early postoperative hemorrhage following aortofemoral bypass occurs in:
A. <1% of cases
B. 1%–2% of cases
C. 2.1%–2.5% of cases
D. 2.6%–3% of cases

Q85. Aortofemoral bypass for juxtarenal aortic occlusion may require suprarenal aortic clamping. The incidence of postoperative renal failure following arterial reconstruction for juxtarenal aortic occlusion with suprarenal clamping is:
A. Similar to infrarenal clamping
B. Higher than infrarenal clamping
C. Lower than infrarenal clamping
D. Postoperative renal failure only occurs following supraceliac clamping

Q86. Groin complications following aortofemoral bypass are seen in:
A. 10% of patients
B. 15% of patients
C. 20% of patients
D. 25% of patients

Q87. The incidence of ureteral injury during aortofemoral bypass reconstruction is:
A. <1%
B. 1.1%–1.5%
C. 1.6%–2%
D. 2.1%–2.5%

Q88. The incidence of retrograde ejaculation following aortoiliac surgery is:
A. 1%–3%
B. 3%–9%
C. 10%–12%
D. 13%–15%

Q89. Seven years after an aortofemoral bypass, an exposed synthetic graft in the groin is seen in a patient. The patient had a previous sartorius myoplasty. Which muscle flap will provide the most satisfactory coverage for the exposed graft in the groin all this time?
A. Rectus femoris
B. Gracilis
C. Tensor fascia latae
D. External oblique

Q90. A 62-year-old man undergoes an uneventful aortobifemoral bypass graft for significant intermittent claudication symptoms of both lower extremities. Preoperative ABI on the right was 0.52 and 0.34 on the left. Preoperative CTA showed infrarenal aortic occlusion with a thrombosed 3.5-cm AAA with occlusion of both common iliac arteries and thrombosed aneurysmal hypogastric arteries (1.8 cm each). In the recovery room he complains of weakness of the right leg primarily involving the right thigh muscles. The most likely cause of this deficit is:
A. Interruption of the artery of Adamkiewicz
B. Intraoperative hypotension
C. Suprarenal aortic clamping
D. Interruption of pelvic arterial supply

Q91. A descending thoracic aorta to femoral bypass graft is best indicated for:
A. Juxtarenal aortic occlusion in a 46-year-old man with bilateral hip claudication and erectile dysfunction
B. Infrarenal aortic occlusion and bilateral iliac artery occlusion with rest pain and history of prior lymphadenectomy
C. A 6-cm infrarenal AAA with bilateral iliac artery occlusion with a history of ileostomy
D. Failed prior aortobifemoral bypass graft in a symptomatic 48-year-old woman with graft occlusion just below the renal arteries with a history of multiple celiotomies for Crohn disease

Q92. An absolute contraindication for a descending thoracic aortofemoral bypass graft is:
A. Remote history of myocardial infarction
B. Remote history of multiple celiotomies
C. Left ventricular ejection fraction of 50%
D. Circumferential distal descending thoracic aortic calcification

Q93. Descending thoracic aortofemoral artery bypass is planned for a 64-year-old man with a prior history of suprapubic cystostomy for bladder neck obstruction. The right limb of the thoracic aortofemoral bypass graft should be brought:

A. Behind the recuts abdominus muscle in the space of Retzius
B. Left descending thoracic aorta to femoral bypass with simultaneous right axillo-femoral graft
C. Right femoral graft limb is brought from the left groin in a suprapubic subcutaneous tunnel and anastomosed to the common femoral artery as in a standard crossover femoral-femoral graft
D. Right femoral limb brought through the obturator foramen and anastomosed to the proximal superficial femoral artery

Q94. The most common cause of acute aortic occlusion is:
A. Saddle embolism
B. In situ thrombosis
C. Occluded aortoiliac graft
D. Occlusion of aortic limbs of EVAR

Q95. Seven years following left common iliac artery stenting, a 61-year-old man develops worsening left flank pain. Urinalysis is negative. There is no history of renal stones. The next best option in diagnosis is:
A. Duplex imaging of the left common iliac artery
B. CTA of the abdominal aorta and iliac arteries
C. MRA of the abdominal aorta and iliac arteries
D. Computed tomography urogram

Q96. A 46-year-old man presented to the emergency room with acute myocardial infarction and underwent coronary artery bypass graft for triple-vessel coronary artery disease and intraaortic balloon insertion via the left common femoral artery. At the time of deployment of the intraaortic balloon, left common iliac artery stenting was performed in order to gain access into the aorta because of severe stenosis of the left common iliac artery. However, the stent projected 2.5 cm above the aortic bifurcation. The patient presented to the vascular surgery clinic 6 weeks later with ischemic rest pain of the right foot. A TASC D lesion with flush occlusion of the right common iliac artery and occlusion of the right external iliac artery was confirmed by CTA. An ipsilateral approach for right iliac intervention was unsuccessful (right common femoral artery access). The next best option for revascularization for the right lower extremity is:

A. Aortobifemoral bypass graft

B. Right iliac artery stenting via left common femoral approach

C. A crossover femoral-femoral graft

D. Placement of a kissing stent in the right common iliac artery and stenting of the right external iliac artery with left brachial access

Q97. As compared to aortofemoral bypass grafting, iliac stenting for iliac artery occlusive disease (TASC C&D) has:

A. Better primary patency

B. Longer length of stay in the hospital if complications develop

C. Equivalent primary patency

D. Inferior primary patency but equivalent secondary patency

Q98. Stent grafts as compared to bare-metal stents for management of iliac artery occlusive disease are preferable in:

A. Patients with flush occlusions

B. Patients with a large amount of thrombus

C. Patients with eccentric plaque with severe calcification involving 75% of the circumference of the artery

D. Stent grafts for iliac artery occlusive disease at the origin of the common iliac artery do not need a kissing balloon angioplasty/stent for contralateral common iliac artery disease

Q99. Symptomatic iliac artery in-stent restenosis at 1 year occurs at a frequency of:

A. 5%

B. 10%

C. 12%

D. 15%

Q100. During iliac stenting for a calcified TASC D lesion, the patient became diaphoretic and complained of nausea with minimal abdominal discomfort. Blood pressure dropped to 90 mmHg from 130 mmHg systolic but became stable with 1 liter of NS infusion. What is the next immediate step in management of this patient?

A. Immediate noncontrast CT scan of the abdomen and pelvis

B. Obtain stat EKG

C. Contrast angiography

D. Increase the fluid administration and start vasopressors

Q101. A 62-year-old woman undergoes left common iliac artery stenting for a near-occlusion of a 2.5-cm segment of the proximal common iliac artery. After removal of the sheath, she experiences pain in the left lower quadrant with stable vital signs. Her postprocedure hemoglobin/hematocrit did not show any change from the preprocedure study. There is no palpable hematoma in the groin, and vital signs remain stable. The most likely diagnosis is:

A. Iliac artery rupture

B. Rectus sheath hematoma

C. Psoas hematoma

D. Vasovagal response

Q102. The most common complication following iliac stenting for occlusive disease is:

A. Rupture of the iliac artery

B. Distal embolization

C. Arterial dissection

D. Stent misadventure

Q103. A 75-year-old woman with symptoms of intermittent claudication on walking 50 yards has near-occlusion of the infrarenal aorta near the origin of the inferior mesenteric artery. There is no history to suggest symptoms of mesenteric ischemia. The best management strategy is:

A. Aortofemoral grafting

B. Open aortic reconstruction

C. Covered stent

D. Bare-metal stent

Q104. A 60-year-old woman with a history of Addison disease has symptomatic near-occlusion of the distal aorta with involvement of the origin of both common iliac arteries (70% stenosis). The best management option is:

A. Aortobifemoral graft

B. Aortoiliac endarterectomy

C. Bare-metal stent in the distal aorta with two kissing stents in the common iliac artery

D. Bilateral kissing, covered, balloon-expandable stents from the distal abdominal aorta extending into each common iliac artery

Q105. The greatest predictor of postintervention complications for aortoiliac occlusive lesions is:

A. Age greater than 70

B. Interventions for acute ischemia

C. Female gender

D. Age greater than 80, patients with critical limb ischemia, and TASC C&D lesions

RATIONALE 1–105

1. RATIONALE

In most patients undergoing open abdominal aortic aneurysm repair without associated common iliac aneurysm or iliac artery occlusive disease, a tube (aorto-aortic) graft is preferred. In patients with associated common iliac aneurysm, the aortobilateral common iliac bypass graft is reconstructed following partial removal of the aorta and common iliac aneurysmal wall (anterior wall). In patients with a large common iliac artery aneurysm, where origin of the external iliac and hypogastric artery is splayed apart, it is almost impossible to create a distal anastomosis incorporating both external iliac artery origin and hypogastric artery origin. In this situation the iliac limb is anastomosed to the hypogastric artery in an end-to-end fashion and the external iliac artery is sutured end-to-side to a Dacron graft, or an interposition graft to the external iliac artery is performed. After restoring flow to one hypogastric artery, the contralateral hypogastric artery may be safely ligated. Femoral anastomosis should be avoided whenever possible, as it is associated with an increased incidence of groin wound complications and late development of femoral anastomotic aneurysm.

Correct Answer   **A** Increased incidence of surgical site infection and late development of anastomotic aneurysm

Reference

Shepard, A. D. (2017). Open nonruptured infrarenal aortic aneurysm repair. In S. S. Hans, A. D. Shepard, & H. R. Weaver (Eds.), *Endovascular and open vascular reconstructions: a practical approach* (pp. 197–204). Boca Raton, FL: CRC Press.

2. RATIONALE

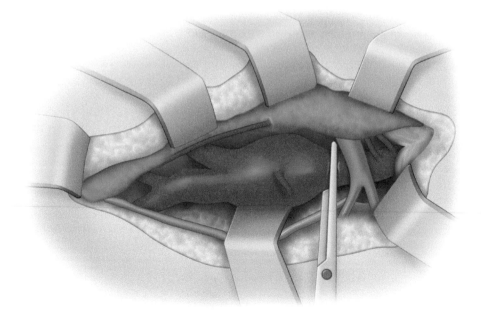

Left flank retroperitoneal exposure of infrarenal AAA with left kidney in its anatomical position.

In a patient with a large-diameter juxtarenal abdominal aortic aneurysm (AAA) with COPD, the left retroperitoneal approach is preferable. In most patients undergoing repair of AAA using the left retroperitoneal approach, the patient is positioned in a modified right lateral decubitus position with the shoulders positioned at 70 degrees to the table and the hips rotated as far posteriorly as possible. For infrarenal AAA repair, the left flank incision is carried back into the 11th intercostal space. For repair of a juxtarenal AAA, exposure of the pararenal aorta is carried with an incision extending to the 10th intercostal space. The peritoneum often overlying the transversalis fascia is stripped away from the abdominal wall, and the musculature is followed to the peritoneal sac and its contents are retracted anteriorly. This plane is developed superficial to the lumbodorsal fascia (the posterior extension of the transversalis fascia) behind the left kidney so that left kidney and ureter are also reflected anteriorly. The lumbar branch of the left renal vein crossing over the aorta proximally is a reliable landmark, with the left renal artery identifiable just above and proximally. In patients with a retroaortic left renal vein, it is necessary to leave the kidney "down" in its normal anatomical position and expose the aorta anterior to the kidney to avoid ligating the left renal vein.

Correct Answer   **C** Left retroperitoneal approach with left kidney remaining in its anatomical position

Reference
Shepard, A. D. (2017). Open nonruptured infrarenal aortic aneurysm repair. In S. S. Hans, A. D. Shepard, & H. R. Weaver (Eds.), *Endovascular and open vascular reconstructions: a practical approach* (pp. 197–204). Boca Raton, FL: CRC Press.

3. RATIONALE

From the Danish Vascular Registry and the Danish Ventral Hernia Database (2007–2012), 2597 patients (838 aortic occlusive disease and 1759 AAA repair) underwent open aortic reconstruction, and the cumulative risk of hernia was 10.4% after 6 years of follow-up. The study found that high body mass index and AAA repair were independent risk factors for a subsequent incisional hernia surgery in patients undergoing aortic reconstructive surgery. Retroperitoneal incision for aortic aneurysm repair may result in injury to the 11th intercostal nerve, which may result in paresthesia in about 30% patients and a "bulge" in the lateral abdominal wall with muscle atrophy in 7%–15%. A genetic predisposition to weakened connective tissue causing the aorta to expand and a subsequent hernia to develop is hypothesized as a common pathophysiological entity in the two diseases. Patients undergoing AAA repair have a 1.6-fold higher risk of subsequent hernia repair than patients undergoing reconstruction for aortoiliac occlusive disease.

Correct Answer   **C** 10%–15%

Reference
Henriksen, N. A., Helgstrand, F., Vogt, K. C., et al. (2013). Risk factors for incisional hernia repair after aortic reconstructive surgery in a nationwide study. *J Vasc Surg, 57*(6), 1524–1530, e1521–1523. PMID: 23548175

4. RATIONALE

Clinically significant colon ischemia occurs in 1%–2% of patients following open repair of AAA with a 50%–75% mortality. Mortality can be as high as 90% if the bowel resection is required for infarction. Colon ischemia is far more common than small bowel ischemia. Early postoperative diarrhea, melena, hematochezia, and persistent metabolic acidosis mandate definitive diagnostic aids such as fiberoptic sigmoidoscopy. Risk factors include ligation of a large inferior mesenteric artery in the presence of a meandering mesenteric artery (arc of Riolan), superior mesenteric artery, and celiac artery occlusive disease. Atheroembolism or retractor blade injury to SMA and prior colon resection are contributing factors for interstitial ischemia. Patients with associated significant SMA stenosis in the presence of large mesenteric collaterals or a large-sized inferior mesenteric artery may need reimplantation of the inferior mesenteric artery into the prosthetic graft using a Carrel patch technique or preoperative stenting of the superior mesenteric artery. Once the diagnosis of colon ischemia is confirmed by fiberoptic sigmoidoscopy or colonoscopy, the patient should be adequately resuscitated and started on intravenous antibiotics targeted towards intestinal microorganisms. If ischemia is localized to mucosa and muscularis mucosa, the patient can be managed conservatively, whereas full-thickness infarction will require emergent laparotomy and bowel resection. In patients with ischemia limited to mucosa and muscularis mucosa, late stricture may develop.

Correct Answer   **B** 1%–2% of patients

Reference
Chaikof, E. L., Dalman, R. L., Eskandari, M. K., et al. (2018). The Society for Vascular Surgery practice guidelines on the care of patients with an abdominal aortic aneurysm. *J Vasc Surg, 67*(1), 2–77.e72. PMID: 29268916

5. RATIONALE

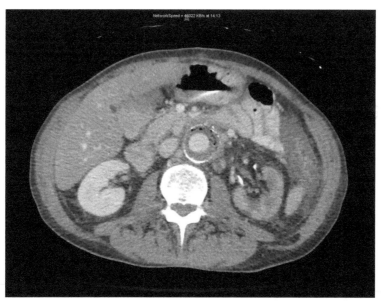

Gas bubbles in the aneurysm sac are indicative of a graft infection.

Graft infections occur in less than 1% of patients undergoing elective repair for unruptured AAA. An aortic prosthetic graft is at risk of infection at the time of implantation or later by a hematogenous spread. Aortic graft infections are difficult to diagnose, as the patient may present with nonspecific symptoms such as generalized weakness, malaise, anorexia, and unexplained weight loss. Occasionally, the patient may present with overt sepsis. Common pathogens include *Staphylococcus aureus* and *Staphylococcus epidermidis*. The laboratory and diagnostic studies are often nondiagnostic. Leukocytosis with a shift to the left, elevated C-reactive protein, and sedimentation rates are often present.

Correct Answer   A <1% of patients

Reference
Hallett, J. W., Jr., Marshall, D. M., Petterson, T. M., et al. (1997). Graft-related complications after abdominal aortic aneurysm repair: reassurance from a 36-year population-based experience. *J Vasc Surg, 25*(2), 277–284; discussion 285–276. PMID: 9052562

6. RATIONALE

Due to the increased use of endovascular repair for infrarenal AAA, most patients requiring open AAA in contemporary vascular practice have juxtarenal or pararenal AAAs. To obtain satisfactory proximal exposure, the left renal vein may need to be ligated and divided medial to the adrenal and gonadal veins if transperitoneal repair is selected. Depending on the quality of the aorta just below the renal arteries, suprarenal, infrarenal, or inter-renal control is obtained. Division of the left renal vein followed by the reanastomosis does not offer any advantage in terms of renal function status on a long-term basis as compared to its ligation. Ligation of the left renal vein is associated with an increased incidence of AKI and renal function deterioration in the early postoperative phase. However, long-term renal function does not seem to be affected. Supraceliac control or proximal aortic balloon occlusion is rarely necessary during repair of even a large juxtarenal AAA.

Correct Answer   A Ligation of the left renal vein medial to the gonadal and adrenal vein

Reference
Pandirajan, K., Katsogridakis, E., Sidloff, D., et al. (2020). Effects of left renal vein ligation during open abdominal aortic aneurysm repair on renal function. *Eur J Vasc Endovasc Surg, 60*(6), 829–835. PMID: 32912760

7. RATIONALE

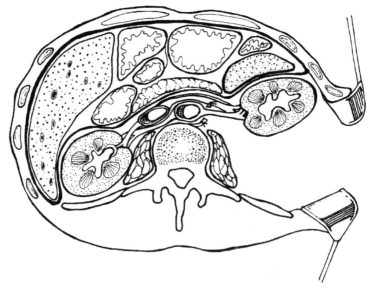

Left retroperitoneal exposure of abdominal aorta with anterior mobilization of the left kidney.

Choosing an appropriate site for proximal control is one of the most important determinations of operative success with proximal AAA repair. The more proximal the aortic clamp, the greater strain on the myocardium and the greater renal/visceral ischemic burden. It is also important to avoid clamping the diseased aorta with an increased risk of renal/visceral and lower extremity atheroembolism. When the origin of the SMA is too close to the renal arteries, supraceliac clamping is preferable because aorta at that site is reliably the least diseased. A left flank approach through the 9th or 10th intercostal space (ICS) is preferable for repair of a suprarenal abdominal aortic aneurysm. Positioning of the patient begins in a modified left thoracotomy position. The incision begins just below the umbilicus at the lateral border of the left rectus sheath and carried obliquely into the chest via the 9th or 10th ICS. The diaphragm is divided circumferentially beginning at the costal margin approximately 2 cm from its lateral attachments to avoid injury to the branches of the phrenic nerve. A mechanical retractor system, the Integra Omni-Tract (Integra Life Science Co., Plainsboro, NJ), is key to good exposure. A retroperitoneal plane posterior to the left kidney is developed, and the left kidney with peritoneal sac and its contents are retracted to the patient's right. The lumbar branch of the renal vein (LRV) is carefully sought as it crosses over the aorta and is divided, providing a guide to the location of the left renal artery. The left diaphragmatic crus are divided along the long axis of the aorta, and this is facilitated by insertion of the left index finger under the crus on top of the aorta. This step helps in exposure of the SMA and celiac artery. Investing fascia over the aorta is divided, and the surgeon's index finger is passed just anterior to and posterior to the aorta to allow passage of the vascular clamp. Extraluminal control is less cumbersome than intraluminal control with balloon occlusion catheters. Control of the right common iliac artery can be safely obtained using intraluminal control during a retroperitoneal approach.

Correct Answer   **D** Left flank retroperitoneal approach through the left 10th intercostal space

Reference

Shepard, A. D. (2018). Proximal abdominal aortic aneurysm repair. In S. S. Hans, A. D. Shepard, H. R. Weaver, P. G. Bove, & G. W. Long (Eds.), *Endovascular and open vascular reconstruction: a practical approach* (pp. 213–219). Boca Raton, FL: CRC Press.

8. RATIONALE

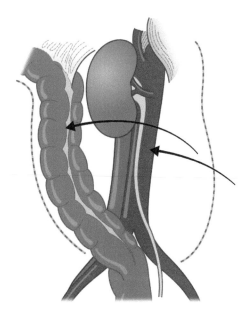

Medial visceral rotation for exposure of the entire abdominal aorta.

Most aortic surgeons prefer exposure of the proximal abdominal aorta using a left retroperitoneal flank approach. Exposure of the more proximal abdominal aorta can also be obtained through a midline incision using medial visceral rotation (MVR). With MVR, peritoneal reflection lateral to the left colon and spleen is incised from the sigmoid colon cephalad to the aortic hiatus. A retrorenal vein is developed, and the spleen, pancreas, and left kidney are retracted medially to provide exposure of the entire abdominal aorta from the aortic hiatus to its bifurcation. The major disadvantage of this approach is the lack of access to the distal descending thoracic aorta, a high incidence of splenic injury (20%), and pancreatitis. In most instances, a supraceliac clamp placement is appropriate, and intraluminal control is more cumbersome in a patient during laparotomy.

Correct Answer   A Clamp placement at the supraceliac level

Reference
Shepard, A. D. (2018). Proximal abdominal aortic aneurysm repair. In S. S. Hans, A. D. Shepard, H. R. Weaver, P. G. Bove, & G. W. Long (Eds.), *Endovascular and open vascular reconstruction: a practical approach* (pp. 213–219). Boca Raton, FL: CRC Press.

9. RATIONALE

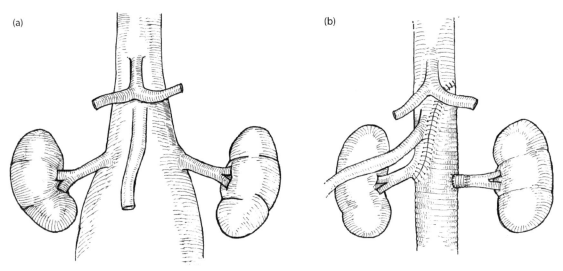

(a)   (b)

Proximal aortic reconstruction with lateral beveled anastomosis, incorporating SMA and right renal artery with either bypass to or reimplantation of the left renal artery. This is commonly performed when there is a significant aortic wall between two renal arteries: (a) suitable for this reconstruction, (b) post-reconstruction.

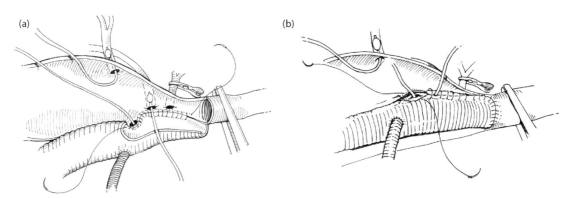

(a)   (b)

Lateral beveled proximal anastomosis to repair an extent IV thoracoabdominal aneurysm. Demonstrating placement of perfusion catheters in the SMA and both renal arteries with construction of an aortic suture line along the posterior wall. Bulldog clamp on the celiac artery. Complication of anterior wall suture line.

Acute kidney injury (AKI) is one of the most commonly reported complications of paravisceral AAA repairs. Minimizing visceral clamp time is critical. Before clamping, hemodynamics should be optimized. Mannitol (25 g) is administered 15–20 minutes before aortic cross-clamping. Inflation of a small (4 or 5 Fr) balloon-tipped occlusion catheter within the orifice of the right renal artery can block the passage of debris into the renal artery. When prolonged (>30 minutes) renal ischemia times are anticipated or in patients with preexisting CKD, cold renal perfusion to reduce metabolic demands consisting of 250 cc of 1°C Ringer's lactate solution (plus methylprednisolone, mannitol, and heparin) is infused into each kidney followed by 50 mL every 10–15 minutes for the duration of clamping. Infusion is performed through a balloon-tipped Pruitt perfusion catheter (9 Fr) for larger renal arteries (LeMaitre Vascular, Inc., Burlington, MA) and 4 or 5 Fr catheters for smaller renal arteries. A similar technique can be used for perfusion of the superior mesenteric artery.

Correct Answer C Perfusion of the renal arteries with a solution of cold Ringer's lactate, heparin, mannitol, and methylprednisolone during aortic occlusion

Reference
Kabbani, L. S., West, C. A., Viau, D., et al. (2014). Survival after repair of pararenal and paravisceral abdominal aortic aneurysms. *J Vasc Surg*, *59*(6), 1488–1494. PMID: 24709440

10. **RATIONALE**

Paravisceral aortic reconstruction usually requires a beveled end-to-end anastomosis which incorporates the origin of renal and visceral arteries. How that is performed depends on the relationship of the renal arteries to the aorta. If both renal arteries originate anteriorly with most of the aneurysmal wall extending posteriorly, a posterior bevel is possible. With this reconstruction the aorta is trimmed to leave the two renal arteries, the SMA and, if necessary, the celiac artery, on the anterior tongue of the aorta while the graft is cut to leave the corresponding posterior bevel. In practice, this type of reconstruction is usually not feasible. More commonly the proximal reconstruction is a laterally based beveled anastomosis that is used when the renal arteries are separated by a significant amount of aneurysmal wall. This technique incorporates the right renal artery, SMA, and celiac artery into the graft or, more frequently, bypassed with a small-caliber sidearm graft previously sewn onto the aortic graft (6 mm PTFE). When using a renal graft, it is imperative to carefully rotate (trim the aortic graft) so that the sidearm is appropriately positioned, usually at the 2 o'clock position (SMA at 12 o'clock), as this will prevent subsequent sidearm kinking of the graft. The graft-to-aorta anastomosis is performed with the inclusion technique, taking the first suture bites at the level of the dependent right renal artery and then carrying the suture line up the posterior wall of the aorta and taking double-thickness bites until the transected edge of the aorta is encountered. Single-thickness aortic wall stitches bring the suture line up to the level of the SMA or celiac artery and then down the transected anterior wall. Following appropriate flushing maneuvers, the perfusion catheters are removed and the suture line is secured, allowing sequential flow to the right renal artery to the celiac and the SMA. If the aneurysm extends well above the origin of the celiac artery mandating an end-to-end anastomosis between the graft and the aorta with reimplantation of the celiac artery, the SMA and left renal artery are done as a separate inclusion patch.

Correct Answer   **D** All of the above are acceptable techniques depending on the local anatomy

Reference
Shepard, A. D. (2018). Proximal abdominal aortic aneurysm repair. In S. S. Hans, A. D. Shepard, H. R. Weaver, P. G. Bove, & G. W. Long (Eds.), *Endovascular and open vascular reconstruction: a practical approach* (pp. 213–219). Boca Raton, FL: CRC Press.

11. RATIONALE

The natural history of thoracoabdominal aortic aneurysm is that of progressive enlargement. The mean rate of growth for TAAA is 0.2 cm/year and is accelerated in patients with dissections and connective tissue disorders. The 5-year survival of patients with TAAA is 13%, and aneurysm rupture is the cause of death in nearly 75% of untreated patients. Factors associated with rupture include aneurysm diameter, rapid expansion, COPD, steroid use, female gender, advanced age, and renal insufficiency. Contemporary series indicate that the rupture risk increases substantially as the aneurysm diameter reaches greater than 6 cm or with a growth rate of 10 mm per year. For patients with TAAA secondary to chronic dissection or those with Marfan syndrome, a 5-cm threshold is used.

Correct Answer   **C** 6.0 cm

Reference
Conrad, M. F., & Cambria, R. P. (2008). Contemporary management of descending thoracic and thoracoabdominal aortic aneurysms: endovascular versus open. *Circulation, 117*(6), 841–852. PMID: 18268161

12. RATIONALE

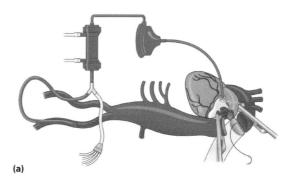

(a)

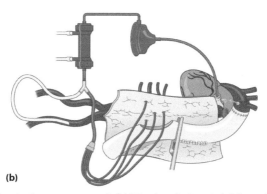

(b)

Legend- Approach to thoracoabdominal aneurysm repair (a) Distal perfusion via left heart bypass (b) Perfusion is maintained by multiple perfusion catheters once reconstruction proceeds distally

Many adjuncts have been recommended to minimize spinal cord ischemia (SCI) after TAAA repair, and only cerebrospinal fluid (CSF) drainage is evidence-based. Intercostal reconstruction had been routinely practiced despite evidence that it is based on retrospective studies. Distal aortic perfusion via left arterial-femoral bypass used in conjunction with motor-evoked potential (MEP) monitoring to dynamically assess SCI during the operation has replaced epidural cooling as the principal cord-protective strategy in patients with type I–III TAAA. Preservation of continuous perfusion of the pelvis (hypogastric artery) is logical and prudent. The addition of MEP monitoring enables the surgeon to depend on objective criteria for direct selective intercostal reconstruction and replaces the subjective application of intercostal reimplantation.

Correct Answer   C Distal aortic perfusion with intraoperative motor evoked potential monitoring

Reference
Conrad, M. F., & Cambria, R. P. (2008). Contemporary management of descending thoracic and thoracoabdominal aortic aneurysms: endovascular versus open. *Circulation*, *117*(6), 841–852. PMID: 18268161

13. RATIONALE

Distal perfusion through atrial femoral bypass and maintenance of distal perfusion pressure at 60–70 mmHg via a centripetal, motorized pump is simple and requires a low dose of systemic heparin. Atrial femoral bypass is initiated by cannulation of the left inferior pulmonary vein, and the arterial return is via the left common femoral artery. Liberal use of atrial femoral bypass for patients with type I–III TAAA is based on the concept of the spinal cord collateral network, emphasizing the importance of pelvic/hypogastric vessels and a selective approach toward intercostal reconstruction. Continuous perfusion of mesenteric circulation during reconstruction of the visceral aortic segment is desirable. This can be accomplished with either a Y connection from the atrial femoral bypass circuit or with in-live mesenteric shunting from the proximal graft after completion of proximal anastomosis.

Correct Answer **D** 60–70 mmHg

Reference

Conrad, M. F., & Cambria, R. P. (2008). Contemporary management of descending thoracic and thoracoabdominal aortic aneurysms: endovascular versus open. *Circulation, 117*(6), 841–852. PMID: 18268161

14. RATIONALE

As the number of comorbid conditions increases, so does the overall operative risks of repair of TAAA. Many series have reported that the presence of coronary artery disease, COPD, and renal insufficiency increases mortality. Preoperative renal insufficiency is the most powerful predictor of postoperative renal failure. Minimizing renal ischemic times, use of cold perfusate, avoiding intraoperative hypotension, and treating stenotic lesions with either bypass or open stent placement reduce renal injury. Postoperative renal dysfunction negatively affects short- and long-term survival.

Correct Answer **A** 30 cc

Reference

Conrad, M. F., & Cambria, R. P. (2008). Contemporary management of descending thoracic and thoracoabdominal aortic aneurysms: endovascular versus open. *Circulation, 117*(6), 841–852. PMID: 18268161

15. RATIONALE

SCI is the most devastating nonfatal complication associated with TAAA reconstruction. The pathogenesis of SCI after aortic replacement is multifactorial, but ultimately results from an ischemic insult caused by temporary or permanent interruption of the spinal cord blood supply. SCI manifests along a clinical spectrum from complete flaccid paraplegia to varying degrees of paraparesis. The degree of SCI directly predicts long-term survival after TAAA repair. Patients with incomplete deficits often recover reasonable function and have a long-term survival like those without SCI. Patients with an SCI deficit score of 1 rarely live beyond the first year. The incidence of dialysis-dependent renal failure following open repair of thoracoabdominal aortic aneurysm is 2%–3%.

Correct Answer **D** Type I–III thoracoabdominal aortic aneurysm and urgency of operation

Reference

Conrad, M. F., & Cambria, R. P. (2008). Contemporary management of descending thoracic and thoracoabdominal aortic aneurysms: endovascular versus open. *Circulation, 117*(6), 841–852. PMID: 18268161

16. RATIONALE

Mesenteric ischemia during and after open TAAA repair has a reported incidence of about 2.5% with a 62% mortality. Mortality is substantially higher if the ischemia is not discovered and corrected intraoperatively or immediately postoperatively. The exact manifestation of ischemia depends on the involved vascular distribution. Celiac malperfusion may vary from clinically nonsignificant to fulminant hepatic failure, pancreatitis, or duodenal necrosis, depending on the patient's anatomy, collateral supply, and preexisting visceral disease. Superior mesenteric artery malperfusion most commonly manifests as bowel ischemia. Visceral reconstruction is preferably performed by an inclusion patch (type II and III) or within the distal (type I) or proximal (type IV) anastomoses. Any intrinsic visceral disease may compromise aortic reconstruction at the time of operation. This may include transaortic orificial eversion endarterectomy and/or stenting. A rapidly escalating vasopressor or inotrope requirement, worsening metabolic acidosis, and rising serum lactate despite adequate volume resuscitation raise the suspicion of mesenteric ischemia both intraoperatively and postoperatively. If clinical diagnosis is strongly suspected in the immediate postoperative period, prompt re-exploration should be carried out.

Correct Answer   C 2%–3%

Reference
Achouh, P. E., Madsen, K., Miller, C. C., et al. (2006). Gastrointestinal complications after descending thoracic and thoracoabdominal aortic repairs: a 14-year experience. *J Vasc Surg, 44*(3), 442–446. PMID: 16950413

17. RATIONALE

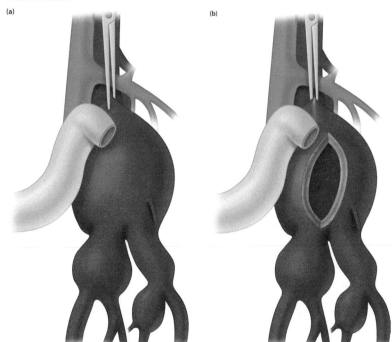

(a) Inflammatory AAA with adherent third and fourth portion of the duodenum. (b) Opened AAA with duodenum remaining attached to duodenum wall.

Inflammatory abdominal aortic aneurysms (AAAs) are uncommon and occur with a frequency from 3% to 10% of surgically repaired AAAs. Inflammatory AAAs occur at a younger age with familial tendency and occur more commonly in men with a history of nicotine abuse in the vast majority of patients. Most patients present with abdominal or back pain, weight loss, and increased sedimentation rate. Inflammatory aortic aneurysms are usually isolated to the infrarenal segment of the abdominal aorta within a characteristic inflammatory cuff of periaortitis and perianeurysmal fibrosis encasing the aneurysm wall, which enhances with contrast. At surgical exploration, a pearly white, glistening aortic wall with dense adhesions to the duodenum (mainly third portion) can be seen. Ureters are often adherent in the retroperitoneal space to the inflammatory abdominal aortic aneurysm and may result in hydronephrosis. The dense inflammatory reaction extends from just below the origin of the renal arteries to just above the common iliac artery bifurcation.

Correct Answer   **B** Duodenum and ureter

Reference
Pennell, R. C., Hollier, L. H., Lie, J. T., et al. (1985). Inflammatory abdominal aortic aneurysms: a thirty-
year review. *J Vasc Surg, 2*(6), 859–869. PMID: 4057444

18. RATIONALE

The primary key to the operation is wide exposure. Preincisional placement of ureteral stents has been recommended. Early division of the left renal vein (not mandatory) prevents undesired bleeding during renal vein dissection and provides better proximal exposure in patients undergoing abdominal aortic aneurysm repair using the transperitoneal approach. The ligament of Treitz should be carefully mobilized, but the third portion and proximal fourth portion of the duodenum should be left attached to the aneurysmal wall and after proximal and distal clamping, opening the anterior wall of the aneurysm with the attached duodenal wall like a trap door, which is retracted toward the right, will help to prevent an injury to the duodenal wall.

Correct Answer   **B** The third and proximal fourth portions of the duodenum should be left attached to the aneurysmal wall

Reference
Tang, T., Boyle, J. R., Dixon, A. K., & Varty, K. (2005). Inflammatory abdominal aortic aneurysms. *Eur J Vasc Endovasc Surg, 29*(4), 353–362. PMID: 15749035

19. RATIONALE

Major venous injury due to open aortic reconstruction is significantly more common during the repair of ruptured AAA as compared to repair of intact AAA. Risk factors associated with major venous injury during open aortic reconstruction are:

A. Periarterial inflammation
B. Repair of associated iliac artery aneurysm

In inflammatory AAA there is significant periarterial inflammation. There is increased risk of iliac/femoral vein thrombosis following repair of iliac vein injury, and patients should have evaluation by duplex venous study to rule out deep venous thrombosis.

Correct Answer   **D** Duplex venous study of the right lower extremity

Reference

Hans, S. S., Vang, S., & Sachwani-Daswani, G. (2018). Iatrogenic major venous injury is associated with increased morbidity of aortic reconstruction. *Ann Vasc Surg*, *47*, 200–204. PMID: 28887236

20. RATIONALE

Accurate positioning of the aortic stent graft ensures a proper landing zone, length, and undisturbed perfusion to the aortic branch vessels. Preoperative planning and imaging may predict optimal fluoroscopic visualization angles, utilized to eliminate parallax during deployment. Aortogram with device in place just prior to deployment is important to perform, as additional rigidity of the device on the wires may alter aortic alignment. Some devices such as the C3 Gore Excluder may allow for unidirectional repositioning after partial deployment or proximal recapturing, which can allow for level and orientation adjustments. Once fully deployed, graft repositioning may not be possible due to the radial forces of the stent and/or proximal fixation struts, as the stent graft becomes fixed in place in most endografts. If deployment is too low, a proximal aortic cuff can be placed. If major branches of the aorta such as renal, celiac, and SMA are at risk of malperfusion due to partial or complete coverage, left brachial access should be obtained to assist with cannulation of the vessels at risk so that either stenting or snorkeling with proximal extensions may be performed using either bare-metal or covered stents if needed.

Correct Answer   D Bare-metal, balloon-expandable stent using left brachial access into the left renal artery

Reference

Cuff, L., & Lu, J. (2021). Complications of endovascular repair of infrarenal abdominal aortic aneurysm. In S. S. Hans (Ed.), *Vascular and endovascular complications — a practical approach* (pp. 62–67). Boca Raton, FL: CRC Press.

21. RATIONALE

The use of a marker catheter for accuracy of limb measurement during deployment of the iliac limb of a stent graft, especially in the presence of tortuous anatomy, is mandatory. If partial or complete coverage of the internal iliac artery occurs, ipsilateral wire access into the internal iliac artery may allow for distal limb extension, and internal iliac artery stenting that extends into the external iliac artery may permit retrograde pelvic perfusion via the snorkel technique. However, there is a risk of late type IB endoleak with use of this technique.

Correct Answer   D Ipsilateral wire access into the right hypogastric artery via the right femoral artery with distal limb extension and internal iliac artery stenting that extends into the external iliac artery to permit retrograde perfusion via the snorkel technique

Reference

Cuff, L., & Lu, J. (2021). Complications of endovascular repair of infrarenal abdominal aortic aneurysm. In S. S. Hans (Ed.), *Vascular and endovascular complications — a practical approach* (pp. 62–67). Boca Raton, FL: CRC Press.

22. RATIONALE

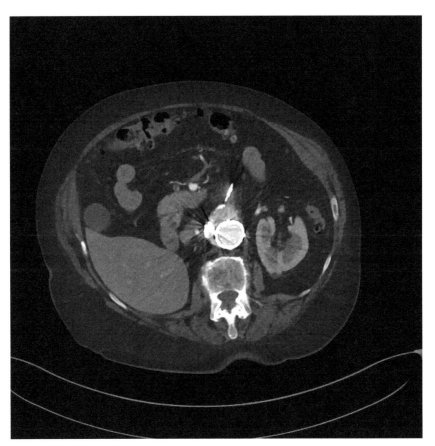

Type IA endoleak.

A type IA endoleak may develop when there is suboptimal wall apposition of the stent graft at the seal zone. In the case of type IA endoleak refractory to balloon angioplasty, a deployment of the balloon-expandable Palmaz stent (Cordis Corporation, Bridgewater, NJ) with its high radial force allows better apposition of the stent graft to the aortic intima. Another useful technique for management of type IA endoleak is to mechanically anchor the stent graft to the landing zone using the Heli-Fx endovascular system (Aptus Endo Systems, Inc., Sunnyvale, CA). In cases where the graft is deployed flush with the lowest renal artery and appears well opposed to the aortic wall, observation is reasonable in a few instances, as there may be resolution of type IA endoleak at 1-month follow-up CT scan. Despite adjunctive intraoperative maneuvers, type IA endoleaks may persist and must be carefully monitored. Persistent type IA endoleaks may need branched or fenestrated endograft if anatomy permits; otherwise, explantation of the endograft and open repair may be the only option available.

Correct Answer   B Consider a large bare-metal stent (Palmaz) or endostapling

Reference

Millen, A. M., Osman, K., Antoniou, G. A., et al. (2015). Outcomes of persistent intraoperative type Ia endoleak after standard endovascular aneurysm repair. *J Vasc Surg*, *61*(5), 1185–1191. PMID: 25656591

23. **RATIONALE**

Early graft limb occlusion is usually due to kinking of the graft or excessive infolding of the graft. Catheter-directed thrombolysis or mechanical thrombectomy followed by relining of the previously placed limb with a covered stent in the distal end can be extended to just above the common iliac bifurcation. If that's not feasible, coil embolization of the right hypogastric artery with extension of the iliac limb to the external iliac artery may be required. In general, it is preferable to avoid extension of the graft to the external iliac artery, as this is a predictor of late graft limb occlusion. Small-diameter external iliac artery and landing zone of the endograft into the external iliac artery at the time of index procedure are independent risk factors for graft occlusion.

Correct Answer **B** Thrombolysis and relining the endograft and extension of the graft to the right external iliac artery with coil embolization of the hypogastric artery

Reference

Bogdanovic, M., Stackelberg, O., Lindström, D., et al. (2021). Limb graft occlusion following endovascular aneurysm repair for infrarenal abdominal aortic aneurysm with the Zenith alpha, excluder, and endurant devices: a multicentre cohort study. *Eur J Vasc Endovasc Surg*, *62*(4), 532–539. PMID: 34266764

24. **RATIONALE**

The conventional approach that type II endoleak without sac enlargement can be safely observed has been recently challenged. The Japanese Committee for Stent Graft Management Registry data showed that the cumulative incidence rates of abdominal aortic aneurysm (AAA)–related mortality, rupture, sac enlargement, and reintervention were higher in patients with persistent type II endoleak. Specifically, the cumulative incidence rates of rupture and AAA-related mortality increased to 2% at 10-year follow-up. Older age, female gender, dilated proximal neck, proximal neck diameter, and chronic kidney disease are independent positive correlates of sac enlargement. These results suggest that persistent type II endoleaks are not benign. considering their long-term implications. The role of preoperative and intraoperative embolization of the side branches of the AAA to reduce incidences of type II endoleak is not well defined. In patients with significant sac enlargement due to type II endoleak from a patent IMA, superior mesenteric artery cannulation followed by advancement of the microcatheter over the microwire with the marginal artery of Drummond or the arc of Riolan and accessing the origin of the inferior mesenteric artery with deployment of microcoils will help in resolution of IMA-associated type II endoleak. Translumbar sac endoleak should be considered if a microcatheter technique via SMA is not successful.

Correct Answer **D** Coil embolization of the inferior mesenteric artery via the superior mesenteric artery using a microcatheter

Reference

Seike, Y., Matsuda, H., Shimizu, H., et al. (2022). Nationwide analysis of persistent type II endoleak and late outcomes of endovascular abdominal aortic aneurysm repair in Japan: a propensity-matched analysis. *Circulation*, *145*(14), 1056–1066. PMID: 35209732

25. RATIONALE

Endovascular juxtarenal aortic aneurysm repair incurs a longer operative time and higher doses of radiation and intravenous contrast than standard EVAR. Perioperative complications for custom fenestrated endografts (FEVAR) and chimney/snorkel parallel grafting (ch. EVAR) were studied in a meta-analysis for juxtarenal aneurysm repair. For FEVAR, cardiac complications occurred in 3.7%, pulmonary complications in 2.3%, sepsis in 0.6%, and ischemic stroke in 0.3%. For ch. EVAR, cardiac complications occurred in 7.4%, pulmonary in 3.2%, and ischemic stroke in 3.2%. The higher incidence of ischemic stroke is due to upper extremity vascular access with additional manipulation of wires and catheters in the transverse arch of the thoracic aorta.

Correct Answer   C 3%–3.5%

Reference

Katsargyris, A., Oikonomou, K., Klonaris, C., et al. (2013). Comparison of outcomes with open, fenestrated, and chimney graft repair of juxtarenal aneurysms: are we ready for a paradigm shift? *J Endovasc Ther, 20*(2), 159–169. PMID: 23581756

26. RATIONALE

There are several leak points related to the bridging stents that are unique to fenestrated and branch type aortic repairs (B/FEVAR). This primarily includes type III leaks from the graft-branch interface and type IC leak from the branch-target vessel interface. With appropriate sizing and planning, these are relatively uncommon. In a series of 650 patients undergoing B/FEVAR with 1679 total branches, the rates of branch-related endoleak requiring intervention were 2.5% for renal, 3.9% for SMA, and 2.8% for celiac branches. Accurate diagnosis of those leaks is made difficult by the proximal location of the branches within the main body of the graft, as they occur early and simultaneously with type IA endoleak on both angiography and CT scan.

Correct Answer   C 2%–3%

References

1. Mastracci, T. M., Greenberg, R. K., Eagleton, M. J., & Hernandez, A. V. (2013). Durability of branches in branched and fenestrated endografts. *J Vasc Surg, 57*(4), 926–933; discussion 933. PMID: 23433817
2. Swerdlow, N. J., McCallum, J. C., Liang, P., Li, C., O'Donnell, T. F. X., Varkevisser, R. R. B., & Schermerhorn, M. L. (2019). Select type I and type III endoleaks at the completion of fenestrated endovascular aneurysm repair resolve spontaneously. *J Vasc Surg, 70*(2), 381–390. PMID: 30583892

27. RATIONALE

A prospective multicenter trial to evaluate the safety and effectiveness of the Zenith fenestrated graft (Cook Medical, Bloomington, IN) for the treatment of juxtarenal AAAs looked at 67 patients with a total of 178 visceral arteries requiring incorporation with small fenestrations in 118, scallops in 51, and large fenestrations in 9, with technical success in all (100%). Of a total of 129 renal arteries targeted by a fenestration, there were 4 (3%) renal artery occlusions and

12 (9%) stenoses. Fifteen patients (22%) required secondary intervention for renal artery with type I endoleak in one patient. At 5 years, patient survival was 91% ± 4% and freedom from major adverse events was 79% ± 6%. Primary and secondary patency of targeted renal arteries was 81% ± 5% and 97% ± 2%.

Correct Answer **B** 22% of patients

Reference

Oderich, G. S., Greenberg, R. K., Farber, M., et al. (2014). Results of the United States multicenter prospective study evaluating the Zenith fenestrated endovascular graft for treatment of juxtarenal abdominal aortic aneurysms. *J Vasc Surg*, *60*(6), 1420–1428.e1421–1425. PMID: 25195145

28. RATIONALE

Evaluation of the use of intraoperative guidance by means of C-arm cone-beam computed tomography (CBCT) and the use of postoperative CBCT in patients undergoing FEVAR in 40 patients revealed a significantly lower dose of contrast with no significant difference in operative time or fluoroscopy time. Postdeployment CBCT is of sufficient quality to evaluate successful aneurysm exclusion and for detection of early complications after FEVAR.

Correct Answer **C** Lower contrast dose

Reference

Dijkstra, M. L., Eagleton, M. J., Greenberg, R. K., et al. (2011). Intraoperative C-arm cone-beam computed tomography in fenestrated/branched aortic endografting. *J Vasc Surg*, *53*(3), 583–590. PMID: 21129898

29. RATIONALE

Iliac artery aneurysm occurs in 40% of patients with abdominal aortic aneurysms. Approximately 80% affect the common iliac artery, with 20% involving the right internal iliac artery. External iliac artery aneurysms are extremely rare. Iliac aneurysms are usually diagnosed incidentally and are asymptomatic in most instances. Some iliac aneurysms can cause abdominal pain with obstructive symptoms involving the GI tract and GU tract, pelvic vein obstruction, and limb ischemia. Limb ischemia may occur secondary to acute thrombosis of the aneurysm. Rupture of iliac aneurysms is associated with significant morbidity and mortality. The expansion rate of common iliac aneurysms has been reported at 0.5–1.5 mm/yr in those less than 3 cm diameter as compared with 2.5–2.8 mm/yr in those measuring greater than 3 cm. The reported incidence of rupture of hypogastric aneurysm is high (38%–49%). The threshold for repair of common iliac aneurysm is 3.5 cm or larger and for hypogastric aneurysm is 3.0 cm.

Correct Answer **B** Common iliac artery, hypogastric artery, external iliac artery

Reference

Sandhu, R. S., & Pipinos, II. (2005). Isolated iliac artery aneurysms. *Semin Vasc Surg*, *18*(4), 209–215. PMID: 16360578

30. RATIONALE

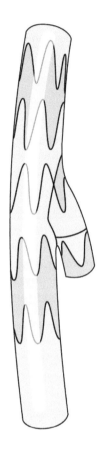

Straight iliac branch device.

In patients with isolated common iliac aneurysms with adequate proximal and distal landing zones (10–15 mm), the aneurysm can be excluded with a covered stent or endograft limb. However, if there is a concomitant AAA or the landing zone is less than 10–15 mm, a bifurcated endograft is required. If the common iliac aneurysm extends to its bifurcation, a variety of options exist to obtain a distal seal. Optimally, antegrade flow is maintained in the internal iliac artery to prevent symptoms of pelvic ischemia.

The common techniques used are:

A. Coil embolization/plug with endograft extension into the external iliac artery
B. Bell-bottom iliac limb
C. IBD
D. Snorkel technique
E. External iliac artery to internal iliac artery bypass with endograft extension
F. Combined open and endovascular approach

When considering IBD, the aortic-to-iliac bifurcation length must be >5 cm, common iliac bifurcation inner diameter >16 mm, internal iliac artery diameter >5–12 mm, with a landing zone of >10 mm, and minimal proximal common iliac diameter of 17 mm. In terms of the placement, a 16 Fr Gore drySeal Flex introducer sheath is advanced over a Cook Lundquist extra stiff wire guided in the contralateral side. A buddy catheter is introduced via the 16 Fr sheath, and an Indy snare is advanced in the contralateral 12 Fr sheath. The Cook tracer metro wire guide is snared establishing through and through femoral access. The IBE is loaded into the Lundquist guide wire and the IBE is advanced into position over both wires. Limited contrast angiography can be obtained through the 16 Fr ipsilateral sheath to demonstrate the level of the aortic bifurcation. The iliac branch portal is deployed 1–1.5 cm above the iliac bifurcation to aid in the internal iliac artery cannulation. The 12 Fr sheath is advanced up and over the iliac bifurcation. The sheath is positioned at the distal end of the iliac portal. A buddy catheter and guide wire are used to catheterize the internal iliac artery. The IBE is introduced and deployed in the internal iliac artery, and angioplasty is performed with a 14-mm angioplasty balloon while the external iliac stent portion of the device is deployed. The delivery catheter is removed and kissing balloon angioplasty is performed for the external iliac artery. In patients with internal iliac artery aneurysms after deployment of IBD, the sheath is advanced and the anterior division is excluded using an Amplatzer plug or coil. The posterior division of the internal iliac artery is catheterized. A proximal stent is placed into the posterior branch, and a self-expanding stent graft is placed in the posterior division. Freedom from IBD occlusion is reported to be 83%–86% at 5 years.

Correct Answer   **C** Iliac branch device (IBD)

Reference
Fargion, A. T., Masciello, F., Pratesi, C., et al. (2018). Results of the multicenter pELVIS Registry for isolated common iliac aneurysms treated by the iliac branch device. *J Vasc Surg, 68*(5), 1367–1373. e1361. PMID: 30072046

31. **RATIONALE**

Abdominal compartment syndrome (ACS) develops as a result of increased intraabdominal pressure secondary to massive fluid administration associated with ongoing hemorrhage and reperfusion of the splanchnic bed. As a result of increased intraabdominal pressure, there is decreased venous return due to compression of the IVC resulting in decreased cardiac output. The compression of the kidneys results in a decrease in renal blood flow and oliguria. There is increase in the airway pressure with a decrease in pulmonary compliance. Intraabdominal pressure >20 mmHg develops in 50% of patients, and of those 20% develop multiple organ failure following open repair of ruptured AAA. Medical therapy includes neuromuscular blockade, positive PEEP, albumin, and diuretics. Dilutional coagulopathy tends to occur in the first 24 hours following repair. After 24 hours of repair, decompressive laparotomy should be considered. In some patients with ACS the abdomen should be kept open, avoiding adhesions between the intestines and abdominal wall. Vacuum-assisted wound closure followed by delayed primary fascial closure is often necessary.

Correct Answer   **C** 20%

Reference
Bjorck, M. (2012). Management of the tense abdomen or difficult abdominal closure after operation for ruptured abdominal aortic aneurysms. *Semin Vasc Surg, 25*(1), 35–38. PMID: 22595480

32. **RATIONALE**

SCI in the form of paraplegia or paraparesis is more common following open repair of ruptured AAA than unruptured AAA. This is often related to prolonged hypotension. It may also result from interruption of the blood supply to the spinal cord due to the abnormally low origin of the blood supply to the spinal cord (artery of Adamkiewicz) or embolization into the hypogastric artery. The incidence of SCI following repair of ruptured AAA varies from 0.26% to 0.74%. The incidence is much lower in patients undergoing an abdominal aortic aneurysm repair for unruptured AAA. Recovery from neurological function is usually poor.

Correct Answer   **A** <1% of patients

Reference
Gialdini, G., Parikh, N. S., Chatterjee, A., et al. (2017). Rates of spinal cord infarction after repair of aortic aneurysm or dissection. *Stroke, 48*(8), 2073–2077. PMID: 28655811

33. RATIONALE

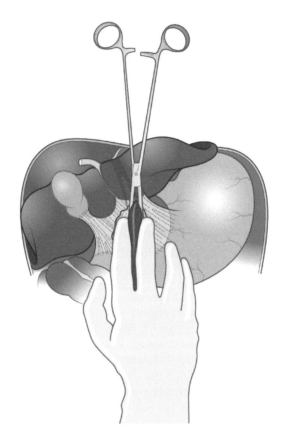

Exposure of the supraceliac aorta.

In patients with profound hypotension, free rupture is suspected, and obtaining rapid proximal control is of paramount importance to avoid circulatory collapse; therefore, anesthetic induction and intubation should be withheld until the incision is ready to be made. Induction of general anesthesia relieves pain, relaxes the abdominal wall musculature, and releases the sympathetic tone, which are all protective mechanisms to maintain blood pressure. In most patients with small- to moderate-sized periaortic hematoma, blunt finger dissection around the aortic neck aids in positioning of the proximal clamp. However, in patients with extensive retroperitoneal hematomas and shock, proximal control at the supraceliac level is preferable. The left lobe of the liver is retracted toward the right following division of the left triangular ligament.

The dissection is done via an opening made in the gastrohepatic omentum. The esophagus with the NG tube is retracted to the left with a Penrose drain. Deep blades of the surgical retractor system are inserted to expose the proximal abdominal aorta through the aortic hiatus in the diaphragm. The muscular fibers of the crus are separated with the help of long Metzenbaum scissors, and a 5- to 6-cm-long opening is made in the right crus. The index and the middle fingers of the right hand are introduced through the opening in the crus, and fascia surrounding the lower descending thoracic aorta is divided. A long-angled aortic clamp is guided with the left hand to be applied to the supraceliac aorta. Although balloon occlusion can be obtained using femoral artery access, in many patients the arteries are extremely tortuous, and passage of the wire can be difficult and valuable time may be lost. Balloon occlusion using brachial artery access is difficult to achieve because of the large size of the balloon in a small artery.

Correct Answer **C** Laparotomy and supraceliac control

Reference
Hans, S. S., & Huang, R. R. (2003). Results of 101 ruptured abdominal aortic aneurysm repairs from a single surgical practice. *Arch Surg, 138*(8), 898–901. PMID: 12912750

34. **RATIONALE**

In a patient with injury to the left renal vein medial to the gonadal and adrenal vein, the injured vein can be divided and ligated. But in patients with injury lateral to the gonadal and adrenal veins, ligation will result in renal vein thrombosis and loss of function of the left kidney. Even if the injury is medial to the gonadal vein and adrenal vein, lateral venorgraphy in a hemodynamically stable patient should be carried out. Ligation of the left renal vein medial to the adrenal and gonadal vein results in renal deterioration in the early postoperative period, but long-term renal function is not affected. Since this patient's blood pressure is relatively low, one should complete the proximal anastomosis and then perform lateral repair of the injured left renal vein, as attempting repair of the lacerated vein may result in further blood loss with persistent hypotension and potential for multiple organ dysfunction.

Correct Answer **D** Vascular clamps on either side of the left renal vein and repair after proximal aortic anastomosis is completed

Reference
Pandirajan, K., Katsogridakis, E., Sidloff, D., et al. (2020). Effects of left renal vein ligation during open abdominal aortic aneurysm repair on renal function. *Eur J Vasc Endovasc Surg, 60*(6), 829–835. PMID: 32912760

35. **RATIONALE**

Warshaw and O'Hara reported a 12% incidence of acute pancreatitis following open repair of intact AAA and 20% following repair of ruptured AAA. Duodenal obstruction occurs from the mass effect due to significant enlargement of the pancreas and from hematoma in the paraduodenal area.[1] Postoperative amylase, lipase levels, and CT scan of the abdomen should be obtained if the patient has persistent ileus following open repair of AAA. Nasogastric tube placement, management of adequate volume status, and total parenteral nutrition are usually required. Reoperation may be necessary if duodenal obstruction does not resolve with conservative management.[2]

Correct Answer **C** Open repair of ruptured AAA

References
1. Warshaw, A. L., & O'Hara, P. J. (1978). Susceptibility of the pancreas to ischemic injury in shock. *Ann Surg, 188*(2), 197–201. PMID: 686887
2. Hans, S. S. (1989). Pancreatitis and duodenal obstruction after aortic surgery. *Am Surg, 55*(3), 177–179. PMID:2919843

36. RATIONALE

Dilutional coagulopathy is due to dilution along with consumption of platelets during massive transfusion and resuscitation with a large volume of crystalloids. Crystalloids do not contain adequate coagulation factors. Adequate fibrinogen levels are essential in managing dilutional coagulopathy. After excessive hemodilution, fibrin clots are more prone to fibrinolysis because major antifibrinolytic proteins are decreased. Fresh-frozen plasma, platelet concentrates, and cryoprecipitate are considered to be the mainstay of hemostatic therapies. In disseminated intravascular coagulopathy, clotting factors are decreased with elevation of PTT and PT and increased in fibrin split products. In primary fibrinolysis there is a decrease in serum fibrinogen, and fibrin degradation products are increased with elevated D-dimer. Fibrin split degradation products are normal in dilutional coagulopathy, but Hct and platelets are slightly low with slight elevation of PTT and PT.

Correct Answer **C** Dilutional coagulopathy

Reference
Weiss, G., Lison, S., Spannagl, M., & Heindl, B. (2010). Expressiveness of global coagulation parameters in dilutional coagulopathy. *Br J Anaesth, 105*(4), 429–436. PMID: 20693180

37. RATIONALE

A horseshoe kidney occurs in approximately 0.25%–0.5% of patients requiring AAA repair. The preferred surgical options for unruptured AAA with a horseshoe kidney in an elective setting are endovascular aneurysm repair or open repair using a left flank retroperitoneal approach. In a hemodynamically stable patient with leaking AAA and horseshoe kidney, endovascular repair is a satisfactory option, but in patients who are hemodynamically unstable and horseshoe kidney was only detected at the time of laparotomy, the isthmus of the horseshoe kidney, if it is thin, can be divided, as it has almost no renal parenchyma. If the isthmus is thick, it should be mobilized with a prosthetic graft brought underneath the isthmus. A medial visceral rotation may be necessary to gain adequate exposure. According to the renal artery anatomy, types of arterial patterns varying from (a) a single renal artery on each side, (b) two renal arteries on each side and one to the isthmus, (c) multiple renal arteries are described in patients with horseshoe kidney. During open repair, preservation of renal arteries of 2 mm or greater in diameter should be considered, as their ligation may lead to ischemia of the renal parenchyma. Renal injury has been reported in 17% of patients undergoing AAA repair in the presence of a horseshoe kidney. Ligation of aberrant renal arteries of <2 mm can be performed without significant risk of renal complications. Reimplantation of accessory renal arteries (>2 mm) into the prosthetic graft can be performed using a Carrel patch technique.

Correct Answer **D** Should be decided by the anatomy of the aneurysm and arterial supply to the horseshoe kidney

Reference
Sachsamanis, G., Charisis, N., Maltezos, K., et al. (2019). Management and therapeutic options for abdominal aortic aneurysm coexistent with horseshoe kidney. *J Vasc Surg*, *69*(4), 1257–1267. PMID: 30591298

38. RATIONALE

Results from the Eurostar Registry consisting of 4901 patients from 113 centers reported a rupture rate of 4.7% for the first year and 0.6% for the second year following endovascular aneurysm repair.

The common features of rupture of AAA in a patient with prior endograft are:

A. Poor compliance and follow-up
B. Stent graft migration
C. Endoleak

In 34 patients in the Eurostar Registry, 39% had no complications prior to the diagnosis of rupture: EVAR was complicated by endoleaks in 20%–25% of patients. Approximately 10% of patients will develop type I endoleak, which is often associated with hostile neck anatomy (short angulated aortic neck with calcified wall, circumferential thrombus at the neck), which prevents a good seal at the proximal neck. Graft migration may occur due to progressive proximal aneurysmal dilatation of the aorta. The decision to perform endovascular or open repair for ruptured AAA in a patient with prior endograft depends on the anatomical findings on CTA of the abdomen and pelvis, and the patient's hemodynamic status and experience of the surgeon.

Correct Answer   D Choice of endovascular versus open repair depends on the findings of the CTA of the abdomen and pelvis and clinical condition of the patient

Reference
Fransen, G. A., Vallabhaneni, S. R., Sr., van Marrewijk, C. J., et al. (2003). Rupture of infra-renal aortic aneurysm after endovascular repair: a series from EUROSTAR registry. *Eur J Vasc Endovasc Surg*, *26*(5), 487–493. PMID: 14532875

39. RATIONALE

Coverage of one and occasionally both renal arteries may be required to facilitate EVAR in patients who are prohibitive risks for open repair. From a vascular quality initiative dataset (2013–2018) analysis, in 2278 patients with ruptured AAA, 2230 had no renal coverage, 30 had single renal artery coverage, and 18 had coverage of both renal arteries. On multivariant regression analysis, bilateral renal artery coverage was associated with increased odds of in-hospital mortality (OR 5.7%), permanent dialysis/30-day mortality (OR 9.5%), and permanent dialysis (OR 47.5%). Single renal artery coverage increased the odds of permanent dialysis/30-day mortality (OR 2.8%). From these observations it was concluded that bilateral renal coverage during repair of ruptured AAA significantly increases in-hospital mortality and lowers the long-term survival. Single renal artery coverage increases the risk of permanent dialysis/30-day mortality primarily as a result of permanent dialysis. It does not significantly affect the in-hospital mortality or 1-year survival and should be considered a viable option in select patients with ruptured AAA with prior EVAR.

Correct Answer   C Single renal artery coverage increases the odds of permanent dialysis/30-day mortality primarily due to the need for permanent dialysis

Reference
Tanious, A., Boitano, L. T., Wang, L. J., et al. (2020). Renal artery coverage during endovascular aneurysm repair for ruptured abdominal aortic aneurysm. *Ann Vasc Surg, 62*, 63–69. PMID: 31201979

40. RATIONALE

The incidence of late open conversion after EVAR should be <5%. The main indications for graft explantation include persistent type IA endoleak despite unsuccessful secondary interventions to correct the endoleak, graft infection, or refractory graft occlusion. The incidence of explant of an endograft is not related to the type of endograft used. Endograft failure <1 year is most commonly due to failure of the proximal seal at the initial procedure and underscores the need to understand the device limitations if used outside the instructions for use (IFU). Late failures are most commonly due to aneurysmal degeneration of the seal zones and device material failure and may occur even after a decade of successful EVAR repair. Emergent repair is most frequently required for infection or rupture. The operative approach is determined by surgeon preference and clinical factors such as suprarenal fixation. Both retroperitoneal and transabdominal approaches can be used, with suprarenal clamping required in most patients. Aortoiliac repair is the most common type of reconstruction after explant of the endograft. Mortality for emergent explant can be as high as 40%. In the elective setting, mortality should be <5%. In patients undergoing explant for graft infection, complete graft removal and replacement with an infection-resistant conduit should be performed. However, partial graft excision can be judiciously employed in patients with instances of sac expansion and rupture secondary to endoleak.

Correct Answer   B 1%–5%

Reference
Turney, E. J., Steenberge, S. P., Lyden, S. P., et al. (2014). Late graft explants in endovascular aneurysm repair. *J Vasc Surg, 59*(4), 886–893. PMID: 24377945

41. RATIONALE

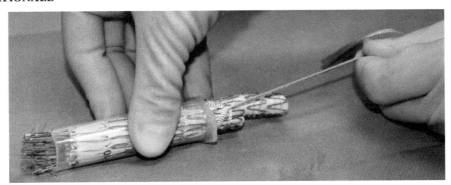

Explantation of the main body of the endograft. Superior movement of syringe barrel with downward traction on the umbilical tape.

It is important to note that complete removal of an endograft with suprarenal fixation can tear the aorta, injure the adjacent renal or visceral artery origins, and prolong suprarenal cross-clamping time. Complete excision of the endograft may necessitate extension of the aortotomy above the level of the renal orifices. When this is required, a beveled anastomosis to incorporate the superior mesenteric artery and right renal artery and left renal artery reimplantation or bypass as necessary should be considered. A retroperitoneal approach simplifies this maneuver. For distal iliac control, a Pruitt occlusion balloon catheter or number 10 arterial dilator is placed and positioned directly into each limb of the aortoiliac endograft to stop retrograde flow. Occasionally, iliac limbs of the stent graft are transected if there is extensive inflammation in the pelvis and are incorporated into the distal anastomosis. Rarely in emergent open repair in the setting of a ruptured aneurysm with the source of rupture due to a type IB endoleak, the proximal endograft can be left in place with the new graft sutured to the prior endograft and extended to the native iliac vessels beyond the prior seal zones. However, most patients with rupture secondary to type IB endoleak can be managed by coil embolization of the ipsilateral hypogastric artery and extension of the iliac limb into the external iliac artery.

Correct Answer   **D** Release of barbs with wire cutter and iced saline in a syringe to collapse the suprarenal segment

Reference

Dubois, L., Harlock, J., Gill, H. L., et al. (2021). A Canadian multicenter experience describing outcomes after endovascular abdominal aortic aneurysm repair stent graft explanation. *J Vasc Surg*, *74*(3), 720–728.e721. PMID: 33600929

42. RATIONALE

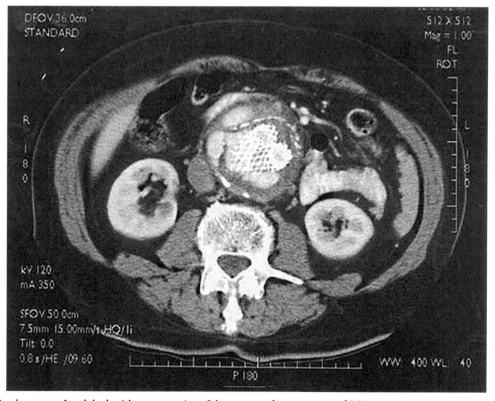

Showing large type I endoleak with extravasation of the contrast due to rupture of AAA.

The Eurostar Registry reported from 1996 to 2000 that 2464 patients were registered with a mean follow-up of 12.19 months, with confirmed rupture in 14 patients. The cumulative risk of rupture was approximately 1% per year.[1] Significant risk factors for rupture were type IA endoleak, type III endoleak, graft migration, and postoperative kinking of the graft. Forty-one patients underwent late conversion to open repair. The cumulative risk of late conversion was approximately 2.1% per year. In this study, first- and second-generation devices were used for EVAR. According to FDA panel reporting on 10,228 U.S. patients who underwent EVAR from 1999 to 2008, only 42% of patients met the most stringent criteria for endovascular repair.[2] Aneurysm sac expansion >5 mm/yr is an independent predictor of later mortality even after adjusting for the presence of endoleak and occurrence of sac intervention.[3] Even in the absence of identifiable endoleak, sac expansion warrants close observation.[3]

Correct Answer **B** Overall incidence of late conversion is 1.9% and delayed risk of rupture is 1% per year

References
1. Harris, P. L., Vallabhaneni, S. R., Desgranges, P., et al. (2000). Incidence and risk factors of late rupture, conversion, and death after endovascular repair of infrarenal aortic aneurysms: the EUROSTAR experience. European Collaborators on Stent/graft techniques for aortic aneurysm repair. *J Vasc Surg, 32*(4), 739–749. PMID: 11013038
2. Circulatory System Devices Panel Meeting. (2021). FDA executive summary. Retrieved from https://www.fda.gov/media/153647/download
3. Deery, S. E., Ergul, E. A., Schermerhorn, M. L., et al. (2018). Aneurysm sac expansion is independently associated with late mortality in patients treated with endovascular aneurysm repair. *J Vasc Surg, 67*(1), 157–164. PMID: 28865980

43. RATIONALE

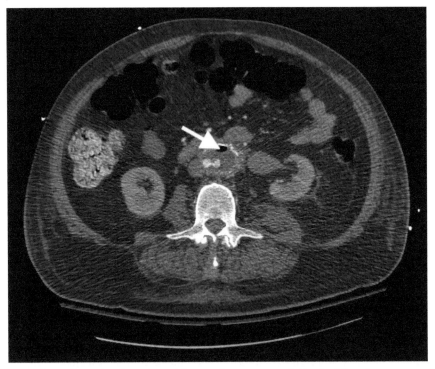

Computed tomography angiography of a patient with secondary aortoenteric fistula. There is gas accumulation within the aneurysm sac in proximity to the bifurcated graft (white arrow pointing to air within the aneurysm sac).

In a hemodynamically stable patient, once the diagnosis is either confirmed or highly suspected, the operating surgeon must decide between two radically different approaches:

A. Staged or sequential extra-anatomic bypass followed by aortic graft excision (infected)
B. Aortic graft excision with in-line aortic graft replacement with one of the following conduits:
    I. Femoral vein (venous autograft)
   II. Cryopreserved arterial allograft
  III. A new prosthetic graft with antimicrobial impregnation (rifampin)

Extensive debridement of the aortic wall and inflammatory tissue with omental coverage is essential. Staged extra-anatomic bypass and graft excision is reserved for patients with multiple comorbidities. If cryopreserved allograft is not available, a rifampin-impregnated Dacron graft is a good alternative. The cryopreserved allograft is placed in such a way that lumbar arteries are anterior. In good- to moderate-risk patients, when planning arterial allograft or rifampin-impregnated Dacron graft, availability of 3 mm of the aortic neck below the renal arteries is sufficient to achieve a satisfactory proximal anastomosis.

Correct Answer   **B**   Cryopreserved arterial allograft

Reference
Fatima, J., Duncan, A. A., de Grandis, E., et al. (2013). Treatment strategies and outcomes in patients with infected aortic endografts. *J Vasc Surg, 58*(2), 371–379. PMID: 23756338

44. RATIONALE

Following a long midline incision, the supraceliac aorta is controlled by mobilization of the left lobe of the liver to the right by division of the triangular ligament and gastroesophageal junction to the left and separating the right crus of the diaphragm. Distal control is obtained at the level of the iliac vessels or distal graft anastomosis. Any omentum encountered is preserved for use as a pedicle flap. Proximal control is moved from the supraceliac to the infrarenal location expeditiously to reduce the visceral/renal ischemic time. Before placement of the proximal clamp, the patient is given an appropriate dose of heparin and intravenous mannitol. The duodenal defect is debrided and closed primarily transversely. Distal anastomosis to the common iliac artery bifurcation is preferable. If a groin anastomosis becomes necessary, attempts should be made to preserve retrograde flow to at least one hypogastric artery. Emergent endovascular stent graft placement in a patient with bleeding secondary to aortoenteric fistula as a "bridge" to definitive surgical repair may be considered in high-risk patients.

Correct Answer   **B**   Supraceliac via midline laparotomy

Reference
Kakkos, S. K., Bicknell, C. D., Tsolakis, I. A., & Bergqvist, D. (2016). Editor's choice — management of secondary aorto-enteric and other abdominal arterio-enteric fistulas: a review and pooled data analysis. *Eur J Vasc Endovasc Surg, 52*(6), 770–786. PMID: 27838156

45. RATIONALE

There is no definite consensus for the appropriate length of treatment with antibiotics to be used for endograft infections with or without aortoenteric fistula. Most vascular and infectious disease specialists recommend 6 weeks of treatment with intravenous antibiotics and then transition to lifetime oral suppressive antibiotics. The rate of reinfection after treatment for aortoenteric fistula after open aortic surgery is significant at 24% and 41% at 1 and 2 years, respectively. These results are not based on type of reconstruction and were similar for extra-anatomic and in situ repair.

Correct Answer   D 6 months/possibly lifelong

Reference

Batt, M., Jean-Baptiste, E., O'Connor, S., et al. (2011). Early and late results of contemporary management of 37 secondary aortoenteric fistulae. *Eur J Vasc Endovasc Surg, 41*(6), 748–757. PMID: 21414817

46. RATIONALE

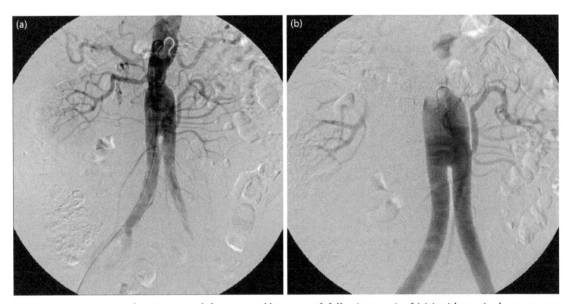

Postoperative aortogram showing patent left aortorenal bypass graft following repair of AAA with tear in the aorta near the origin of left renal artery.

Operative repair of juxtarenal AAA can be technically challenging. In the absence of the need to visualize the right distal common iliac artery, a left flank retroperitoneal approach is being increasingly used for open repair of proximal complex AAAs, repeat aortic surgery, AAA in the presence of horseshoe kidney, hostile abdomen, or inflammatory AAA. In the presence of aortic laceration at the origin of the left renal artery, a satisfactory option is to ligate the renal artery near its origin and reconstruct a prosthetic bypass using a 6-mm PTFE prosthesis with origin of the graft from the main body of the prosthetic graft or the left limb of the prosthetic graft (proximally) using end-to-side anastomosis and an end-to-end anastomosis to the spatulated left renal artery distally. Renal artery reconstruction at the time of open repair of paravisceral aneurysm increases the risk of acute kidney injury and mortality.

Correct Answer   D Bypass graft to the left renal artery with origin from the main body or the left limb of the prosthetic graft (end-to-side) to the left renal artery with end-to-end anastomosis distally

Reference
Wooster, M., Back, M., Patel, S., Tanious, A., Armstrong, P., & Shames, M. (2017). Outcomes of concomitant renal reconstruction during open paravisceral aortic aneurysm repair. *J Vasc Surg*, *66*(4), 1149–1156. PMID: 28648481

47. RATIONALE

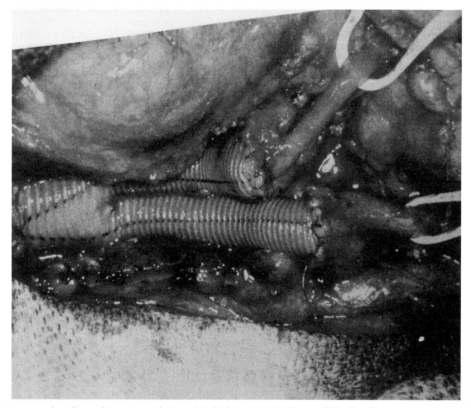

Silastic loop around each renal artery supplying pelvic kidney near the iliac graft limb to iliac artery anastomosis.

Careful evaluation of the preoperative imaging is important to identify and then plan for reconstruction of the renal arteries supplying the pelvic kidney. The pelvic kidney may be rotated with its pelvis lying inferiorly, and some patients with pelvic kidney and horseshoe kidney may have multiple renal arteries as opposed to a single renal artery on each side. Various methods such as temporary shunt, in situ renal perfusion, and use of an axillofemoral graft as alternative to maintaining blood supply to the pelvic kidney during aortic clamping have been proposed. The use of cold renal perfusion reduces renal metabolic demands. A solution containing 250 mL of 1% Ringer's lactate plus methyl prednisolone, mannitol, and heparin is infused in the renal artery using irrigating balloon catheters or a balloon-tipped Pruitt perfusion catheter. A custom-made fenestrated graft has been described to be used in the highest-risk patients. Renal arteries and ureters should be carefully identified during open repair. Systemic heparization before aortic cross-clamping, use of ice cold saline renal perfusion, and reestablishment of arterial flow are important steps to preserve renal function in the pelvic kidney. During distal anastomosis of iliac limbs of the prosthetic graft, each renal artery to the pelvic kidney is incorporated in the distal anastomosis.

Correct Answer   D Reimplantation of renal arteries supplying the pelvic kidney incorporating in the aortobiiliac graft reconstruction

Reference
Majumder, B., Perera, A. H., Browning, N., et al. (2017). Fenestrated endograft as a new perspective for the treatment of infrarenal abdominal aortic aneurysm with a congenital pelvic kidney – a case report and review of literature. *Ann Vasc Surg*, *45*, 266.e261–266.e264. PMID: 28712962

48. RATIONALE

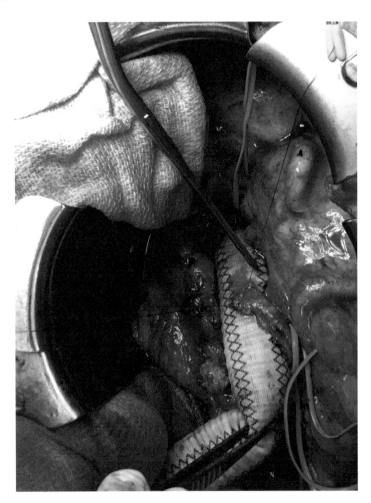

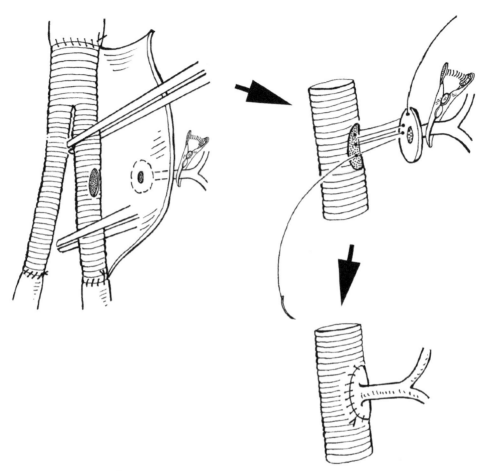

Inferior mesenteric artery reimplantation using a Carrel patch.

Patients undergoing open AAA repair with prior colon resection, severe superior mesenteric artery stenosis, or large inferior mesenteric artery with prominent mesenteric collateral such as arc of Riolan are at a greater risk of developing colon ischemia with the possibility of colon infarction. Standard EVAR with coverage of the IMA will result in ischemic colitis, as the IMA is large and its coverage may result in sigmoid colon ischemia. A fenestrated graft (homemade) can be challenging to design. If the patient has SMA stenosis and a normal-size IMA, SMA stenting should be considered prior to EVAR, provided the superior mesenteric artery stent does not project proximally into the aorta for >1 cm, as it may get dislodged during deployment of the main body of the stent graft. Open repair with reimplantation of the inferior mesenteric artery as a Carrel patch is probably the safest option in this clinical scenario.

Correct Answer   **B** Open repair with inferior mesenteric artery reimplantation

Reference
Hans, S. S. (2020). Abdominal aortic aneurysm repair in a patient with celiac artery occlusion and a large inferior mesenteric artery. In S. S. Hans (Ed.), *Challenging arterial reconstructions: 100 clinical cases* (pp. 15–17). Cham, Switzerland: Springer Nature Switzerland AG.

49. RATIONALE

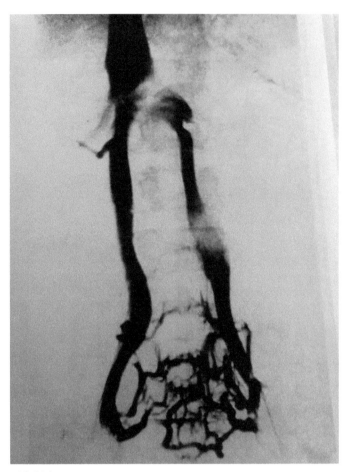

Double IVC in a patient with AAA.

The incidence of a double inferior vena cava is 0.3%–0.5% in the general population. The most common venous anomaly associated with AAA is a retroaortic renal vein as a result of persistence of the dorsal limb during development and a circumaortic venous collar due to persistence of both dorsal and ventral venous limbs. Normally the left renal vein is formed by the persistence of the ventral limb and regression of the dorsal limb of the venous collar. Anomalies of both renal segments of the inferior vena cava are classified as type A-persistent right posterior cardinal vein (retrocaval ureter), type B-persistent right subcardinal vein (normal IVC), type C-persistent left subcardinal vein (left IVC), and type BC-persistent right and left supracardinal and subcardinal veins (double IVC). In most patients with double inferior vena cava, mobilization of the left inferior vena cava, especially at the neck of the aneurysm, is important, as the left-sided vena cava crosses toward the right anteriorly and should be carefully mobilized in order to prevent injury to the vein, which may result in significant hemorrhage. A small tear in the tributary of the inferior vena cava may result in serious intraoperative hemorrhage and hypotension with multiple organ dysfunction. Inadvertent ligation of one of the paired channels will result in thrombosis causing edema of the lower extremity and serious sequelae of venous hypertension.

Correct Answer   B Mobilization of the left-sided inferior vena cava near the aortic neck

Reference

Hans, S. S. (2020). Open repair of abdominal aortic aneurysm in a patient with double inferior vena cava. In S. S. Hans (Ed.), *Challenging arterial reconstructions: 100 clinical cases* (pp. 23–26). Cham, Switzerland: Springer International Publishing AG.

50. RATIONALE

Marrocco-Trischitta et al. reported on 25 patients who underwent open AAA repair in the presence of biopsy-proven cirrhosis of the liver. They did not observe any difference in perioperative complications between cirrhotic patients and controls. However, there was higher intraoperative blood loss, longer operative time, and increased length of stay in patients with liver cirrhosis. From their study they concluded that in patients with compensated cirrhosis of the liver, open AAA repair can be safely performed. However, the reduced life expectancy in cirrhotic patients with MELD score >10 suggests that the repair should not be offered in this group of patients as their life expectancy is short. Patients undergoing open repair for intact AAA have increased operative bleeding, transient liver dysfunction, and increased length of stay but satisfactory survival. Patients presenting with ruptured AAA in the presence of liver cirrhosis have a uniformly poor prognosis.

Correct Answer   B Incidence of perioperative complications in patients with compensated cirrhosis of the liver is similar to those without cirrhosis but there is greater blood loss, increased operative time, and increased length of stay

Reference

Marrocco-Trischitta, M. M., Kahlberg, A., Astore, D., Tshiombo, G., Mascia, D., & Chiesa, R. (2011). Outcome in cirrhotic patients after elective surgical repair of infrarenal aortic aneurysm. *J Vasc Surg, 53*(4), 906–911. PMID: 21215574

51. RATIONALE

Paraplegia following infrarenal aortic reconstruction is rare and is multifactorial, with interruption of the abnormally located greater radicular artery (localized at the level of T9–T12 in 75%, T5–T8 in 15%, and L1–L2 in 10%), as the predominant factor. Atheroembolization, prolonged suprarenal clamping, shock, and interruption of pelvic arterial circulation are other important factors in causing spinal cord ischemia. In this patient the most probable cause of paraplegia was lack of antegrade flow into both hypogastric arteries. In the presence of thrombosed left hypogastric artery aneurysm, ligation of the right hypogastric artery effectively resulted in loss of arterial supply to the conus medullaris. In this patient a separate bypass from the right limb of the graft to the hypogastric artery after resection of the right hypogastric aneurysm should have been performed in order to maintain antegrade arterial flow to at least one hypogastric artery. Gloviczki et al. described six types of ischemic injuries to the spinal cord, with type I representing complete infarction of the dorsal spinal cord, manifesting as complete motor and sensory loss distal to the lesion, and type VI with infarction of the posterior one-third of the cord with preservation of motor function but with loss of proprioception and loss of sense of vibration. The remaining types (type II to type V) represent varying degrees of neurological deficits in the lower extremities.

Correct Answer   D Interruption of hypogastric arterial flow

Reference

Gloviczki, P., Cross, S. A., Stanson, A. W., et al. (1991). Ischemic injury to the spinal cord or lumbosacral plexus after aorto-iliac reconstruction. *Am J Surg, 162*(2), 131–136. PMID: 1862833

52. RATIONALE

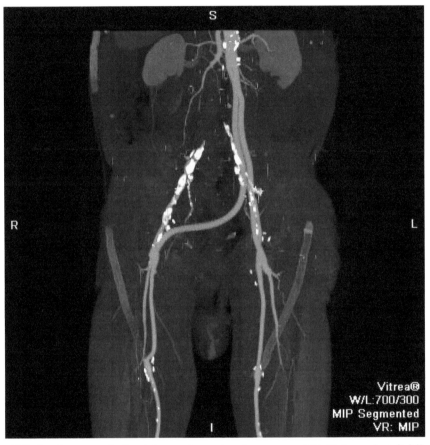

Postoperative CTA showing patent in-line left aortofemoral and crossover right iliofemoral graft following remote removal of infected aortofemoral graft.

The incidence of prosthetic aortic graft infection ranges from 0.6% to 3%.[1] Management options in patients with aortic graft infections include explantation of the graft and reconstruction by extra-anatomic bypass (axillofemoral), rifampin-soaked prosthetic graft, and cryopreserved aortic allograft. In situ autologous aortoiliac/femoral reconstruction using superficial femoral veins and popliteal veins have been championed by Clagett et al. Selection of revascularization strategy depends on the type of bacterial flora isolated from the graft, extent of graft infection, and presence or absence of aortoenteric fistula. Charlton Ouw et al. reported on 28 patients with infected infrarenal abdominal aortic graft with in situ reconstruction in 79% of patients using a prosthetic graft, cadaver homograft, and native femoral-popliteal veins with in-hospital mortality of 7% and reinfection rate of 25%.[2]

Correct Answer   **C** Aortofemoral reconstruction using a left flank retroperitoneal approach with bilateral groin incisions with a prosthetic graft as a conduit

References
1. Chung, J., & Clagett, G. P. (2011). Neoaortoiliac System (NAIS) procedure for the treatment of the infected aortic graft. *Semin Vasc Surg, 24*(4), 220–226. PMID: 22230677
2. Charlton-Ouw, K. M., Sandhu, H. K., Huang, G., et al. (2014). Reinfection after resection and revascularization of infected infrarenal abdominal aortic grafts. *J Vasc Surg, 59*(3), 684–692. PMID: 24239115

53. RATIONALE

Results from the GLOBAL STAR database (2007–2010) from experienced institutions in the UK evaluated 318 patients from 14 countries with deployment of a fenestrated aortic graft. The primary procedural success rate was 99%, perioperative mortality was 4.1%, and intraoperative target vessel loss was 0.6%.[1] Fenestrated endovascular aneurysm repair (FEVAR) is an independent predictor of the need for postoperative transfusion.[1] FEVAR promotes positive infrarenal neck remodeling and greater sac shrinkage compared with standard endovascular aneurysm repair.[2]

Correct Answer   **A** Using a fenestrated endograft

References
1. Early results of fenestrated endovascular repair of juxtarenal aortic aneurysms in the United Kingdom. (2012). *Circulation, 125*(22), 2707–2715. PMID: 22665884
2. Teter, K., Li, C., Ferreira, L. M., Ferrer, M., et al. (2022). Fenestrated endovascular aortic aneurysm repair promotes positive infrarenal neck remodeling and greater sac shrinkage compared with endovascular aortic aneurysm repair. *J Vasc Surg, 76*(2), 344–351.e341. PMID: 35276266

54. RATIONALE

The natural history of type II endoleaks is not well defined. It has been demonstrated that in approximately 20% of patients, early type II endoleaks may persist, and persistent type II endoleaks are associated with the need for secondary interventions, sac enlargement, and rupture of AAA. Delayed type II endoleaks are more likely to be associated with sac enlargement as compared to early type II endoleaks. A significant number of patients require multiple interventions for type II endoleaks. Coil embolization via the superior mesenteric artery, iliolumbar artery, or direct (translumbar) sac embolization are effective modalities for managing type II endoleaks. A patient with type II endoleak and a rapid sac growth rate should raise the suspicion of possible delayed type I or type III endoleak.

Correct Answer   **B** 6%–8%

Reference
Sarac, T. P., Gibbons, C., Vargas, L., et al. (2012). Long-term follow-up of type II endoleak embolization reveals the need for close surveillance. *J Vasc Surg, 55*(1), 33–40. PMID: 22056249

55. RATIONALE

Most experts agree that in patients presenting with a ruptured EVAR with suitable anatomy, EVAR is preferable to open repair. A multicenter trial (IMPROVE) from 29 centers in the UK and one in Canada randomized 613 patients with ruptured AAA: 316 to EVAR as the first strategy (if aortic morphology was suitable; open repair if not) and 297 to open repair. At 1 year, all-cause mortality was 41.5% for the endovascular group and 45.1% for the open repair group. There was no survival benefit for the endovascular group over 1 year but it offered patients faster discharge and better quality of life. The reintervention rate was similar in both groups. Several other single-institution studies showed that EVAR for ruptured AAA is a suitable treatment option, but its costs are prohibitive.

Correct Answer   **C** 45% for open repair, 41% for EVAR

Reference

Powell, J. T., Sweeting, M. J., Thompson, M. M., et al. (2014). Endovascular or open repair strategy for ruptured abdominal aortic aneurysm: 30 day outcomes from IMPROVE randomised trial. *BMJ*, *348*, f7661. PMID: 24418950

56. RATIONALE

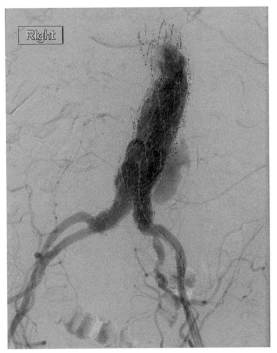 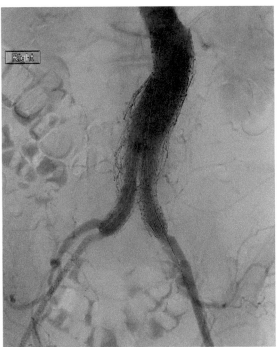

Type III endoleak repaired with a relining EVAR stent graft. Images are intraoperative angiography before (left) and after (right) relining stent graft placement.

Maleux et al. reported a 2.1% incidence of type III endoleaks in 965 patients undergoing EVAR from 1995 to 2014. In most cases the underlying mechanism was disconnection of the stent graft components (56%) and a fabric defect in the remaining 44%.[1] Type III endoleaks may result in rupture of AAA or occasionally in aortoduodenal fistula. CT angiography is the best imaging modality for detection of type III endoleaks, though plain abdominal films can confirm a disconnection of a stent graft limb and its components. Treatment consists of placement of a covered stent across the separated graft components. If there is a fabric tear at the flow divider, relining with conversion of the graft to aortobiiliac configuration is a better option.

The FDA sent a notification (Oct. 28, 2019) regarding the greater risk of type III endoleak with the Endologix AFX and Endologix STRATA device with close follow-up mandatory in patients where those devices were deployed.[2]

Correct Answer   B 2%–3% of patients

References
1. Maleux, G., Poorteman, L., Laenen, A., et al. (2017). Incidence, etiology, and management of type III endoleak after endovascular aortic repair. *J Vasc Surg, 66*(4), 1056–1064. PMID: 28434700
2. Update on Risk of Type III Endoleaks with Use of Endologix AFX Endovascular AAA Graft System. (2022). U.S. Food and Drug Administration Safety Report. Retrieved from Inactive Link—https://www.fda.gov/medical-devices/safety-communications/update-endologix-afx-endovascular-aaa-graft-systems-and risk-and-type-iii-endoleak-fda-safety#publications

57. RATIONALE

Rupture of AAA in a patient with a prior endograft remains a lethal problem. It has been reported that an existing endograft provides neither acute nor 1-year survival benefit after ruptured abdominal aortic aneurysm repair. Cho et al. reported 20% mortality of abdominal aortic aneurysm in a patient with prior endovascular repair and 38.1% with open repair ($P = 0.27$) in patients who had rupture of an abdominal aortic aneurysm with prior endovascular repair. Similar several other retrospective studies showed similar mortality in patients with ruptured AAA with prior endografts and those who had de novo rupture of abdominal aortic aneurysm.

Correct Answer   D Provides neither acute nor 1-year survival benefit

Reference
Cho, J. S., Park, T., Kim, J. Y., et al. (2010). Prior endovascular abdominal aortic aneurysm repair provides no survival benefits when the aneurysm ruptures. *J Vasc Surg, 52*(5), 1127–1134. PMID: 20674248

58. RATIONALE

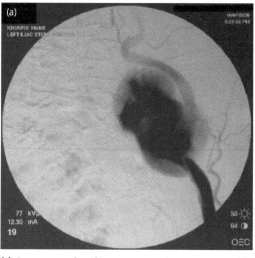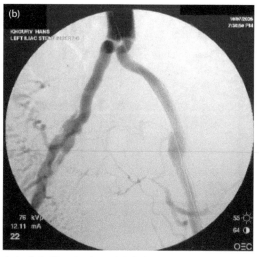

(a) Large saccular iliac anastomotic aneurysm with kink in left iliac limb and left hypogastric artery occlusion.
(b) Exclusion of aneurysm using iliac limb endograft.

In a population-based study (1959–1990), Hallet et al. reported on 307 patients who had undergone open AAA repair, and 9.4% had a graft-related complication. They reported a para-anastomotic false aneurysm (3%) at a follow-up of 6.1 years, three at the proximal anastomoses and the remaining six at the iliac/femoral anastomosis. Femoral anastomotic aneurysms are more common than iliac anastomotic aneurysms. Whenever anatomically feasible, endografting of the iliac and aortic anastomotic aneurysm is preferable to open repair. The iliac anastomotic aneurysm may be saccular and have associated redundancy of the iliac limb of the prosthetic graft and may require brachial access with snaring of the guide wire from the femoral approach as the wire tends to coil in a large aneurysmal sac. If the hypogastric artery is patent in a patient with a large anastomotic iliac aneurysm, it should be coil embolized or an Amplatzer plug be used to prevent retrograde flow into the aneurysm sac.

Correct Answer **B** Endovascular repair using a covered stent by left femoral and brachial access with coil embolization of hypogastric artery if patent

Reference
Hallett, J. W., Jr., Marshall, D. M., Petterson, T. M., et al. (1997). Graft-related complications after abdominal aortic aneurysm repair: reassurance from a 36-year population-based experience. *J Vasc Surg, 25*(2), 277–284; discussion 285–276. PMID: 9052562

59. RATIONALE

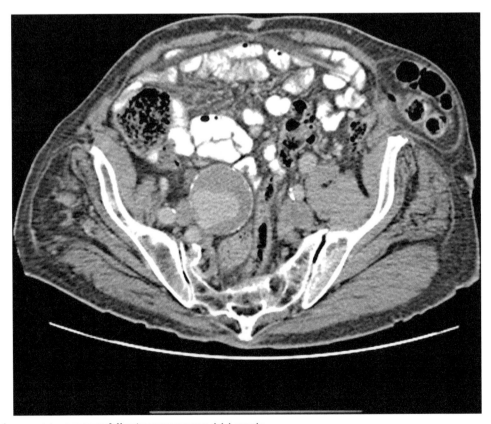

Large hypogastric aneurysm following remote open AAA repair.

Preservation of a hypogastric artery is almost impossible in patients with a large hypogastric aneurysm. Open repair is difficult because of its location deep in the pelvis, with surrounding venous structures, and as ligation of the branches of the hypogastric artery is usually necessary. Endovascular repair is preferable by first performing the coil embolization of the hypogastric branches (anterior and posterior) followed by endograft coverage of the origin of the hypogastric artery. Endografting of a hypogastric artery aneurysm is usually not feasible because of the difficulty in obtaining satisfactory landing zones proximally and distally. The risk of rupture of hypogastric artery aneurysm >3 cm in diameter is estimated to be 38% with a mortality of 50%–60%. Implantation of IBD devices for the treatment of hypogastric artery aneurysm in selected cases can yield good technical results with a high primary patency and low rate of perioperative complications. However, there is a higher rate of reintervention during midterm follow-up. Ipsilateral femoral access is preferable, as gaining access to the ipsilateral iliac artery from contralateral access is difficult, if not impossible, in patients with prior aortoiliac grafts.

Correct Answer   D Ipsilateral femoral access with placement of coils in the outflow branches of hypogastric artery and a covered stent across the outflow of the hypogastric artery

Reference
Kliewer, M., Plimon, M., Taher, F., et al. (2019). Endovascular treatment of hypogastric artery aneurysms. *J Vasc Surg, 70*(4), 1107–1114. PMID: 31147136

60. RATIONALE

Spinal cord ischemia (SCI) is one of the most dreaded complications of thoracic aortic endovascular intervention, occurring in up to 10% of patients.

Factors that contribute to the risks of development of SCI are:

A. Length of aortic coverage
B. Prior aortic surgery (open and endovascular)
C. Occluded vertebral arteries and internal iliac arteries
D. Intraoperative hypotension
E. Perioperative anemia

Preoperative planning should carefully consider the necessary length of coverage of the thoracic aorta. A proximal seal of at least 20 mm of healthy parallel-walled aorta is appropriate. If the coverage of the subclavian artery is necessary to achieve this, staged or concomitant revascularization to preserve the collateral flow to the left vertebral arteries is recommended by performing the left subclavian artery transposition into the left common carotid artery or subclavian-to-carotid bypass. Distally, a 20-mm seal is also desirable. Coverage of robust intercostals (if detected by CTA) that can be spared is desirable while still maintaining an adequate seal. Cerebrospinal fluid (CSF) drainage, if the length of the thoracic aorta to be covered is 20 cm or greater or in other high-risk settings, should be placed preoperatively. Intraoperatively once the device is deployed, CSF drainage can be initiated by simultaneously increasing the mean arterial pressure to >90 mmHg. CSF drainage can be performed (up to 10–20 cc per hour) to maintain an intracranial pressure of 10 mmHg or less.

Correct Answer   B Prior aortic surgery (open and endovascular)

Reference

Ullery, B. W., Cheung, A. T., Fairman, R. M., et al. (2011). Risk factors, outcomes, and clinical manifestations of spinal cord ischemia following thoracic endovascular aortic repair. *J Vasc Surg*, *54*(3), 677–684. PMID: 21571494

61. **RATIONALE**

Consensus guidelines from both the United States and Europe recommend TEVAR for:

A. Traumatic aortic injury and pseudoaneurysm
B. Penetrating aortic ulcer (>20 mm in diameter and 10-mm neck)
C. Intramural hematoma
D. Complicated type B aortic dissection
E. Thoracic aortic aneurysm >5.5 cm in transverse/AP dimension

Contraindications to TEVAR are limited mostly to anatomical considerations, inadequate proximal distal seal zones, or inadequate access vessels. Connective tissue disorders and contaminated fields are relative contraindications for TEVAR.

Correct Answer C TEVAR has a mortality of 19% and open repair 33%

Reference

Cheng, D., Martin, J., Shennib, H., et al. (2010). Endovascular aortic repair versus open surgical repair for descending thoracic aortic disease a systematic review and meta-analysis of comparative studies. *J Am Coll Cardiol*, *55*(10), 986–1001. PMID: 20137879

62. **RATIONALE**

A meta-analysis of nearly 9000 patients undergoing TEVAR looked at the calculated incidence of retrograde type A aortic dissection, which was observed to be 2.5% of patients, with associated mortality of 37%.

Retrograde aortic dissection may be increased when TEVAR is used:

A. Among patients with Marfan syndrome
B. For acute/chronic dissection
C. With more proximal landing zones (zone 0–2)
D. When the proximal diameter is oversized >15%
E. When aggressive wire manipulation or balloon molding is performed

Correct Answer C 2.5% of patients

Reference

Chen, Y., Zhang, S., Liu, L., et al. (2017). Retrograde type A aortic dissection after thoracic endovascular aortic repair: a systematic review and meta-analysis. *J Am Heart Assoc*, *6*(9):e004649. PMID: 28939705

63. **RATIONALE**

Posterior circulation strokes occur in approximately 3.1% of patients following TEVAR and typically occur in the context of coverage of the left subclavian artery. In more than 20% of aneurysms and dissections requiring endovascular repair, it is necessary to cover the left subclavian artery to achieve an adequate proximal seal. The left subclavian artery perfuses the brain via the left vertebral artery, which is dominant in over 60% of patients. Coverage of the left subclavian artery without its revascularization dramatically increases the risk for posterior circulation stroke (>5%) as compared to <2% with preoperative revascularization.

Anatomical factors that increase the risk of posterior circulation stroke include:

A. Dominant left vertebral artery in the setting of left subclavian artery coverage
B. Aberrant, hypoplastic, or absent right subclavian artery
C. Left vertebral artery terminating in the posterior inferior cerebellar artery
D. Anomalous origin of the left vertebral artery from the aortic arch

If there is a compelling reason to avoid preoperative revascularization of the left subclavian artery, it is necessary to demonstrate a patent right vertebral artery in continuity with a patent circle of Willis.

Correct Answer **B** 3%–3.5% of patients

Reference
Feezor, R. J., Martin, T. D., Hess, P. J., et al. (2007). Risk factors for perioperative stroke during thoracic endovascular aortic repairs (TEVAR). *J Endovasc Ther, 14*(4), 568–573. PMID: 17696634

64. RATIONALE

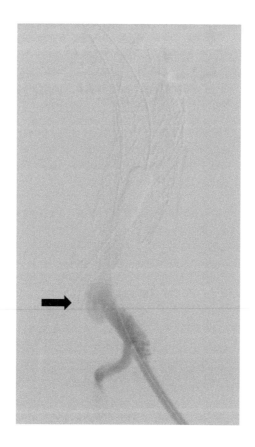

Iliac artery rupture.

Access artery injuries include iliac artery dissection, rupture, and thrombosis. Transfemoral access is feasible in only 70% of cases undergoing TEVAR. Thrombosis of the access arteries occurs in the setting of inadequate intraoperative anticoagulation and an occlusive or near-occlusive sheath.

Factors associated with access artery dissection and rupture include:

A. Inadequate iliac artery diameter
B. High-grade and/or long-segment stenosis
C. Severe calcification
D. Tortuosity of iliac arteries

For access, the iliac artery diameter must be 7 mm or greater. When these concerns are identified preoperatively, it is advisable to consider adjunctive measures to mitigate the risk of access artery injury. Specifically, small iliac diameter may be overcome with the use of serial hydrophilic dilators as long as there is no concomitant severe calcification. Open or endovascular conduits should also be considered. Open conduits may utilize the use of either an aortic or a common iliac proximal anastomosis exposure via a retroperitoneal approach. Endovascular conduits typically span from the common iliac to distal external iliac or even common femoral artery; a 12-mm-diameter graft is selected due to the additional friction imparted, as compared to the diameter of the native iliac artery.

Correct Answer   **C** Severe calcification

Reference
Jackson, B. M., Woo, E. Y., Bavaria, J. E., & Fairman, R. M. (2011). Gender analysis of the pivotal results of the Medtronic Talent Thoracic Stent Graft System (VALOR) trial. *J Vasc Surg, 54*(2), 358–363, 363.e351. PMID: 21397440

65. **RATIONALE**

A type IA or type IB endoleak should be treated intraoperatively. In a large international registry of patients undergoing TEVAR, the incidences of type IA or type IB was <1%. These endoleaks are the result of inadequate oversizing or implantation of the device in an unintended segment where the aortic diameter is larger than expected. Careful preoperative planning based on high-quality axial imaging with adherence to IFU should help prevent this complication. Adjunctive measures to enhance the precision of deployment such as rapid ventricular pacing or use of adenosine to temporarily halt the aortic impulse can be implemented. If type IA or type IB endoleak is identified on completion of the aortogram, balloon molding of the seal zone or extension of coverage with additional components should be performed. Balloon molding of the proximal seal should be avoided in cases of TEVAR performed for aortic dissection.

Correct Answer   **A** <1%

Reference
Tsilimparis, N., Debus, S., Chen, M., et al. (2018). Results from the study to assess outcomes after endovascular repair for multiple thoracic aortic diseases (SUMMIT). *J Vasc Surg, 68*(5), 1324–1334. PMID: 29748101

66. RATIONALE

Perioperative stroke as a complication of TEVAR occurs in 3%–5% of cases with an associated mortality of 16%–20%. Most are embolic strokes and may occur inadvertently as a result of endovascular manipulation in the arch and ascending aorta. While the incidence of clinically significant stroke is low, postoperative diffusion-weighted MRIs show small "silent" embolic strokes in as many as 60% of TEVAR patients. A prior history of stroke is associated with at least fivefold higher odds of stroke. History of coronary artery disease, renal failure, and female gender also increase the incidence of stroke. Longer operative times and inadequate anticoagulation are other factors that may be associated with perioperative strokes in patients undergoing TEVAR. Perioperative hypotension and anemia also contribute to stroke by reducing intracranial perfusion pressure. Intraoperative blood loss greater than 800 cc is also associated with increased stroke risk. Analysis of the Eurostar Registry showed that a "shaggy aorta" was associated with a 30-fold increase in the odds of perioperative stroke. Extending the coverage to the left common carotid (zone 1) or left subclavian (zone 2) in order to obtain an adequate seal is associated with an increased risk of perioperative stroke either due to malperfusion or embolization.

Correct Answer **B** 3%–5% of cases

Reference

Leurs, L. J., Bell, R., Degrieck, Y., et al. (2004). Endovascular treatment of thoracic aortic diseases: combined experience from the EUROSTAR and United Kingdom Thoracic Endograft registries. *J Vasc Surg, 40*(4), 670–679; discussion 679–680. PMID: 15472593

67. RATIONALE

To obtain a distal seal during performance of TEVAR, intentional coverage of the celiac artery was performed in 4% of cases from a large reported series. Manifestations of foregut ischemia are variable, including ischemic pancreatitis, perforated gastric ulcer, splenic infarction, acalculus cholecystitis, shock liver, and multiorgan failure resulting in mortality. Adequate evaluation of the mesenteric circulation is imperative prior to intentional coverage of the celiac artery. In patients with an ectatic visceral segment, postoperative mesenteric ischemia may result from the distal migration of the endograft with inadvertent coverage of the celiac artery. In patients where the distal seal is tenuous due to ectasia, alternative strategies such as fenestrated or branched endovascular aneurysm repair may be a better option to avoid a serious complication of foregut ischemia. Clinically significant foregut ischemia has been reported in up to 12% of patients following TEVAR.

Correct Answer **B** 0%–12% of patients

Reference

Rose, M. K., Pearce, B. J., Matthews, T. C., et al. (2015). Outcomes after celiac artery coverage during thoracic endovascular aortic aneurysm repair. *J Vasc Surg, 62*(1), 36–42. PMID: 25937603

68. RATIONALE

In acute type B aortic dissection, great care should be taken to ensure deployment of the endograft in the true lumen, with catastrophic consequences if deployed in the false lumen, namely malperfusion of the critical branch vessel and death. Therefore, identification of the true and false lumen is of paramount importance. Even with open exposure of the femoral artery, it may be difficult to identify the true and false lumen even on inspection. Given that multiple fenestrations exist even if the true lumen is definitively assessed in the groin, that may not ensure that the guide wire will remain in the true lumen as it is advanced cephalad. Therefore, careful evaluation of preoperative CTA, intravascular ultrasound, and angiography via the sheath at the level of each branch vessel is necessary.

Correct Answer   D Careful evaluation of preoperative CTA, use of intravascular ultrasound, and intraoperative angiography at the level of each branch vessel

Reference
Han, S. M., Gasper, W. J., & Chuter, T. A. (2016). Endovascular rescue after inadvertent false lumen stent graft implantation. *J Vasc Surg, 63*(2), 518–522. PMID: 25595403

69. RATIONALE

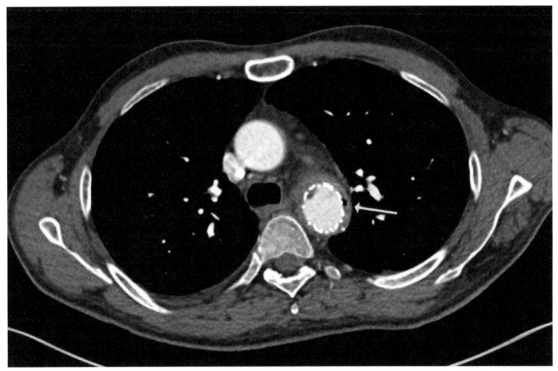

Gas in the aneurysm sac post-stent graft for traumatic thoracic aortic rupture.

In a large systemic review of EVAR and TEVAR infections, the mean time to presentation ranged from 115 to 991 days with incidence of <1%. Diagnosis is usually confirmed by the presence of perigraft inflammation or air. Mechanisms of graft infection include seeding from a bloodstream infection, contamination from an infection in an adjacent structure, or a break in the sterile technique at the time of implantation. The most frequently isolated microorganisms were staphylococcal species (30.1%), streptococcus (14.8%), and fungus (9.2%). Most patients (90%) require stent graft removal and in situ reconstruction or extra-anatomical bypass and a secondary endovascular procedure. The survival rate is higher in the patients with infected EVAR (58%) than TEVAR (27% $P = 0.000$). Patients with aortoenteric fistula (AEF) have the worst prognosis. Consultation with an infectious disease specialist for consideration of long-term treatment of antibiotics and/or antifungals should be obtained.

Correct Answer   A <1%

Reference
Li, H. L., Chan, Y. C., & Cheng, S. W. (2018). Current evidence on management of aortic stent-graft infection: a systematic review and meta-analysis. *Ann Vasc Surg, 51*, 306–313. PMID: 29772328

70. RATIONALE

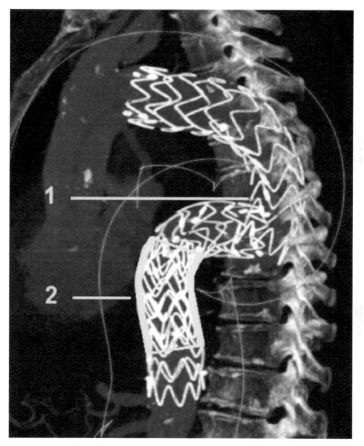

Migration of thoracic aortic stent graft with component separation.

As thoracic endografts are subject to a more forceful aortic impulse than infrarenal endografts, over a long period this may result in device migration (>10 mm) or component separation. The incidence of migration has been reported at 7% in a series of 123 patients over a median follow-up of 3 years and associated incidence of type I or type III endoleak of 44%.

Risk factors for graft migration include:

A. Neck angulation >60 degrees
B. Neck length <15 mm
C. Inadequate overlap between components (<5 cm)
D. Extreme tortuosity in the thoracic segment

In patients with dissection and associated aneurysm, the aortic wall may be diseased over a long segment and subject to progressive degeneration, which can manifest as either dilatation or elongation of the aorta, which in turn, can cause loss of the proximal/distal seal, device migration, or both. Bird beaking/lack of apposition to the aortic wall along the lesser curvature has been associated with device migration. The bird beak effect was significantly more frequent after traumatic aortic rupture treatment. Aortic angle of greater than 50 degrees is predictive of bird beak occurrence.

Correct Answer   C 7%

Reference
Geisbüsch, P., Skrypnik, D., Ante, M., et al. (2019). Endograft migration after thoracic endovascular aortic repair. *J Vasc Surg*, *69*(5), 1387–1394. PMID: 30553729

71. RATIONALE

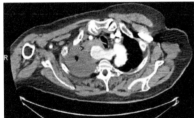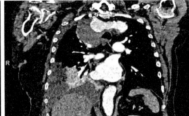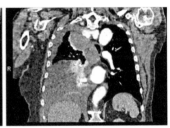

CTA of the chest showing ruptured large right aberrant subclavian aneurysm with hemothorax (2018).

The symptoms of aberrant subclavian artery are most often related to the development of aneurysmal disease occurring at its origin. The aneurysm develops in 60% of cases and is known as Kommerell diverticulum. Verzini et al. reported the results from a multicenter registry (2007–2013) from seven centers in Italy with the findings that the mean diameter of 4.2 cm is an indication for repair. Most patients had hybrid intervention, with a TEVAR covering the origin of the right subclavian artery and carotid-to-subclavian bypass or transposition on both sides in most patients in order to achieve an adequate landing zone and the prevent bird-beaking phenomenon seen in the tight "gothic arch." There are several options available to address this dilemma: the first option of simply covering the necessary branch has the potential for increased risk of stroke and in the instance of extended descending aorta coverage, spinal cord ischemia. Another option in the current era is to involve a snorkel for at least one of the arch vessels. In the future, branched endovascular aortic repair may be a better option than TEVAR, but this may result in endoleaks with subsequent risk of rupture.

Correct Answer   D 4 cm or greater in AP/transverse diameter

Reference
Verzini, F., Isernia, G., Simonte, G., et al. (2015). Results of aberrant right subclavian artery aneurysm repair. *J Vasc Surg*, *62*(2), 343–350. PMID: 26211377

72. RATIONALE
Current guidelines suggest repair for:

A. All symptomatic descending thoracic aortic aneurysm (TAA) patients
B. Asymptomatic patients with aneurysm diameter ≥55–60 mm

C. Rapidly extending aneurysm

D. In Marfan syndrome or in a patient with positive family history of descending thoracic aortic aneurysm with a diameter of ≥50 mm

Open surgical repair is more durable in younger patients and is mandatory in patients with aneurysms resulting from chronic dissection. Simultaneous abdominal and thoracic aneurysms are seen in 20%–25% of patients.

Correct Answer   **C** Open repair

Reference

Hiratzka, L. F., Bakris, G. L., Beckman, J. A., et al. (2010). 2010 ACCF/AHA/AATS/ACR/ASA/SCA/SCAI/ SIR/STS/SVM guidelines for the diagnosis and management of patients with Thoracic Aortic Disease: a report of the American College of Cardiology Foundation/American Heart Association Task Force on Practice Guidelines, American Association for Thoracic Surgery, American College of Radiology, American Stroke Association, Society of Cardiovascular Anesthesiologists, Society for Cardiovascular Angiography and Interventions, Society of Interventional Radiology, Society of Thoracic Surgeons, and Society for Vascular Medicine. *Circulation*, *121*(13), e266–e369. PMID: 20233780

73. RATIONALE

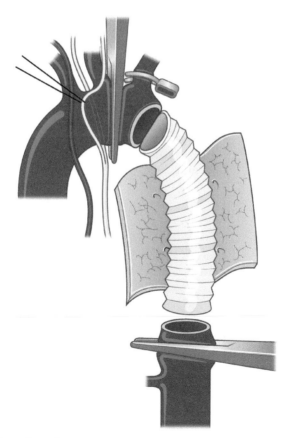

Open repair of descending thoracic aortic aneurysm.

For an isolated descending thoracic artery aneurysm, the patient is placed in a right lateral decubitus position with the left thorax upwards. At the discretion of the surgeon, a lumbar spinal drain is used to prevent spinal cord ischemia (SCI). A left posterolateral thoracotomy is performed, and the left chest is entered via the fourth intercostal space if the transverse aortic arch is to be intervened upon or via the eighth intercostal space for the distal descending thoracic aortic aneurysm thoracic. The left femoral vessels are exposed using a transverse inguinal incision for cannulation in readiness for cardiopulmonary bypass (CPB). The descending thoracic aorta is mobilized for resection. When a large aneurysm that contains debris is mobilized, atheromatous emboli can travel retrograde to the cranial vessels; therefore, the aorta should not be touched until an appropriate time of circulatory arrest. If there is insufficient room to cross-clamp the aorta proximally, cardiopulmonary bypass with deep hypothermic circulatory arrest (DHCA) is usually recommended. Otherwise, left heart bypass or femoral artery–femoral vein bypass (partial CPB) techniques can be used. This does not necessitate circulatory arrest. When CPB is performed, 2–3 units of autologous blood are withdrawn for later reinfusion. After heparinization, a venous cannula is inserted under transesophageal echography (TEE) guidance into the right atrium using a Seldinger technique via the left common femoral vein. The left common femoral artery is isolated, and an 8-mm Dacron graft is sewn in an end-to-side manner via a transverse arteriotomy for arterial return. When the long segments of the aorta are to be replaced, the distal clamp is initially set at approximately T5 to maintain lower intercostal artery perfusion; the distal clamp is then repositioned at the distal thoracic aorta when constructing the distal anastomosis. After proximal and distal anastomoses are constructed, the intercostal arteries are reattached, if felt necessary, by isolating a segment of the graft. Alternatively, the intercostal artery patch reimplantation can occur before the distal anastomosis to reduce the SCI time. The clamps are removed, and the CPB is stopped when the patient is normothermic. The left femoral artery is primarily repaired. Hemostasis is assured with protamine sulfate and autologous blood. The native aneurysm is closed over the graft to separate from adjacent viscera, chest tubes are placed, and thoracotomy and groin wounds are closed.

Correct Answer A Posterolateral thoracotomy via 8th intercostal space

Reference
Patel, H. J., Shillingford, M. S., Mihalik, S., et al. (2006). Resection of the descending thoracic aorta: outcomes after use of hypothermic circulatory arrest. *Ann Thorac Surg*, *82*(1), 90–95; discussion 95–96. PMID: 16798196

74. RATIONALE

The most common complication following open descending thoracic aortic aneurysm repair is postoperative respiratory failure. Risk factors for postoperative respiratory failure include active cigarette smoking, COPD, coronary artery disease, chronic kidney disease, or bleeding complications. Early ambulation and incentive spirometry in addition to ensuring tobacco cessation prior to surgery are important strategies to decrease the incidence of respiratory failure. Intraoperative intercostal nerve cryoablation reduces narcotic use and postoperative pain, thus leading to deep inspiration and expiration following thoracotomy and help reduce the incidence of respiratory failure.

Correct Answer B Respiratory failure

Reference
Patel, H. J., Shillingford, M. S., Mihalik, S., et al. (2006). Resection of the descending thoracic aorta: outcomes after use of hypothermic circulatory arrest. *Ann Thorac Surg*, *82*(1), 90–95; discussion 95–96. PMID: 16798196

75. RATIONALE

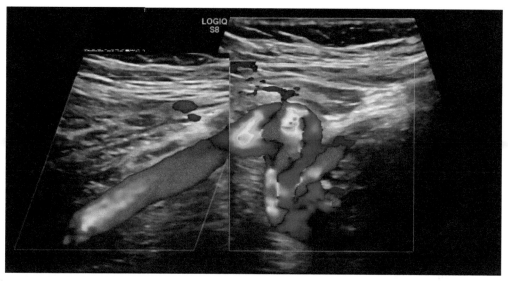

Duplex imaging showing partially thrombosed subclavian and axillary artery aneurysm with tortuosity.

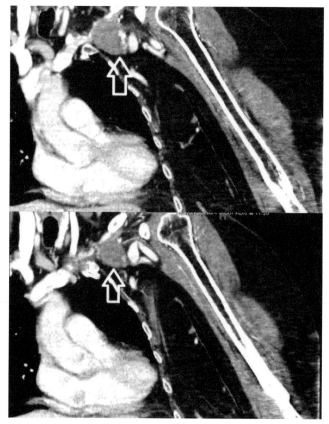

CTA showing large subclavian and axillary artery aneurysm with tortuosity.

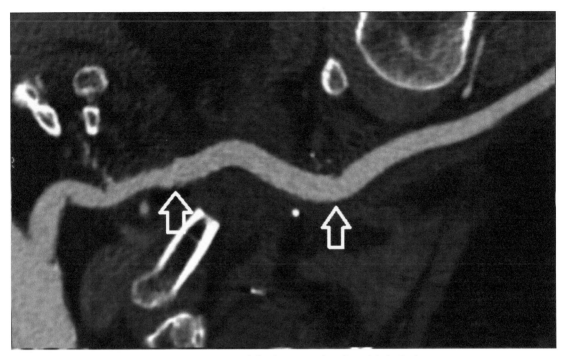

Postoperative CTA showing patent interposition graft (within arrows) and partial claviculectomy.

The majority (39%) of subclavian artery aneurysm (SAAs) are located in the proximal segment (39%). The middle segment accounts for 25% and the distal segment 24%, with associated involvement of the proximal axillary artery. Indications for subclavian artery aneurysm repair include size >2 cm, symptoms, or size >1.5 cm and concurrent operation for other aortic pathology. Proximal aneurysms are mostly caused by atherosclerotic disease, collagen disorders, trauma, and infection. The middle-segment SAAs are mainly caused by collagen disorders and trauma. Distal SAAs are mostly described in relation to thoracic outlet syndrome or as a consequence of blunt or penetrating trauma. Most patients present with a pulsating mass and shoulder pain. Other symptoms include pain from embolization before local compression, embolization, thrombosis, and rupture. Duplex ultrasound scanning for distal SCCA, CTA, and catheter-based angiography are often necessary prior to open repair. Despite the increasing interest in endovascular repair of the aneurysm, open repair of the subclavian artery is preferable and requires thoracotomy. For repair of proximal SAAs, sternotomy with or without supraclavicular and transclavicular/infraclavicular incision with partial resection of the clavicle may be necessary. The majority of subclavian artery aneurysm and nearly all aberrant subclavian artery aneurysms can now be repaired using a TEVAR-based approach without the need for sternotomy or thoracotomy.

Correct Answer **A** To prevent thromboembolic complications

Reference
Andersen, N. D., Barfield, M. E., Hanna, J. M., et al. (2013). Intrathoracic subclavian artery aneurysm repair in the thoracic endovascular aortic repair era. *J Vasc Surg, 57*(4), 915–925. PMID: 23375432

76. RATIONALE

Recurrent laryngeal nerve is the most common nerve to be injured during open repair of a subclavian artery aneurysm, resulting in hoarseness. Stent graft repair is being increasingly utilized, but these options are dependent on the anatomical characteristics of the aneurysm and vascular access. Traumatic subclavian artery aneurysm and iatrogenic subclavian artery aneurysm are best repaired using endovascular techniques. Patency of the reconstruction following endovascular repair may further improve with the development of better stent grafts, as in-stent stenosis and thrombosis were reported in an early series.

Correct Answer **B** Recurrent laryngeal

Reference

Vierhout, B. P., Zeebregts, C. J., van den Dungen, J. J., & Reijnen, M. M. (2010). Changing profiles of diagnostic and treatment options in subclavian artery aneurysms. *Eur J Vasc Endovasc Surg,* *40*(1), 27–34. PMID: 20399124

77. RATIONALE

Most aneurysms involving the upper extremity arteries are posttraumatic or secondary to connective tissue disorders or congenital in origin. These aneurysms are relatively uncommon and account for <1% of all peripheral artery aneurysms. Chronic repetitive trauma from the use of crutches can cause aneurysmal degeneration in the proximity arteries (axillary and high brachial) in the upper extremity. All symptomatic true and all pseudoaneurysms in axillary and brachial artery distribution should be repaired. Brachial and radial artery pseudoaneurysms may be secondary to vascular access for coronary or peripheral arteriography with or without associated intervention. Mycotic pseudoaneurysms have also been reported in patients with a history of intravenous drug abuse. During repair of axillary and brachial artery aneurysms, the median nerve needs to be protected, as the median nerve lies lateral to the brachial artery in the upper arm. However, the nerve crosses the artery from the lateral to medial side as it descends. Just before it enters the forearm, the medial nerve passes between the tendons of the biceps brachii and brachialis.

Correct Answer **A** <1%

Reference

Gray, R. J., Stone, W. M., Fowl, R. J., Cherry, K. J., & Bower, T. C. (1998). Management of true aneurysms distal to the axillary artery. *J Vasc Surg,* *28*(4), 606–610. PMID: 9786253

78. RATIONALE

All symptomatic true or pseudoaneurysms involving the axillary and brachial artery should be repaired. The most common presentation of axillary and brachial artery aneurysms is distal embolization resulting in hand ischemia. Patients may also present with neurological symptoms associated with brachial plexus (axillary artery) or median nerve (brachial artery) compression. Pseudoaneurysm due to infection can be safely ligated due to abundant collaterals. Asymptomatic true aneurysms should be repaired if equal to or greater than 2 cm in the transverse/AP diameter. Primary repair, resection with end-to-end anastomosis, patch angioplasty, and interposition graft are many options for repair depending on the anatomy and local findings at the time of repair.

Correct Answer   **D** >2 cm

Reference
Gray, R. J., Stone, W. M., Fowl, R. J., Cherry, K. J., & Bower, T. C. (1998). Management of true aneurysms distal to the axillary artery. *J Vasc Surg, 28*(4), 606–610. PMID: 9786253

79. RATIONALE

The overall reported mortality rate of elective aortobifemoral bypass (ABF) ranges from 1% to 4% with a 10-year primary patency nearing 80%. However, 10%–20% of patients experience some form of graft failure, including limb stenosis, thrombosis, infection, and degenerative pseudoaneurysms. A subset of these patients (1%–3%) present with bilateral limb occlusion. The optimal treatment for occluded aortobifemoral graft includes limb thrombectomy (selected cases) axillobifemoral bypass, thoraco-bifemoral bypass, or redo-aortobifemoral bypass graft. Patients undergoing repeat aortobifemoral bypass have higher procedure complexity as compared to primary aortobifemoral bypass, as evidenced by greater operative time, greater blood loss, and need for adjunctive procedures. However, similar perioperative morbidity, mortality, and mid-term survival as compared to primary aortobifemoral bypass have been reported. Patients undergoing repeat aortobifemoral bypass graft require extensive dissection of the profunda femoris artery to obtain adequate outflow, and there is frequent need for concomitant infrainguinal bypass more often in patients presenting with tissue loss.

Correct Answer   **A** <5%

Reference
Scali, S. T., Schmit, B. M., Feezor, R. J., et al. (2014). Outcomes after redo aortobifemoral bypass for aortoiliac occlusive disease. *J Vasc Surg, 60*(2), 346–355.e341. PMID: 24657290

80. RATIONALE

Aortic access can be obtained in a repeat aortobifemoral bypass using a retroperitoneal approach through a curvilinear left posterolateral incision extending from the midline halfway between the umbilicus and the pubic bone to the 8th or 9th intercostal space with hips as flat as possible. The retroperitoneal tunnels are created by reflecting the viscera to the right and performing blunt dissection between the right and left femoral incision. The right retroperitoneal tunnel occurs cephalad to the bladder and allows the limb of the graft to course as a gentle arc. Patients with difficulty in creating right retroperitoneal tunnel should have a left aortofemoral bypass performed, and a simultaneous crossover femoral-femoral bypass is performed using a suprapubic subcutaneous tunnel to avoid injury to the ureter and iliac veins during tunneling of the right limb of the graft. Midline celiotomy with an infra-mesocolic approach has also been used; however, because of the scarring in prior aortic dissection near the renal arteries, there is a greater chance of injury to important structures and increased blood loss.

Correct answer   **C** Left flank retroperitoneal approach

Reference

Scali, S. T., Schmit, B. M., Feezor, R. J., et al. (2014). Outcomes after redo aortobifemoral bypass for aortoiliac occlusive disease. *J Vasc Surg*, *60*(2), 346–355.e341. PMID: 24657290

81. RATIONALE

Mortality of aortobifemoral bypass ranges from 1% to 3.6%, and it increases with concomitant complication and with mortality as low as 0.5% with no complications, 10% with one major complication, and up to 36% with three or more major complications. Complications and mortality were significantly higher in patients with increasing age, presence of tissue loss, baseline renal insufficiency (threefold risk of death), and coronary artery disease (twofold risk of death). Medical complications (cardiac, pulmonary) are more common (15%) than surgical complications. Prevention and treatment of medical complications are largely mitigated with appropriate patient selection and meticulous anesthetic management and optimal postoperative critical care.

Correct Answer   D 20%

Reference

Bredahl, K., Jensen, L. P., Schroeder, T. V., et al. (2015). Mortality and complications after aortic bifurcated bypass procedures for chronic aortoiliac occlusive disease. *J Vasc Surg*, *62*(1), 75–82. PMID: 26115920

82. RATIONALE

Aortobifemoral bypass has excellent early patency (85%–92% at 5 years) and late patency (80%–85% at 10 years). Graft thrombosis is the most commonly encountered late complication and is usually due to progression of atherosclerotic disease. Correction of the disease at the origin of the profunda femoris artery is important to maintain long-term patency. If there is stenosis at the origin of the profunda femoris artery, a concomitant profundoplasty should be performed or a graft-femoral anastomosis should be carried down to the profunda femoris artery past the orificial disease. There is no difference in long-term patency between end-to-end versus end-to-side proximal anastomosis. Bilateral limb thrombosis or complete graft occlusion is significantly less common than single-limb thrombosis and may be due to an inflow problem. Early graft thrombosis requires operative thrombectomy and repair of the underlying technical issue or, rarely, an infrainguinal reconstruction to improve the outflow. Unilateral graft limb thrombosis may present as intermittent claudication due to the presence of collateral flow, but up to 20%–25% of patients may present with acute critical limb ischemia. Long-term patency after revision is approximately 68% with an 85% limb salvage rate.

Correct Answer   B Primary patency 85%–92% at 5 years and 80%–85% at 10 years

Reference

Brewster, D. C. (2014). Aortofemoral bypass for atherosclerotic aortoiliac occlusive disease. In James C. Stanley, Frank Veith, Thomas W. Wakefield (Eds.), *Current therapy in vascular and endovascular surgery*, (5th ed., pp. 418–422). Philadelphia, PA: Elsevier Saunders.

83. RATIONALE

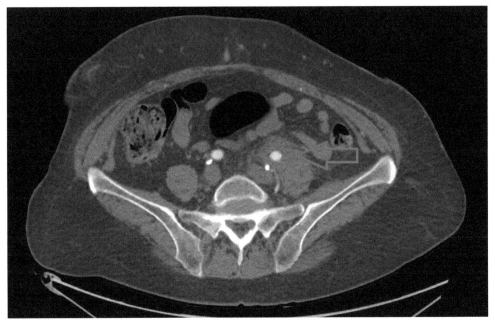

CTA showing perigraft (left) collection indicative of infection.

Aortic graft infection is a rare (0.2%–5%) but devastating complication of aortofemoral reconstruction. It is generally a result of inoculation of bacteria from elsewhere in a patient at the time
of surgery, most often from the skin, but the microorganisms can also be seeded in the postoperative period as a result of skin breakdown. Contact between the graft and the gastrointestinal
tract can also result in infection. The average time from the index operation to symptomatic
infection ranges from 41 to 62 months and is associated with a high mortality (40%) and limb
loss (11%) with a reinfection rate of 18% if not treated adequately. Concomitant or nosocomial
infection, particularly bloodstream, septicemia, urinary tract infection, and surgical site infection, are strong predictors of late graft infection. Patients with a graft infection can present with
fulminant sepsis, and many indolent infections can be difficult to diagnose. The groin incision
may demonstrate erythema or a draining sinus tract. Patients may exhibit abdominal or back
pain. There may be leukocytosis with elevated inflammatory markers. Imaging may demonstrate gas or heterogeneous fluid around the graft. The principles of treatment are complete
graft excision and debridement of local infected tissue. Reconstructive options include extra-
anatomic bypass graft and several methods of in-line bypass such as cryopreserved allograft,
rifampin-bonded prosthetic Dacron graft, and autologous vein using a neo-aortoiliac system
(NAIS). Each procedure has its advantages and disadvantages. The treatment should be based
on virulence of infection, urgency of the operation, and general medical condition of the
patient. Graft preservation may be considered in a limited subset of circumstances. Patients
who present with focal infection, such as those in whom infection is limited to one limb or in
the groin with low-virulence bacteria and no systemic signs of sepsis, have been treated successfully with antibiotics without total graft excision. Elderly frail patients with a hostile abdomen may also be considered for graft-preservation therapy with serial surgical debridement,
segmental vascular reconstruction ideally with an autologous (vein) conduit, use of antibiotic-
impregnated beads, and long-term parental antibiotics. Infections with more virulent organisms such as *Pseudomonas* and MRSA require complete graft excision.

Correct Answer   A 3.5–5 years

Reference
Calligaro, K. D., Veith, F. J., Yuan, J. G., et al. (2003). Intra-abdominal aortic graft infection: complete or partial graft preservation in patients at very high risk. *J Vasc Surg, 38*(6), 1199–1205. PMID: 14681612

84. RATIONALE

The incidence of early postoperative hemorrhage following aortofemoral bypass is in the range of 1%–2%. Intraoperative hemorrhage is avoided by familiarity with and knowledge of anatomy and preoperative imaging with evaluation of anomalous venous anatomy such as retroaortic left renal vein, left-sided, or duplicated inferior vena cava. Inferior mesenteric vein, adrenal vein, gonadal, lumbar, and iliac veins are also at risk of injury. Close attention should be paid to preoperative medications such as antiplatelets or anticoagulants and stopped according to the guidelines (7–10 days for clopidogrel, 5 days for warfarin, 2–3 days for apixaban). Those with a mechanical valve or high CHAZD2-VASC score should be considered for bridging with heparin. During proximal aortic anastomosis, use of pledgets and bioglue (Cryolife, Kennesaw, GA) for thin and tenuous aortic walls is useful to obtain satisfactory hemostasis. Reinforcement sutures should be placed with the aortic clamp in place, as pulsatile flow without clamping may result in an increase in the size of the needle hole when the suture is being placed.

Correct Answer   B 1%–2% of cases

Reference
Brewster, D. (2018). Aortofemoral bypass. In J. Fischer (Ed.), *Fischer's mastery of surgery* (7th ed., pp. 2332–2343). Wolters Kluwer Health, UK.

85. RATIONALE

Progression of aortoiliac atherosclerosis eventually results in abdominal aortic occlusion just below the level of the renal arteries. A small number of patients may have thrombosed small abdominal aortic aneurysms with thrombus extending to just below the origin of the renal arteries. Chronic occlusion of the abdominal aorta may occur at the (a) juxtarenal level, (b) at the level of the inferior mesenteric artery, and (c) at the aortic bifurcation. Suprarenal clamping in patients with juxtarenal aortic occlusion did not show any impairment of renal function as compared to those undergoing infrarenal clamping. This may be due to the short duration of renal ischemia, which is required in this group of patients to complete the proximal anastomosis.

Correct Answer   A Similar to infrarenal clamping

Reference
West, C. A., Jr., Johnson, L. W., Doucet, L., et al. (2010). A contemporary experience of open aortic reconstruction in patients with chronic atherosclerotic occlusion of the abdominal aorta. *J Vasc Surg, 52*(5), 1164–1172. PMID: 20732782

86. RATIONALE

Groin complications comprising lymphocele, hematoma, local wound dehiscence, and infection are seen in 20% of patients and will require operative intervention in 6.8% of patients. Most will occur within the first 3 months. Patient factors predisposing to groin complications include

(a) increased BMI, (b) diabetes mellitus, and (c) reoperation in the groin. The most common complication is a seroma/lymphocele. A seroma occurs when there is dead space and/or a reaction to a foreign body such as graft. The inflammatory response within the surrounding tissue leads to transudate of serous fluid with a straw-colored appearance with a consistency similar to that of pleural fluid. A lymphocele occurs when the lymphatic channels are not appropriately ligated or cauterized during dissection of the groin, resulting in lymph collection. Clinically, both are similar as a soft, compressible, bulging mass in the groin without any overlying changes in the skin. In contrast, hematoma appears more heterogenous on duplex imaging, with seroma and lymphocele appearing cystic. Surgical wound dehiscence can be superficial or deep, and management is dictated by concomitant infection and depth of involvement. Type I is limited to skin necrosis, superficial wound dehiscence, or local infection. Type II includes deep wound dehiscence. Type III involves the underlying graft. Treatment involves meticulous dissection, suture ligation of any lymphatic vessel, use of transverse incision in the groin, and use of topical negative pressure wound therapy using a self-contained dressing consisting of a sponge and occlusive dressing placed over a closed incision and connected to a portable vacuum device that maintains a subatmospheric pressure that decreases the amount of fluid in the wound bed with minimal external contamination. These are applied for 5–7 days and have decreased the rate of wound infection from 20% to 5.11%. Small asymptomatic seromas can be safely observed. Larger seromas within skin breakdown should be drained, preferably in the operating room. For suspected lymphocutaneous fistula, injection of isosulfan or methylene blue in the foot will help identify the disrupted lymphatic channels. Excisional wound debridement is performed in many patients who may also need sartorius myoplasty to obtain adequate tissue coverage. Antibiotics are not necessary unless there is cellulitis or signs of local infection. Wound complications lengthen the overall recovery from weeks to months and increase the risk for graft infection and thrombosis.

Correct Answer   C 20% of patients

Reference
Hasselmann, J., Björk, J., Svensson-Björk, R., & Acosta, S. (2020). Inguinal vascular surgical wound protection by incisional negative pressure wound therapy: a randomized controlled trial-INVIPS trial. *Ann Surg, 271*(1), 48–53. PMID: 31283565

87. **RATIONALE**
Ureteral injury occurs in <1% of the time in association with aortofemoral reconstruction. It is often related to difficult dissection of the iliac vessels due to inflammatory reaction in the common iliac arteries around the atherosclerotic plaque. It may also occur during creation of the retroperitoneal tunnels and closure of the posterior retroperitoneum. Injuries typically involve the distal ureter. Graft limbs that are inadvertently placed superficial to the ureter (anterior) during the tunneling may lead to ureteral compression and occasionally ureteroarterial fistula. Ureteral obstruction in properly placed graft limbs can be due to an inflammatory response as well. Distal ureteral injuries will require direct reimplantation of the ureter into the bladder. Most ureteral injuries (50%–70%) are not identified at the time of surgery. In suspected cases of ureteral injury with subsequent formation of urinoma on CT scan, delayed scans using CT-intravenous pyelogram, if positive, will demonstrate enhancement of the fluid collections suggestive of ureteral leak. These patients will require ureteral stenting and nephrostomy. The vascular surgeon should obtain a urology consult in patients with suspected ureteral injury during the index operation. Incidentally discovered asymptomatic postoperative hydroureter/hydronephrosis following aortofemoral reconstruction usually resolves spontaneously and rarely needs intervention.

Correct Answer   A <1%

Reference
Wright, D. J., Ernst, C. B., Evans, J. R., et al. (1990). Ureteral complications and aortoiliac reconstruction. *J Vasc Surg*, *11*(1), 29–35; discussion 35–27. PMID: 2296102

88. RATIONALE

Retrograde or dry ejaculation occurs in 3%–9% of patients undergoing aortoiliac surgery and is due to injury to T11–L3 sympathetic nerve fibers anatomically located at the aortic bifurcation, left side of the distal aorta, and left common iliac artery. Between 25% and 37% of patients develop new-onset erectile dysfunction after aortobifemoral bypass, which is usually thought to be iatrogenic in most patients. It is important for the surgeon to assess the patency of the hypogastric artery as well as obtain an accurate history of erectile dysfunction preoperatively. Minimal dissection in the area of the aortic bifurcation, left common iliac artery, and maintaining antegrade flow to at least one hypogastric artery should help in minimizing the risk of erectile dysfunction and retrograde ejaculation.

Correct Answer   B 3%–9%

Reference
Brewster, D. (2018). Aortofemoral bypass. In J. Fischer (Ed.), *Fischer's mastery of surgery* (7th ed., pp. 2332–2343). Wolters Kluwer Health.

89. RATIONALE

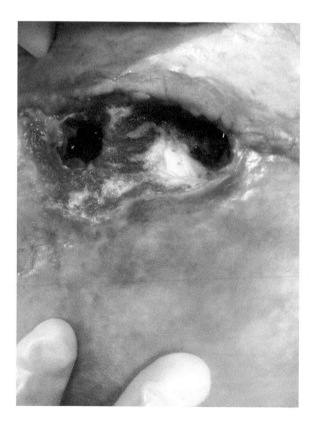

Exposed PTFE of left groin.

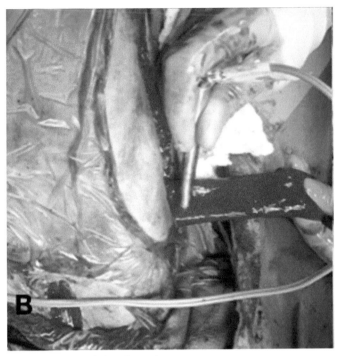

Gracilis muscle flap bloodflow checked with doppler probe.

In a patient with suspected graft limb infection with a prior history of aortobifemoral graft with severe comorbidities, a conservative approach using parenteral antibiotics, excisional debridement, muscle flap, and negative pressure wound therapy should be considered so that the graft is surrounded by healthy noninfected tissue. This treatment involving preservation of the graft should only be considered in those patients where there is no suspicion or diagnosis of bleeding at the anastomotic suture line as well as no evidence of infection with gram-negative bacteria such as *Pseudomonas* which may lead to anastomotic disruption. Sartorius muscle flap is the most used flap for coverage of exposed graft in the groin. In patients where the sartorius is not available, a retroflexed gracilis muscle flap is a suitable alternative to provide tissue coverage in the groin. Morasch et al. performed a gracilis muscle flap in 18 patients with failure of flap in only 2 patients at a mean follow-up of 40 ± 10 months. Other muscle flap choices such as rectus femoris and tensor fascia latae should be considered in patients where the gracilis flap cannot be used. Rectus femoris muscle flap is preferred if the excposed graft in the groin is above the level of the inguinal ligament which may occur following crossover femoral-femoral graft reconstruction.

Correct Answer   **B** Gracilis

Reference
Morasch, M. D., Sam, A. D., 2nd, Kibbe, M. R., et al. (2004). Early results with use of gracilis muscle flap coverage of infected groin wounds after vascular surgery. *J Vasc Surg*, *39*(6), 1277–1283. PMID: 15192569

90. RATIONALE

Right thigh muscle weakness probably represents ischemia/infarction of the right lumbosacral nerve root (type III) with asymmetric neurological deficits – a type of spinal cord ischemia. In this type of arterial reconstruction, a separate bypass to at least one hypogastric artery from the limb of the prosthetic graft should be performed to avoid disruption of the arterial supply. The prognosis is much better than with type I or type II spinal cord ischemia. In this patient, thrombosis of bilateral hypogastric aneurysms precluded a separate bypass to the hypogastric artery.

Correct Answer **D** Interruption of pelvic arterial supply

Reference

Gloviczki, P., Cross, S. A., Stanson, A. W., et al. (1991). Ischemic injury to the spinal cord or lumbosacral plexus after aorto-iliac reconstruction. *Am J Surg, 162*(2), 131–136. PMID: 1862833

91. RATIONALE

Descending thoracic aortofemoral artery bypass is best indicated for patients with multiple prior abdominal operations with extensive intraabdominal scarring, prior infrarenal aortic reconstruction, and history of infected aortic prosthesis. For patients who can tolerate this operation and have satisfactory cardiopulmonary status and a relatively healthy normal descending thoracic aorta, this procedure is superior to the alternative reconstruction such as axillofemoral bypass because of its superior 5-year cumulative patency rate of 81% versus 63% for axillofemoral bypass. Axillobifemoral bypass graft is usually reserved for high-risk patients with limb-threatening ischemia. Preoperative evaluation includes risk stratification, nuclear cardiac stress testing, and pulmonary function testing. Echocardiography should be performed to detect any valvular lesion and assess the left ventricular function. CTA of the chest, abdomen, and pelvis with bilateral lower extremity runoff should be obtained to ensure that the distal thoracic aorta is suitable for proximal anastomosis and vessels for distal anastomosis are satisfactory.

Correct Answer **D** Failed prior aortobifemoral bypass graft in a symptomatic 48-year-old woman with graft occlusion just below the renal arteries with a history of multiple celiotomies for Crohn disease

Reference

Sapienza, P., Mingoli, A., Feldhaus, R. J., et al. (1997). Descending thoracic aorta-to-femoral artery bypass grafts. *Am J Surg, 174*(6), 662–666. PMID: 9409593

92. RATIONALE

Contraindications to descending thoracofemoral bypass include aneurysmal or occlusive disease of the descending thoracic aorta with severe calcification as an absolute contraindication. Inability to tolerate single-lung ventilation is also an absolute contraindication. Relative contraindications include moderate to severe chronic obstructive pulmonary lung disease or prior thoracotomy with residual dense adhesions. Before starting the operation, the patient, anesthesiologist, and the surgeon should discuss the operative plan with risks, benefits, complications, and recovery. The patient is placed on the operating table with a vacuum bean bag extending from shoulders to the proximal thigh. After introduction of general anesthesia and placement of a double-lumen, endotracheal tube, the left hemithorax is elevated 45–65 degrees while maintaining the pelvis as flat as possible. The left arm is supported on an arm cradle, helping to extend the lower thorax and avoid a brachial plexus injury.

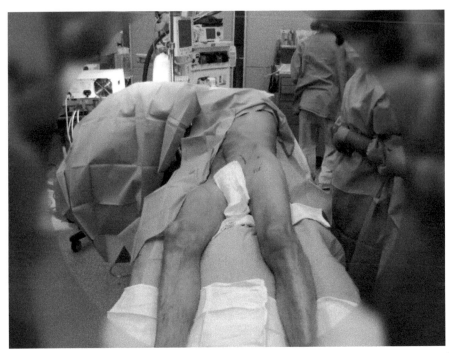

Patient positioned in a right side down thoracoabdominal position with the left arm in a supportive arm cradle and hips as flat as possible to facilitate exposure of both groins.

Correct Answer   D Circumferential distal descending thoracic aortic calcification

Reference
Criado, E., Johnson, G., Jr., Burnham, S. J., et al. (1992). Descending thoracic aorta-to-iliofemoral artery bypass as an alternative to aortoiliac reconstruction. *J Vasc Surg, 15*(3), 550–557. PMID: 1538513

93. RATIONALE

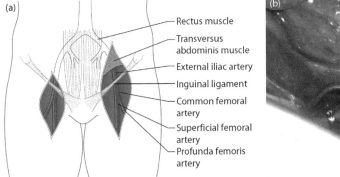

(a)

- Rectus muscle
- Transversus abdominis muscle
- External iliac artery
- Inguinal ligament
- Common femoral artery
- Superficial femoral artery
- Profunda femoris artery

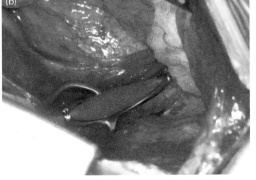

(b)

(a) Standard groin exposure with left incision extending 10 cm above the inguinal ligament and an additional 10-cm incision through the aponeurosis of the external and internal oblique muscles on the left, extending parallel to the inguinal ligament and approximately 2 cm cephalad to its caudal border. (b) A partially occluding aortic clamp is preferred because it helps maintain antegrade blood flow through the aorta during the proximal anastomosis, potentially limiting the magnitude of ischemia to the lower torso, visceral vessels and anterior spinal artery.

The procedure is started with exposure of the femoral artery bifurcation on both sides to reduce the length of time of exposure of viscera in the chest. The chest cavity is opened to minimize the associated heat loss. The left groin incision is extended proximally approximately 10 cm above the inguinal ligament, and the retroperitoneum is accessed at that site to facilitate the creation of the tunnel connecting the left groin to the left thorax. A 10-cm-long incision is made through the aponeurosis of the external and internal oblique muscles on the left, extending parallel to the inguinal ligament. The internal oblique muscle fibers are separated in their direction, and the transverse abdominal muscle and transverse fascia are opened in the lateral aspect of the incision. The retroperitoneal space is then entered medial to the iliac crest; this is the caudal end of the tunnel for passage of the graft. A posterolateral thoracotomy through the 8th intercostal space is performed to expose the descending thoracic aorta. After entering the pleural cavity, the left lung is deflated. Two "figure-of-eight" sutures are placed in the center of the diaphragm to retract the diaphragm. The inferior pulmonary ligament is taken down. The pleura around the distal descending thoracic aorta is incised and approximately 6 cm of the aorta above the diaphragm is exposed, and after the site for proximal anastomosis is selected, the intercostal arteries are preserved. A retroperitoneal tunnel is created to pass the graft limbs from the thorax to the groin. A 2-cm access incision is made in the posteromedial aspect of the left diaphragm over the ribs through the open thoracic incision. The location of the aortotomy and the exit site through the diaphragm must be aligned carefully to avoid lateral kinking of the graft. The left hand dissects the left retroperitoneal space through the left retroperitoneal incision, aiming cephalad medial over the extrailiac vessels and psoas major muscle. Posterior to the left kidney and posteromedial to the spleen a long tunneler is guided through the tunnel and used to pass the umbilical tape, facilitating the passage of the graft.

Correct Answer   **C** Right femoral graft limb is brought from the left groin in a suprapubic subcutaneous tunnel and anastomosed to the common femoral artery as in a standard crossover femoral-femoral graft

Reference
Pippinos, I., & Hernandez, H. (2017). Thoracofemoral bypass. In G. Long, M. Weaver, P. Bove, & S. S. Hans (Eds.), *Endovascular and open vascular reconstruction: a practical approach* (pp. 307–311). Boca Raton, FL: CRC Press.

94. RATIONALE

From a Swedish Nationwide Vascular Database (1994–2014) 715 cases of acute aortic occlusion were identified with a mean age of 60.7 years; 50.5% were women. The cause was in situ thrombosis (64.1%), saddle embolus (21.3%), and occluded graft/stent/stent graft (14.7%). Patients with saddle embolism were older (mean age 74.3 years) and a with preponderance of women (62.1%). The most common methods for revascularization were thromboembolectomy (32%), thrombolysis (22.4%), axillary-bifemoral bypass (18.9%), and aortobiiliac/bifemoral bypass (18.2%). In situ thrombosis was mostly treated with bypass surgery, and embolus treated with embolectomy. Endovascular techniques to treat acute aortic occlusion are becoming more frequent. The amputation rate was 8.6% and mortality was 19.9% within 30 days of surgery, with mortality highest in embolectomy group (30.9%).

Correct Answer   **B** In situ thrombosis

Reference
Grip, O., Wanhainen, A., & Björck, M. (2019). Acute aortic occlusion. *Circulation, 139*(2), 292–294. PMID: 30615512

95. RATIONALE

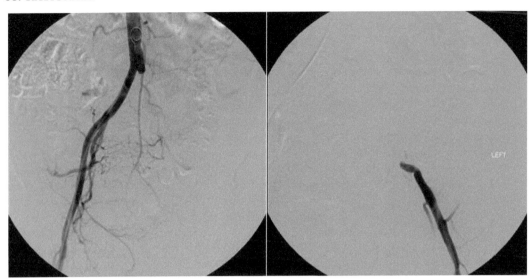

Diagnostic angiography for intermittent claudication demonstrating left common iliac artery (CIA) occlusion extending into the left external iliac artery (EIA) with distal reconstitution.

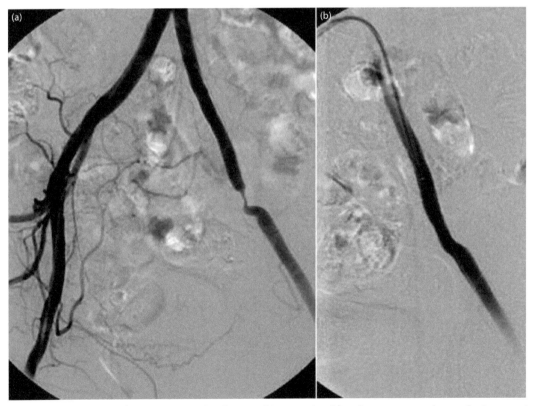

Left external iliac artery (EIA) stenosis 9 months after initial intervention (a) and status post-endovascular intervention with angioplasty and self-expanding stent (b).

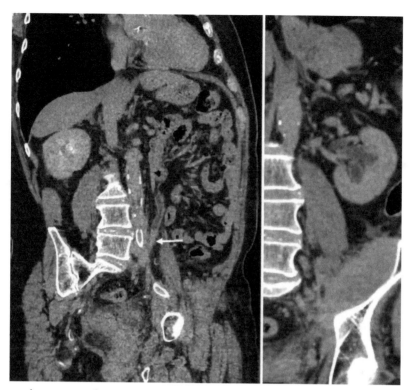

Computed tomography urogram demonstrating left hydroureteronephrosis from persistent fibrosis approximately 2 years after initial stenting of left common iliac artery (CIA) and subsequent stenting of left external iliac artery (EIA). Arrow indicates transition point of ureter at level of persistent fibrosis.

It is extremely uncommon to develop left lower quadrant flank pain years after left iliac stenting unless there is concern for aneurysmal disease. Ureteral complications after open aortoiliac reconstruction have been well documented in the literature, but ureteral complications following iliac stenting are uncommon. Those were first described in 2014 with the development of left hydronephrosis 2 months following iliac artery stenting in the Japanese literature. In this patient moderate left ureteral hydronephrosis developed in close proximity to the left common iliac stent without any abnormalities in the right kidney and right ureter. The patient was treated by robotic-assisted ureterolysis and omental wrap. There was a dense scar tissue forming an inflammatory rind adherent to the left common iliac artery. In open aortoiliac reconstruction during tunneling of the graft, which is tunneled posterior to the ureter, it can result in scar tissue with involvement of the ureter resulting in hydronephrosis. This type of hydronephrosis rarely requires intervention and really does not progress. In this patient, because of significant pain in the left flank and extensive scar tissue formation, ureterolysis became necessary.

Correct Answer   **D** Computed tomography urogram

Reference

Hans, S. S., Lee, M. M., & Jain, N. (2020). Ureteral stenosis following iliac artery stenting. *J Vasc Surg Cases Innov Tech*, 6(3), 469–472. PMID: 32923750

96. RATIONALE

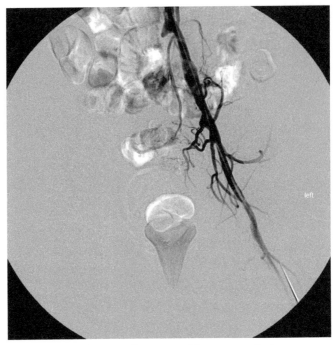

Aortogram via left femoral artery access showing right common iliac artery occlusion.

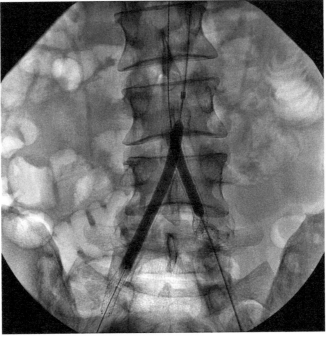

Guide wire crossing the right external iliac artery post-stent angioplasty of the right common iliac stent extending into the distal aorta and kissing balloon in the left common iliac stent.

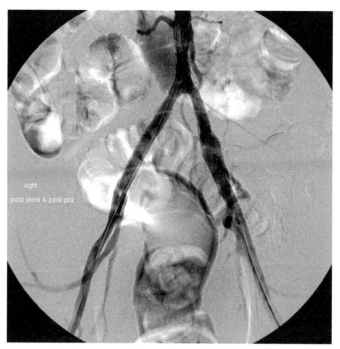

Abdominal and pelvic aortogram showing successful aortoiliac stenting.

Percutaneous revascularization (stenting) for TASC D lesions can be technically challenging, more so in patients who have flush occlusion of the common iliac artery. The presence of concomitant aortic or common femoral artery disease determines the approach to be used for access. The ipsilateral retrograde femoral approach is generally preferred but may not always be successful. The contralateral femoral approach is usually not successful because of lack of support, and in this patient because of the cephalad extension of the common iliac stent, it would have been almost impossible to pass the catheter/sheath up and over from the contralateral approach. In this situation, left brachial access is a suitable option with or without contralateral balloon occlusion of the patent common iliac artery. In some centers, a 6 Fr sheath or larger in the brachial artery necessitates a brachial artery cutdown to prevent brachial artery access complications.

Correct Answer   D Placement of a kissing stent in the right common iliac artery and stenting of the right external iliac artery with left brachial access

Reference

Bechara, C. F., Barshes, N. R., Lin, P. H., & Kougias, P. (2012). Recanalization of flush iliac occlusions with the assistance of a contralateral iliac occlusive balloon. *J Vasc Surg, 55*(3), 872–874. PMID: 22169670

97. RATIONALE

Sachwani et al. reported results of iliac stenting in 103 limbs (100 patients) and compared those with the results of aortofemoral grafting in 101 patients with iliac artery occlusions. Iliac stenting had lower morbidity, shorter hospital length of stay, and equivalent secondary patency as compared to aortofemoral graft reconstruction. However, primary patency was inferior in the iliac stenting group as compared to aortofemoral grafting. At 72 months, the primary patency for aortofemoral bypass was 91% as compared to 73% for iliac stenting ($P = 0.10$). Secondary patency was equivalent with 98% in aortobifemoral group and 85% in the iliac stenting group. The average hospital length of stay was 7 ± 2 days in the aortobifemoral group and 1 ± 0.2 days in the iliac stenting group ($P = 0.001$). There were no periprocedure deaths in the iliac stenting group, and there were four deaths in aortobifemoral group ($P = 0.58$). In patients with iliac artery occlusions with severe calcification, the use of bare-metal stents may result in iliac artery perforation, particularly in patients in whom oversized iliac stents are deployed. Results of PTFE-covered self-expanding stents versus bare-metal stents for chronic iliac artery occlusions revealed a higher midterm patency for covered self-expanding stents.

Correct Answer **D** Inferior primary patency but equivalent secondary patency

Reference
Sachwani, G. R., Hans, S. S., Khoury, M. D., et al. (2013). Results of iliac stenting and aortofemoral grafting for iliac artery occlusions. *J Vasc Surg, 57*(4), 1030–1037. PMID: 23177535

98. RATIONALE

There is a reported higher risk of vessel rupture during angioplasty in patients with eccentric severely calcified stenoses/occlusions in the iliac segment. In order to prevent rupture, the use of covered stents in severely calcified iliac arteries with significant stenosis or occlusions has been advocated by some investigators. Long-term follow-up of the randomized Covered versus Balloon Expandable Stent Trial (COBEST), demonstrated significantly higher patency of covered stents versus bare-metal stents at 5 years. Covered stents may also decrease the risk of distal embolization in calcified complex lesions. During deployment of covered stents, meticulous calculation of the stent length should be taken into consideration to avoid inadvertent coverage of the origin of the hypogastric artery. Intravascular shock wave lithotripsy should be considered in severly calcific lesions prior to angioplasty/stent deployment.

Correct Answer **C** Patients with eccentric plaque with severe calcification involving 75% of the circumference of the artery

Reference
Mwipatayi, B. P., Sharma, S., Daneshmand, A., et al. (2016). Durability of the balloon-expandable covered versus bare-metal stents in the Covered versus Balloon Expandable Stent Trial (COBEST) for the treatment of aortoiliac occlusive disease. *J Vasc Surg, 64*(1), 83–94.e81. PMID: 27131926

99. RATIONALE

Following balloon angioplasty and stenting, an inflammatory response occurs in the host artery with myointimal proliferation and tissue ingrowth. Symptomatic iliac artery in-stent restenosis occurs with a frequency of 10% at 1 year and is probably more common at longer follow-up. In-stent restenosis may be more common in patients with more complex lesions. The treatment options include standard balloon angioplasty, cutting balloon angioplasty, and consideration for placement of a covered stent. Thrombosis may form in a segment of severe in-stent restenosis and will require thrombolysis with use of catheters (McNamara, Angio-Jet) and pharmacomechanical thrombectomy along with tissue plasminogen activator (tPA) administration. Such patients need to be monitored in the critical care unit. Failure to treat thrombus and perform angioplasty for in-stent restenosis may result in distal embolization.

Correct Answer **B** 10%

Reference
Kudo, T., Chandra, F. A., & Ahn, S. S. (2005). Long-term outcomes and predictors of iliac angioplasty with selective stenting. *J Vasc Surg, 42*(3), 466–475. PMID: 16171589

100. RATIONALE

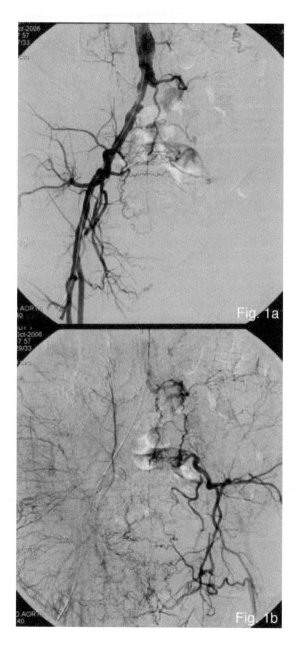

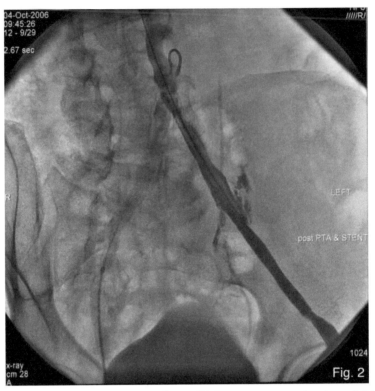

(a) Occlusion of left common and iliac artery TASC-D lesion. (b) Contrast extravasation due to left iliac artery rupture during intervention.

Iliac artery rupture during angioplasty/stenting and during passage of the stent graft during EVAR is an underreported complication. An incidence of 0.8%–0.9% of iliac rupture during iliac artery angioplasty and stenting has been reported. Iliac rupture during stenting presents as back pain, left lower quadrant pain or flank pain, nausea, and a decrease in blood pressure. In the case of small perforations, classic signs may not be present. The major predictors of iliac artery rupture are severe eccentric calcification in the plaque and oversizing of the postangioplasty balloon catheter. Fluid resuscitation and contrast injection to confirm contrast extravasation should be performed immediately along with balloon tamponade and placement of a covered stent at the site of the perforation. If the sheaths are pulled in the recovery room and hypotension occurs, a prompt return to the intervention suite or hybrid OR should be done to evaluate the site of the bleeding with deployment of a covered stent at the site of the perforation. After deployment of a covered stent, a contrast study should be performed to confirm hemostasis. Repairs of perforation closer to the common femoral artery are associated with high procedure success and low morbidity and mortality, whereas perforations closer to the aorta are more treacherous with inferior outcomes.

Correct Answer   C Contrast angiography

Reference
Allaire, E., Melliere, D., Poussier, B., et al. (2003). Iliac artery rupture during balloon dilatation: what treatment? *Ann Vasc Surg, 17*(3), 306–314. PMID: 12712371

101. RATIONALE

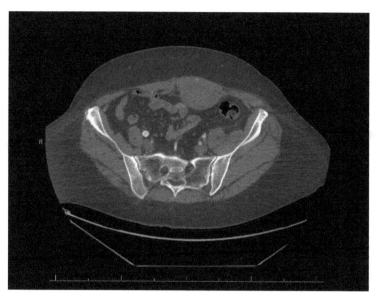

Left rectus sheath hematoma.

Rectus sheath hematoma due to inadvertent perforation of the deep/inferior epigastric artery during arteriography/intervention may occur. Rectus sheath hematoma may also occur following application of the closure device. Predisposing factors include large access sheath size, repeat or multiple punctures of the artery, concomitant use of anticoagulants, advanced age, female gender, and history of hypertension. A non-contrast CT scan is diagnostic unless the hematoma is large and painful. Conservative treatment is usually successful in small- to moderate-sized hematomas. However, in large hematomas with significant pain and discomfort, coil embolization of the deep epigastric artery or operative ligation may be necessary.

Correct Answer   B Rectus sheath hematoma

Reference
Osinbowale, O., & Bartholomew, J. R. (2008). Rectus sheath hematoma. *Vasc Med*, *13*(4), 275–279.
      PMID: 18940904

102. RATIONALE

Distal embolization has been reported with a frequency of 8.8%–24% and is more common following interventions for iliac artery occlusions as compared to those with iliac artery stenoses. In patients with suspected thrombosis within a segment of iliac artery stenosis, consideration should be given to pretreatment with thrombolytic agents or use of a mechanical thrombectomy device. Balloon angioplasty as the primary therapy in such cases is associated with a higher risk of embolization. A variety of stent misadventures such as acute stent thrombosis (stent deployed subintimally), balloon rupture during partial stent deployment, stent migration, stent crush, and compression of the contralateral iliac artery may occur. Acute stent thrombosis should be an extremely rare event, and when it occurs it is usually related to an unrecognized dissection distal to the stent. A rare but dreaded complication of stent implantation is stent infection with septic endarteritis and development of a mycotic pseudoaneurysm.

Correct Answer B Distal embolization

Reference
Timaran, C. H., Stevens, S. L., Freeman, M. B., & Goldman, M. H. (2002). Predictors for adverse outcome after iliac angioplasty and stenting for limb-threatening ischemia. *J Vasc Surg*, *36*(3), 507–513. PMID: 12218974

103. RATIONALE

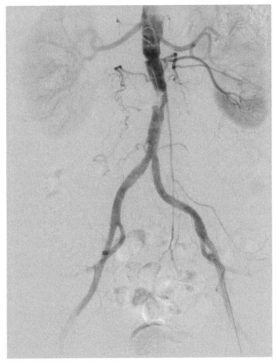

(a) Near-focal occlusion of the infrarenal aorta.

A focal stenosis approaching near occlusion is relatively uncommon and is more prevalent in young women with a history of severe nicotine abuse, hyperlipidemia, and premature ovarian failure. Traditionally, aortic endartectomy and/or aortic bypass grafting have been the standard treatment option for these symptomatic patients. However, open aortic reconstruction has significant morbidity and even mortality. In men, open aortic reconstruction may result in erectile dysfunction and retrograde ejaculation. During the last two to three decades endovascular options have largely supplanted open aortic reconstructions. A technical success of 82% has been reported with deployment of a covered stent. Technical success is defined as residual stenosis of less than 15% or a trans-stenotic systolic pressure gradient of less than 10%. More contemporary series have reported technical success of 91.7%.[1] Use of a covered stent near the origin of the inferior mesenteric artery may result in its occlusion; therefore, the evaluation of the mesenteric circulation by preoperative imaging studies is absolutely necessary to prevent bowel infarction. Since the availability of balloon-expandable covered stents requiring lower-profile sheaths for their deployment, the procedure has become much more simplified. Preangioplasty of the lesion should be avoided in patients suspected of overlying thrombus in order to decrease the likelihood of distal embolization. Spinal cord ischemia has been reported with covered stenting for aortic occlusion.[2]

Correct Answer **C** Covered stent

References
1. Grimme, F. A., Reijnen, M. M., Pfister, K., et al. (2014). Polytetrafluoroethylene covered stent placement for focal occlusive disease of the infrarenal aorta. *Eur J Vasc Endovasc Surg, 48*(5), 545–550. PMID: 25218651
2. Hans, S. S., Ngo, W., & McAllister, M. (2014). Paraplegia after aortic and superior mesenteric artery stenting for occlusive disease. *Ann Vasc Surg, 28*(2), 492.e417–499. PMID: 24295883

104. RATIONALE

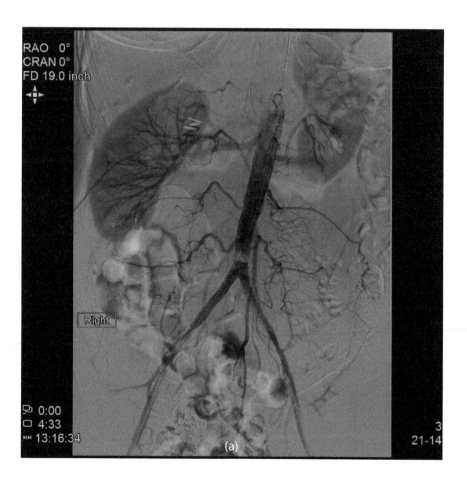

(a)

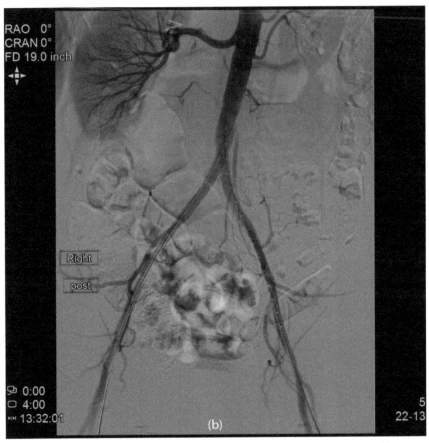

(a) Near-focal occlusion of distal abdominal aorta. (b) Treated with kissing, balloon-expandable covered stents from distal aorta to common iliac arteries.

Open aortic reconstruction in the form of aortoiliac endarterectomy and aortobifemoral grafting is associated with 2%–4.5% 30-day mortality and significant morbidity (15%–20%). Primary patency at 5 years has been reported from 85% to 92% and at 10 years from 80% to 85% in a large series. Patients have an increased length of stay, and it usually takes 10–12 weeks to resume presurgical activities. Endovascular therapy for these types of lesions is highly successful with minimal morbidity and a very short length of hospital stay. Balloon-expandable covered stents in distal abdominal and proximal iliac artery occlusion lesions are preferable because of their stronger radial force. In patients with continued nicotine abuse with small-size arteries, in-stent stenosis may occur, requiring secondary intervention. Long-term data available for the Icast/Advanta V12 device for such lesions appears to be satisfactory.

Correct Answer   D Bilateral kissing, covered, balloon-expandable stents from the distal abdominal aorta extending into each common iliac artery

Reference

Mwipatayi, B. P., Ouriel, K., Anwari, T., et al. (2020). A systematic review of covered balloon-expandable stents for treating aortoiliac occlusive disease. *J Vasc Surg, 72*(4), 1473–1486.e1472. PMID: 32360678

105. RATIONALE

In a multicenter database of 2012 consecutive patients undergoing aortoiliac stenting among 18 centers in Japan (2005–2009), associated factors for periprocedure (30 days) complications were examined. Using multivariate logistic regression analysis, advanced age (>80 years), critical limb ischemia, and Transatlantic Inter-Societal Consensus (TASC II) Class C and D were independently associated with periprocedure complications with adjusted odds ratio and 95% confidence intervals (CI) of 1.9 (1.3–2.9), 2.3 (1.5–3.4), and 2.4 (1.6–3.4), respectively.

Correct Answer **D** Age greater than 80, patients with critical limb ischemia, TASC C&D lesions

Reference

Iida, O., Soga, Y., Takahara, M., et al. (2014). Perioperative complications after aorto-iliac stenting: associated factors and impact on follow-up cardiovascular prognosis. *Eur J Vasc Endovasc Surg, 47*(2), 131–138. PMID: 24611185

SECTION 9: LOWER EXTREMITY ARTERIAL DISEASE

MCQs 1–50

Q1. The optimal management of a leaking femoral anastomotic aneurysm is by:

A. Endovascular approach using brachial and retrograde superficial femoral artery access

B. Direct open repair

C. Open repair with proximal control obtained by a retroperitoneal approach by a transverse incision 2–3 cm above the groin

D. Open repair with proximal balloon occlusion of the ipsilateral graft limb with access from the contralateral graft limb in the groin

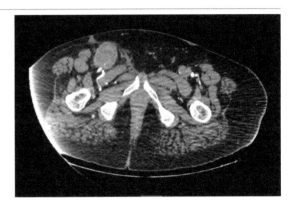

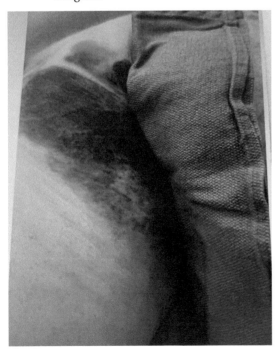

Q2. A 68-year-old man was found to have a 3.2-cm right common femoral artery aneurysm. The incidence of contralateral synchronous femoral aneurysm is:

A. <25%

B. 25%–50%

C. 51%–60%

D. A contralateral femoral artery aneurysm is likely if the patient has AAA

Q3. Popliteal aneurysms present as a rupture in:

A. <2% of patients

B. 3%–7% of patients

C. 8%–10% of patients

D. Rupture of popliteal aneurysm occurs only if the patient sustains trauma

Q4. A 60-year-old man undergoes staged open repair of a popliteal aneurysm. At the time of repair, there was no evidence of synchronous AAA. Which statement reflects the best surveillance strategy?

DOI: 10.1201/9781003389897-9

A. Lifelong surveillance of abdomen (abdominal aortic ultrasound), as AAA may develop years after popliteal aneurysm repair

B. Subclavian artery aneurysm should be suspected

C. Yearly abdominal aortogram

D. If the patient does not have a femoral aneurysm, the chances of developing AAA are low

Q5. The optimal site for femoral anastomosis during performance of a crossover femoral-femoral graft is:

A. Under the inguinal ligament at the junction of the external iliac and common femoral artery

B. Superficial femoral artery

C. Distal common femoral artery

D. Deep femoral artery

Q6. A crossover femoral-femoral graft with inflow on the left is planned in a patient with extensive scarring in the suprapubic area from remote burns. The best alternative to a subcutaneous suprapubic tunnel is:

A. Excision of burn scar and coverage of the prosthetic graft with rectus abdominus flap

B. Tunnel in the prevesical space

C. Excision of burn scar and gracilis muscle flap

D. Consider bilateral axillofemoral bypass graft

Q7. During creation of a crossover femoral-femoral graft in a patient with occlusion of the right limb of EVAR with patent superficial femoral arteries on both sides with near occlusion of right common femoral artery:

A. The distal anastomosis should always be performed to the deep femoral artery

B. Distal anastomosis should always be performed to the superficial femoral artery

C. Distal anastomosis to the proximal common femoral artery

D. Prior to distal anastomosis, a right common femoral endarterectomy with a patch graft is performed, then the distal anastomosis of the femoral-femoral bypass is performed at the site of the distal arteriotomy in the patch graft

Q8. Wound complications following axillo-femoral graft reconstruction are reported in:

A. 5% of patients

B. 10% of patients

C. 15% of patients

D. 20% of patients

Q9. Five-year patency of an axillofemoral bypass graft ranges from:

A. 25%–60%

B. 30%–70%

C. 35%–80%

D. 40%–90%

Q10. Asymptomatic femoral artery pseudoaneurysm following percutaneous arterial access for coronary/peripheral interventions should be treated as the pseudoaneurysm reaches a transverse/AP diameter of:

A. 10–12 mm

B. 13–15 mm

C. 16–20 mm

D. >20 mm

Q11. The incidence of retroperitoneal hemorrhage following femoral artery access is:

A. 0.2%

B. 0.5%

C. 1%

D. 1.5%–2%

Q12. The incidence of arterial perforation following orbital atherectomy for occlusive disease of femoral and popliteal arteries is:

A. <5%

B. 0.5%–1.0%

C. 0.5%–1.5%

D. 0.5%–2.2%

Q13. The incidence of distal embolization following percutaneous intervention of femoral-popliteal arteries is:
- **A.** Similar in patients with critical limb ischemia as compared to those with intermittent claudication
- **B.** Greater in patients with critical limb ischemia as compared to those with intermittent claudication
- **C.** Lower in patients with critical limb ischemia as compared to those with intermittent claudication
- **D.** Distal embolization occurs more frequently with aortoiliac intervention than with femoral-popliteal intervention

Q14. Results of subintimal recanalization of chronic total occlusion of long segment occlusion of femoral-popliteal arteries reveal a primary-assisted patency as well as secondary patency at 1 year to be approximately:
- **A.** 50%
- **B.** 60%
- **C.** 70%
- **D.** 80%

Q15. Antegrade femoral approach for treatment of popliteal and infrapopliteal arterial occlusive disease is best used for patients with:
- **A.** Patients with high BMI
- **B.** Patients with high femoral artery bifurcation
- **C.** Recent closure device application in the common femoral artery
- **D.** Iliac artery tortuosity and with severe calcification at the aortic bifurcation

Q16. The following statement regarding antegrade femoral access best reflects the outcomes:
- **A.** The incidence of femoral artery stenosis or occlusion is higher than retrograde access
- **B.** The incidence of hematoma is higher in patients with antegrade femoral artery access than with retrograde access
- **C.** Most complications following antegrade femoral access require intervention

- **D.** The incidence of groin hematomas with antegrade access is the same as with retrograde access, and most hematomas can be managed conservatively

Q17. The long-term primary and secondary patency of popliteal artery aneurysm exclusion with saphenous vein graft is:
- **A.** 70%–80%
- **B.** 80%–85%
- **C.** 80%–90%
- **D.** 80%–95%

Q18. Popliteal stent graft migration and endoleak following popliteal aneurysm repair are caused by:
- **A.** Insufficient overlap with normal artery in the proximal and distal seal zone
- **B.** Undersizing of the stent
- **C.** Forces due to repetitive knee flexion
- **D.** Insufficient overlap in the proximal and distal seal zone, undersizing of the stent, and due to repetitive knee flexion

Q19. An independent predictor of stent graft thrombosis for the exclusion of popliteal aneurysm using endovascular management is:
- **A.** One-vessel runoff
- **B.** Use of longer stents
- **C.** Use of multiple stents
- **D.** Use of multiple and longer stents

Q20. Regarding endovascular repairs vs. open repair of popliteal aneurysm, the following statement best reflects the outcome:
- **A.** Primary patency of open repair is superior to endovascular repair at 1 year
- **B.** At long-term follow-up (3 years), primary patency of open and endovascular repair is similar
- **C.** At long-term follow-up (3 years) the primary patency of open repair is superior
- **D.** Most endovascular repairs are performed for acute ischemia due to thrombosis of popliteal aneurysms

Q21. During popliteal artery balloon angioplasty for near occlusion of the popliteal artery with one-vessel runoff, there is a dissection flap detected on arteriogram in the distal popliteal artery 2 cm proximal from its distal end. The best management option is:

A. Prolonged low pressure balloon inflation
B. Deployment of a covered stent
C. Deployment of Supera stent
D. Bare-metal self-expandable stent

Q22. Antegrade recanalization of infrapopliteal artery occlusion for critical limb ischemia has a failure rate of:

A. 10%
B. 15%
C. 20%
D. 25%

Q23. The incidence of combined superficial and deep surgical site infection following infrainguinal bypass is:

A. <5%
B. 5%–18%
C. 19%–22%
D. 23%–25%

Q24. Ipsilateral great saphenous vein as a conduit for femoral-infrapopliteal bypass is inadequate in:

A. <5% patients
B. 5%–10% patients
C. 11%–14% patients
D. 15%–20% patients

Q25. The reported 5-year patency of femoral-popliteal bypass using an autologous saphenous vein is:

A. 90% above the knee, 80% below the knee
B. 80% above the knee, 70% below the knee
C. 75% above the knee, 65% below the knee
D. 65% above the knee, 55% below the knee

Q26. The following statement regarding tourniquet occlusion during femoral-infrapopliteal bypass is correct:

A. Should not be used or it may result in irreversible muscle ischemia
B. Improves visualization and avoids clamping of small, calcified target arteries
C. Results in better primary patency
D. Results in better secondary patency

Q27. The incidence of early graft thrombosis (within 30 days) following femoropopliteal bypass is:

A. <5%
B. 5%–10%
C. 11%–15%
D. 16%–18%

Q28. Two weeks following a femoropopliteal bypass with PTFE graft, there is breakdown of the wound in the groin. There is evidence of deep infection with cultures growing *Pseudomonas*. The optimal management consists of:

A. Antipseudomonal antibiotics, excisional debridement in operating room, and negative pressure wound therapy
B. Partial removal of the proximal graft conversion into a composite graft (vein and PTFE), excisional debridement, sartorius myoplasty, and antipseudomonal antibiotics
C. Complete removal of the graft with ex situ revascularization, excisional debridement, and antipseudomonal antibiotics
D. Removal of PTFE graft, use of cryopreserved vein as a new bypass, debridement, and antipseudomonal antibiotics

Q29. A 60-year-old woman presents to the emergency room with a thrombosed left femoropopliteal graft (Rutherford type IIA ischemia) performed with a 7-mm PTFE prosthesis performed 29 months earlier. The best management option is:

A. Open thrombectomy
B. Convert to autologous vein reconstruction
C. Arteriography and thrombolytic therapy
D. Anticoagulation

Q30. Two years following femoral tibial in situ bypass, a severe (70%) focal stenosis near the distal anastomosis is detected on duplex imaging. Optimal management consists of:

A. Open repair with vein patch or bovine pericardial patch
B. Percutaneous angioplasty
C. Interposition vein graft at the distal anastomosis
D. Surveillance with duplex imaging and intervention if the stenosis progresses further

Q31. The most common cause of early (within 30 days) graft thrombosis with the use of the in situ technique for lower extremity bypass is:
A. Retained valve leaflets
B. Residual arteriovenous fistula
C. Inadequate vein segment
D. Infection

Q32. Lower extremity edema following infrainguinal arterial bypass using an autologous vein for chronic limb ischemia occurs in:
A. 10%–20% of patients
B. 21%–35% of patients
C. 36%–49% of patients
D. 50%–100% of patients

Q33. The incidence of lymphatic fistula following lower extremity arterial bypass is:
A. 0.1%–0.5%
B. 0.6%–1.0%
C. 1.1%
D. 2%

Q34. The diagnostic study of choice when groin swelling develops 2 months following femoral tibial bypass using an autologous vein is:
A. Ultrasonography
B. MRI
C. CT scan
D. Lymphography with blue dye (isosulfan)

Q35. During femoral tibial in situ bypass reconstruction for critical limb ischemia, the transected great saphenous vein at the saphenofemoral junction cannot be brought to the common femoral artery. The common femoral artery has 70% stenosis. The most useful adjunct is:
A. Common femoral stent using contralateral access
B. Common femoral atherectomy using contralateral access
C. Common femoral endarterectomy with patch grafting and placement of the proximal anastomosis of the in situ bypass over the distal portion of the patch
D. Interposition prosthetic (PTFE) graft from the common femoral artery to the origin of the in situ vein bypass

Q36. A 68-year-old man with a previous history of multiple arterial constructions including aortobifemoral bypass (AFB) as an index operation presents with bleeding from the left groin. The patient is hemodynamically stable. CTA of the abdomen and pelvis shows normal body and right limb of the graft, but there is evidence of perigraft fluid around the distal 5 cm of the left limb of the AFB. WBC scan shows increased uptake in the groin. The best management option is:
A. Left Axillofemoral graft routed laterally over the iliac crest with distal anastomosis to the mid-superficial femoral artery following removal of the left limb of the AFB
B. Crossover Femoral-Femoral graft following removal of the left left limb of the AFB and with left sided portion of the crossover Femoral-Femoral graft routed laterally over the iliac crest
C. Local debridement of perigraft tissue and sartorius myography
D. Reconstruction with a new graft flush from the origin of the left limb of the AFB with distal anastomosis to the mid-SFA via the obturator canal

Q37. During passage of a graft through the obturator canal during performance of the obturator bypass, the tunneling of the graft in the thigh should be:
A. Posterior to the adductor longus
B. Posterior to the vastus medialis
C. Anterior to the adductor longus
D. Posterior to the gracilis

Q38. A 30-year-old woman is seen in the emergency room with grade 2A acute ischemia. She is in normal sinus rhythm. She does not have a history of atrial fibrillation or coronary artery disease. CTA shows filling defect in the right common femoral artery. Her younger sister had an embolectomy performed 1 year ago. At embolectomy, a lobulated piece of white yellow gelatinous material was removed. The most likely diagnosis is:
A. Paradoxical embolus
B. Embolus from atrial myxoma

C. Adventitious cystic disease of the common femoral artery

D. Angioleiomyoma

Q39. Acute limb ischemia resulting from arterial embolis occurs in:

A. 5%

B. 10%

C. 15%

D. 20%

Q40. A 66-year-old man is scheduled for femoropopliteal bypass for ischemic rest pain controlled by analgesics not amenable for percutaneous intervention. In the preoperative suite he complains of cough and mild shortness of breath. SARS-CoV-2 test is positive. The next best course of action is:

A. Proceed with bypass, taking all the precautions for SARS/CoV-2 patients

B. Postpone the bypass for 2 weeks

C. Postpone the bypass for 4 weeks

D. Postpone the bypass for 7 weeks

Q41. The findings that best differentiate Rutherford classification of category 2a from 2b ischemia are:

A. Intact sensation in 2b

B. Inability to move the muscles in 2a

C. Mottling of the skin in 2b

D. Absence of muscle weakness, minimal loss of motor function (toes) with absent sensory loss, and absence of pain at rest in 2a

Q42. The most common cause of acute aortic occlusion is:

A. Saddle embolism

B. In situ thrombosis

C. Occluded aortoiliac graft

D. Occlusion of aortic limbs of EVAR

Q43. Which of the following conditions is not an absolute contraindication to catheter-directed thrombolysis for acute limb ischemia?

A. Major surgery including arterial bypass graft within 2 weeks

B. Patient with a recent gastrointestinal bleed or a significant risk of bleeding

C. Recent stroke or craniotomy or intraspinal surgery within 4 months

D. Uncontrolled hypertension

Q44. In comparing endovascular peripheral vascular intervention for acute limb ischemia versus chronic limb ischemia, patients with acute limb ischemia had:

A. Lower in-hospital event rates

B. Lower technical failure

C. Lower major amputation

D. Similar mortality compared with their chronic limb ischemia counterparts

Q45. Endovascular versus surgical revascularization for acute limb ischemia (ALI) from a propensity-score matched analysis using a national inpatient sample database showed that endovascular revascularization has a:

A. Higher incidence of major bleeding

B. Higher composite of death/myocardial infarction/stroke

C. Greater need for transfusion

D. Lower composite of death/myocardial infarction/stroke

Q46. Combining catheter-directed thrombolysis (CDT) with percutaneous mechanical thrombectomy (PMT) results in:

A. Delay in clearing the thrombus

B. Increase in the incidence of bleeding complications

C. Lower incidence of myoglobinuria

D. Fasciotomy for compartment syndrome is less frequently required

Q47. The incidence of compartment syndrome as a complication of reperfusion for acute lower limb ischemia is up to:

A. 5%

B. 10%

C. 15%

D. 20%–21%

Q48. Fasciotomy for compartment syndrome of the thigh needs decompression of the:

A. Anterior compartment

B. Adductor (medial) compartment

C. Posterior compartment

D. All three compartments

Q49. **The 5-year patency of an iliofemoral bypass graft is:**
A. 80%
B. 85%
C. 90%
D. 93%

Q50. **A 60-year-old woman with a history of type II diabetes mellitus and hypertension presents with dry gangrene of right big toe with rest pain. She's a current smoker. The ankle-brachial index on the right is 0.40 and the left is 0.8. Arteriogram shows right superficial femoral artery occlusion with reconstitution of the popliteal artery runoff by the anterior tibial artery in continuity with the popliteal artery. Post-tibial artery and peroneal artery are occluded. She has adequate Great saphenous vein. The best management for revascularization is:**
A. Endovascular recanalization using artherectomy
B. Endovascular recanalization using drug eluting stent
C. Right femoral-popliteal bypass using GSV
D. Either endovascular or surgical bypass should give equivalent results

RATIONALE 1–50

1. RATIONALE

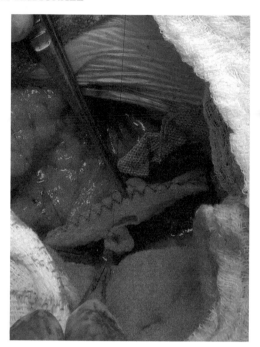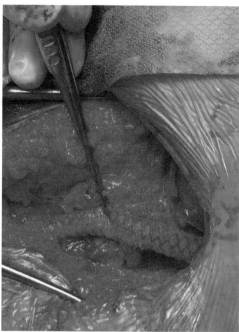

Deep femoral artery with a cuff is being implanted into the interposition graft following repair (resection) of femoral anastomotic aneurysm.

Contained rupture of a femoral anastomotic aneurysm is rare unless the aneurysm is large (larger than 4.5 cm). Femoral anastomotic aneurysms are usually asymptomatic but may present with pain due to compression of surrounding nerves; occasionally, thrombosis of the femoral anastomotic aneurysm may result in acute ischemia of the lower extremity. Most patients require open repair with an interposition graft (Dacron or PTFE) with reimplantation of the deep femoral artery into the graft. Anastomosis of the new interposition graft is done with the proximal end-to-end anastomosis to the remotely placed prosthetic graft and distal anastomosis to the proximal superficial femoral artery. Endovascular options are limited, as maintenance of patency of the profunda femoris artery is important. Recurrent femoral anastomotic aneurysm may occur after repair and is almost three times greater in women than in men.

Correct Answer C Open repair with proximal control obtained by a retroperitoneal approach by a transverse incision 2–3 cm above the groin

Reference

Munie, S. T., Shepard, A. D. (2018). Open repair or femoral and femoral anastomotic aneurysms. In S. S. Hans (Ed.), *Endovascular and open vascular reconstruction: a practical approach* (pp. 263–268). Boca Raton, FL: Taylor & Francis.

2. RATIONALE

Degenerative femoral artery aneurysms are uncommon with a reported incidence of 5 patients per 100,000. Lawrence et al. reported that complications related to femoral artery aneurysms do not occur unless the aneurysm reaches 3.5 cm or greater in maximum AP/transverse diameter. Synchronous femoral and aortic aneurysms occur in 50%–90% of patients, synchronous popliteal aneurysms in 27%–44%, and synchronous contralateral femoral artery aneurysms in 26%–50% of patients.

Correct Answer **B** 25%–50%

Reference
Lawrence, P. F., Harlander-Locke, M. P., Oderich, G. S., et al. (2014). The current management of isolated degenerative femoral artery aneurysms is too aggressive for their natural history. *J Vasc Surg, 59*(2), 343–349. PMID: 24461859

3. RATIONALE

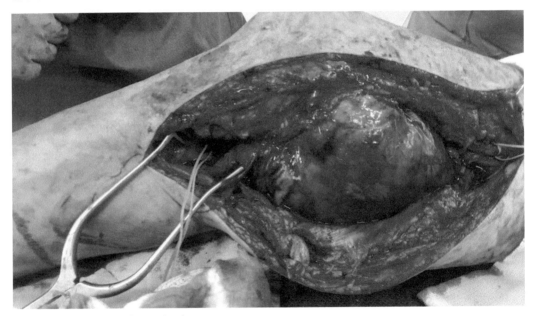

Large popliteal aneursym with contained rupture.

Most popliteal aneurysms are diagnosed as an asymptomatic pulsatile mass behind the knee in a patient with coexisting AAA. The presentation may be due to acute thrombosis of the popliteal aneurysm and may vary from intermittent claudication to severe limb ischemia depending on the status of runoff and collaterals in the knee. Rupture is relatively uncommon and is present in 3%–7% of patients. Other symptoms resulting from popliteal aneurysms include deep venous thrombosis and peroneal nerve palsy. The risk of major amputation is much higher in patients who present with rupture or acute ischemia than those presenting with chronic ischemia. Free rupture is extremely uncommon. Endovascular repair with stent graft in the event of rupture is preferable, but may be technically difficult due to associated tortuosity of the popliteal artery, and open repair with interposition of a PTFE graft or great saphenous vein conduit may be necessary.

Correct Answer **B** 3%–7% of patients

Reference
Pulli, R., Dorigo, W., Troisi, N., Innocenti, A. A., et al. (2006). Surgical management of popliteal artery aneurysms: which factors affect outcomes? *J Vasc Surg, 43*(3), 481–487. PMID: 16520159

4. RATIONALE

Raven et al. reported that among 82 patients with isolated popliteal artery aneurysm at the time of index operation, 23 developed new aneurysms. They also observed that 4.3% of patients treated with vein bypass graft developed a graft aneurysm at late follow-up.[1] Popliteal artery aneurysm has been traditionally managed with open bypass following its exclusion. Endovascular repair has been used during the past 12–20 years with placement of a covered stent graft. Cervin et al., from a series of 592 procedures performed for treatment of popliteal aneurysms, concluded that patency of reconstruction with open repair is superior to endovascular repair, particularly in patients presenting with acute ischemia.[2] Lifelong surveillance may be warranted in patients following repair of popliteal aneurysms, as bilateral popliteal aneurysms are associated with development of abdominal aortic aneurysm at long-term follow-up.

Correct Answer **A** Lifelong surveillance of abdomen (abdominal aortic ultrasound), as AAA may develop years after popliteal aneurysm repair

References

1. Ravn, H., Wanhainen, A., & Björck, M. (2008). Risk of new aneurysms after surgery for popliteal artery aneurysm. *Br J Surg*, *95*(5), 571–575. PMID: 18306151
2. Cervin, A., Tjärnström, J., Ravn, H., et al. (2015). Treatment of popliteal aneurysm by open and endovascular surgery: a contemporary study of 592 procedures in Sweden. *Eur J Vasc Endovasc Surg*, *50*(3), 342–350. PMID: 25911500

5. RATIONALE

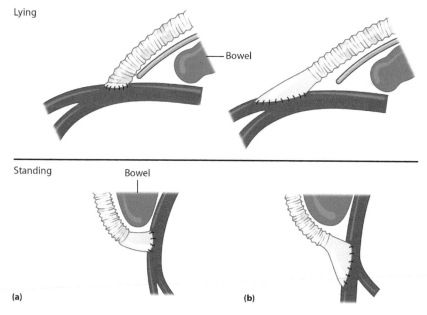

(a) Kinking of the graft anastomosis when placed too close to the inguinal ligament; (b) anastomosis placed further distal on the femoral artery to avoid kinking.

Arteriotomy in the proximal common femoral artery can lead to angulation of the graft with resulting thrombosis. A more distal common femoral arteriotomy, usually over the femoral bifurcation extending into either the superficial femoral artery (if it is patent) or profunda femoris artery (if superficial femoral artery is occluded), can avoid this angulation, thus providing smooth curvature of the origin of the crossover femoral-femoral graft. Oblique arteriotomy extending from the common femoral artery extending into the proximal deep femoral artery lessens the angle of curvature of the graft and is necessary in patients with occlusion of the superficial femoral artery.

Correct Answer C Distal common femoral artery

Reference
Silver, S., & Mohammad, F. (2017). Extra-anatomic reconstruction for aortoiliac occlusive disease. In S. S. Hans & A. D. Shepard (Eds.), *Endovascular and open vascular reconstruction: a practical approach* (pp. 301–306). Boca Raton, FL: CRC Press.

6. **RATIONALE**

In conjunction with stent angioplasty of the iliac inflow vessel, a femoral-femoral bypass offers high-risk patients an alternative to aortobifemoral bypass. After performing the femoral anastomosis of the prosthetic graft at the inflow site, the graft is typically brought in the suprapubic subcutaneous tunnel to the opposite groin. Because of extensive scarring in the suprapubic area, this tunnel may be difficult to create, with potential risk of skin breakdown overlying the prosthetic graft. The retropubic (prevesical space) is an extraperitoneal space located posterior to the symphysis pubis and anterior to the urinary bladder. It is separated from the anterior abdominal wall by the transversalis fascia. In this situation, groin incisions are extended cephalad for 8–10 cm and with a blunt finger dissection after incising the external and internal oblique muscles, the transversalis fascia is opened and retroperitoneal tunnel is created. A simultaneous blunt finger dissection is used to create the second tunnel from the opposite side between the left suprainguinal retroperitoneal space and the right groin that courses immediately to the posterior rectus muscle and both anterior and cephalad to the bladder in the preperitoneal space.

Correct Answer B Tunnel in the prevesical space

Reference
Silver, S., & Mohammad, F. (2017). Extra-anatomic reconstruction for aortoiliac occlusive disease. In S. S. Hans & A. D. Shepard (Eds.), *Endovascular and open vascular reconstruction: a practical approach* (pp. 301–306). Boca Raton, FL: CRC Press.

7. **RATIONALE**

Extensive endarterectomy of the outflow (common femoral artery) in a patient with near occlusion of the common femoral artery may be necessary, followed by patch closure using a bovine pericardial patch. An incision in the patch is performed in its distal portion for creating outflow anastomosis. Anastomosis in the proximal portion of the patch or to the proximal common femoral artery may result in kinking of the graft. Careful closure of the groin incision after satisfactory hemostasis as well as ligation of lymphatic channels is necessary to avoid hematuria and seroma (lymphocele), which may place the graft at risk for infection. Primary patency for crossover femoral-femoral graft for critical limb ischemia has been reported to be 88%, 82%, and 74% at 1, 3, and 5 years, respectively; for patients with intermittent claudication, 93%, 92%, and 90% for the same time period has been reported. Tunnelling injury to the small bowel and bladder has been reported. Finger dissection and keeping the tunnel uniform over a large radius will aid in avoiding visceral injury and kinking of the graft. Risk of injury is higher in patients with a history of radiation, prior pelvic surgery, and patients with inguinal hernia. In patients with suspected groin infection associated with ipsilateral occlusion of the graft limb, the crossover graft can be tunneled superiorly and laterally and anastomosed to the superficial femoral artery in the upper thigh.

Correct Answer   **D** Prior to distal anastomosis, a right common femoral endarterectomy with patch graft is performed, then the distal anastomosis of the femoral-femoral bypass is performed at the site of the distal arteriotomy in the patch graft

Reference
Pursell, R., Sideso, E., Magee, T. R., & Galland, R. B. (2005). Critical appraisal of femorofemoral crossover grafts. *Br J Surg*, *92*(5), 565–569. PMID: 15810055

8. RATIONALE

The operative risk of axillofemoral bypass is significantly lower than aortofemoral bypass, as celiotomy as well as cross-clamping of the aorta is avoided. However, a 15% incidence of wound complication is reported, which includes groin infection, seroma, hematoma, and lymphocele formation. Wound complications are unfavorable prognostic factors for graft infection. Multiple prior surgeries, especially redo exposures, increase the risk of graft infection. The risk of graft infection has been reported to be up to 15% and is more common in patients undergoing the operation for critical limb ischemia. Outcomes are dependent on the indication for the procedure, with significantly poorer results reported in the infection and emergent group. Perigraft seroma with sterile fluid collection around the graft with a pseudocapsule can be diagnosed by duplex imaging and confirmed by CT angiography. Graft thrombosis and failure both in the immediate postoperative period as well as long term are challenging problems. Patients' specific factors such as demographics, comorbidities, hypercoagulative state, quality of inflow, and outflow as well as type of conduit are important factors contributing to graft failure.

Correct Answer   **C** 15% of patients

Reference
Dickas, D., Verrel, F., Kalff, J., & Koscielny, A. (2018). Axillobifemoral bypasses: reappraisal of an extra-anatomic bypass by analysis of results and prognostic factors. *World J Surg*, *42*(1), 283–294. PMID: 28741197

9. RATIONALE

Axillofemoral bypass has a limited patency, and that is the main reason it remains an alternative approach to revascularization in patients who are extremely high risk, with shorter life expectancy and have critical limb ischemia. The 5-year patency of axillofemoral bypass has been reported from 35% to 80%. Factors predicting decreased patency include clinical presentation of arterial occlusive disease (critical ischemia with gangrene/ulcers of toes), graft material (Dacron versus PTFE), and extent of infrainguinal arterial occlusive disease. Multiple studies comparing Dacron to externally supported PTFE grafts have not shown any significant difference between the patency of these two conduits, whereas superficial femoral artery occlusive disease is a predictor of worse outcomes.

Correct Answer   **C**   35%–80%

Reference

Martin, D., & Katz, S. G. (2000). Axillofemoral bypass for aortoiliac occlusive disease. *Am J Surg, 180*(2), 100–103. PMID: 11044521

10. RATIONALE

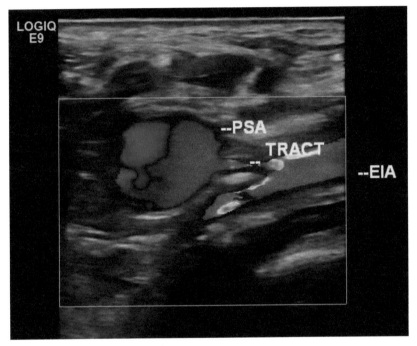

Femoral pseudoaneurysm with a long narrow neck.

Access site complications remain the most encountered complication in peripheral vascular intervention with rates ranging from 3.5% to 8.9%. Advanced age, female gender, high or low body mass index, hypertension, use of antithrombotic therapy, and prolonged procedure time are predictors of access site complications. The incidence of femoral pseudoaneurysm from a prospective study of 1000 patients was 3.8% on postprocedural arterial duplex study with an 8% incidence after intervention and 2% with diagnostic study as large-caliber sheaths are used during intervention as compared to diagnostic studies. Most pseudoaneurysms <10 mm will resolve spontaneously. Large pseudoaneurysms >20 mm often require intervention. Ultrasound-guided compression has been replaced by ultrasound-guided thrombin injection. Thrombin injection is safe with a 2% incidence of distal embolization. A follow-up duplex study is done 24 hours after injection to verify the satisfactory thrombosis of the pseudoaneurysm. Multilobular pseudoaneurysms or patients on anticoagulation may require reinjection. Surgical repair is reserved for rapidly expanding pseudoaneurysms, overlying skin necrosis, limb ischemia, nerve palsy, wide short neck of the pseudoaneurysm, and multiple failed attempts with thrombin injections.

Correct Answer   **D**   >20 mm

Reference

Ortiz, D., Jahangir, A., Singh, M., et al. (2014). Access site complications after peripheral vascular interventions: incidence, predictors, and outcomes. *Circ Cardiovasc Interv, 7*(6), 821–828. PMID: 25389345

11. RATIONALE

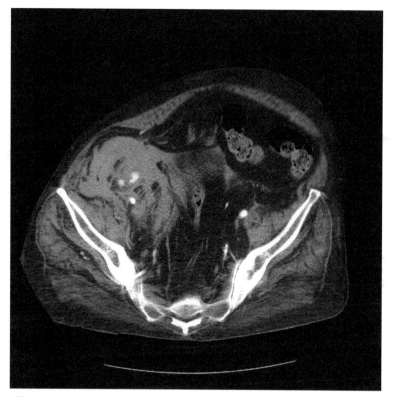

Right retroperitoneal hematoma with active extravasation of the contrast.

The reported incidence of retroperitoneal hemorrhage (RPH) following femoral artery access is 0.5%. Independent predictors of RPH are arterial access above the inferior (deep) epigastric artery, large sheath size, low body weight, female gender, and the concomitant use of glycoprotein IIb/IIIa inhibitors. Retroperitoneal hemorrhage can be insidious, and hemodynamic instability is usually a late sign of ongoing bleeding. Patients in the early stage complain of back or flank pain. If the patient is hemodynamically stable, CT scan of the abdomen and pelvis is obtained with intravenous contrast to assess the retroperitoneum for active extravascularization from the external iliac artery or its branches. Prompt resuscitation with blood and intravenous fluids is the most important intervention, and anticoagulants should be stopped. Refractory hypotension is indicative for immediate endovascular or open repair. For arteriotomies in the distal external iliac artery proximal to the deep epigastric artery using contralateral femoral access, deployment of a covered stent at the site of extravasation can be performed. For arteriotomies in the common femoral artery, endovascular balloon tamponade followed by open repair of the femoral artery is more appropriate.

Correct Answer   **B** 0.5%

Reference

Farouque, H. M., Tremmel, J. A., Raissi Shabari, F., et al. (2005). Risk factors for the development of retroperitoneal hematoma after percutaneous coronary intervention in the era of glycoprotein IIb/IIIa inhibitors and vascular closure devices. *J Am Coll Cardiol*, *45*(3), 363–368. PMID: 15680713

12. RATIONALE

Arterial perforation can occur while advancing wires, catheters, balloons, and stents. On arteriography there is extravasation of the contrast outside the vessel walls. If the perforation happens into an adjacent vein, a fistula with contrast flowing into the venous system is seen. Guide wire perforation is usually self-limited and resolves spontaneously following the reversal of anticoagulation. However, if the perforation happens in a collateral or a side branch of a large-caliber vessel and the arteriotomy is made wider by advancing the catheter over the wire, uncontrolled bleeding can result in a hemodynamic instability, the need for blood transfusion, open repair, and an extended hospital stay. Perforation may also occur in severely calcified arteries when higher pressures are required for angioplasty. Atherectomy has a relatively low rate of perforation in peripheral arteries. Orbital atherectomy has a perforation rate of 0.5%–2.3% in patients with occlusive lesions of femoral/popliteal arteries.

Correct Answer   **D** 0.5%–2.2%

Reference

Swee, W., Wang, J. Y., & Lee, A. C. (2014). Managing perforation of the superficial femoral artery. 2014, 59–68. Retrieved from https://evtoday.com/articles/2014-oct/managing-perforations-of-the-superficial-femoral-artery

13. RATIONALE

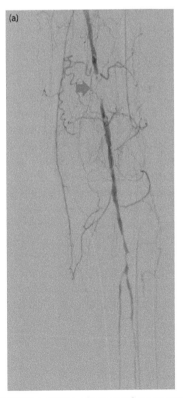
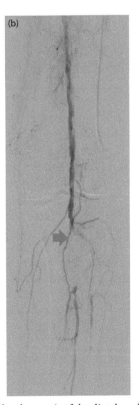
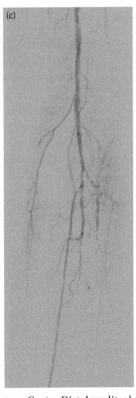

Left: Mid/distal SFA occlusion with severe multifocal stenosis of the distal popliteal artery. *Center:* Distal popliteal artery occlusion probably due to plaque embolization *Right:* Successful revascularization of distal popliteal and superficial femoral artery.

Distal embolization occurs when a plaque or thrombus is dislodged farther distally into the lower extremity arterial system. Its incidence is variable and depends on how embolization is reported. The rate of distal embolization is higher in patients treated for critical limb ischemia as compared to those treated with symptoms of intermittent claudication (3.2% vs. 1.2%). Distal embolization is more likely to occur during infrainguinal vessel procedures as compared to aortoiliac interventions. Patients with femoropopliteal TASC IIC lesions and undergoing treatment of long-segment occlusions have a higher rate of distal embolization. Atherectomy procedures carry a significantly higher incidence of distal embolization as compared with other modalities of percutaneous interventions. Patients who undergo urgent endovascular revascularization have a higher rate of distal embolization compared to elective procedures. The rate of distal embolization also increases with the number of arteries treated, treatment of chronic total occlusions, and treatment of in-stent restenosis. Routine use of distal embolic protection devices or filters is protective.

Correct Answer **B** Greater in patients with critical limb ischemia as compared to those with intermittent claudication

Reference
Shrikhande, G. V., Khan, S. Z., Hussain, H. G., et al. (2011). Lesion types and device characteristics that predict distal embolization during percutaneous lower extremity interventions. *J Vasc Surg*, *53*(2), 347–352. PMID: 21129906

14. RATIONALE

Long-segment subintimal recanalization of chronic total occlusions (CTOs) are frequently associated with postangioplasty dissection. These lesions are typically stented whether they are flow-limiting or not, based on the improved patency rate associated with primary stenting. Despite relatively low primary-assisted patency (68%) and secondary patency (70%) at 1 year, subintimal recanalization limb salvage rates are as high as 92%. This technique therefore represents a satisfactory alternative to surgical bypasses in patients with critical limb ischemia, especially in the absence of a suitable vein or in high surgical-risk patients.

Correct Answer **C** 70%

Reference
Suri, R., Wholey, M. H., Postoak, D., et al. (2006). Distal embolic protection during femoropopliteal atherectomy. *Catheter Cardiovasc Interv*, *67*(3), 417–422. PMID: 16489560

15. RATIONALE

An antegrade femoral approach via the ipsilateral limb allows for intervention of more distal stenoses/occlusions. This approach also enables better control of the guide wires and catheters and does not require the additional length of the guide wires and catheters. This approach is best indicated for use in patients with iliac artery tortuosity or if the aortic bifurcation is known to be heavily diseased because the up and over maneuver is not required during antegrade access. In patients with prior endovascular aneurysm repair for abdominal aortic aneurysm or in patients with acute angle of the aortic bifurcation, the up and over technique may be technically challenging. This approach (antegrade approach) can be more difficult in obese patients. For this approach, it is best to ensure that the proximal common femoral artery is accessed over the femoral head in order to direct the guide wire to enter into the superficial femoral artery.

A distal common femoral artery puncture may direct the wire preferentially to enter the profunda femoris artery. This approach is also helpful in patients with previous aortoiliac stent graft or prosthetic graft, as going up and over the bifurcation of the graft may be technically challenging.

Correct Answer   D Iliac artery tortuosity and with severe calcification at the aortic bifurcation

Reference

Wheatley, B. J., Mansour, M. A., Grossman, P. M., et al. (2011). Complication rates for percutaneous lower extremity arterial antegrade access. *Arch Surg, 146*(4), 432–435. PMID: 21502451

16. RATIONALE

The safety of antegrade femoral access for treating infrainguinal atherosclerotic occlusive disease has been well demonstrated. Antegrade access is more frequently used in the setting of critical limb ischemia (tissue loss). From a large vascular quality initiative sample, the data showed that the incidence of overall hematoma or hematoma requiring intervention in arterial stenosis/occlusion was similar in patients with retrograde femoral access or antegrade femoral access.

Correct Answer   D The incidence of groin hematomas with antegrade access is the same as with retrograde access, and most hematomas can be managed conservatively

Reference

Siracuse, J. J., Farber, A., Cheng, T. W., et al. (2019). Common femoral artery antegrade and retrograde approaches have similar access site complications. *J Vasc Surg, 69*(4), 1160–1166.e1162. PMID: 30527937

17. RATIONALE

When comparing open versus endovascular treatment of a popliteal artery aneurysm (PAA), most studies compare primary, primary assisted, and secondary patency in a longitudinal fashion. The historical gold standard with respect to the treatment of PAA is aneurysm exclusion with saphenous vein graft bypass, which has a documented long-term primary and secondary patency of 80%–95%

A most recent meta-analysis of over 4500 patients did find a significantly lower 1-year primary patency rate (88.3% vs. 81.21%, $p = 0.01$) in the endovascular treatment group, but no clinical adverse sequalae were reported ($p = 0.79$). The endovascular group has a lower wound complication rate and shorter length of stay as compared to the open group. There is a slight tendency of higher stent graft thrombosis and reduced patency after reintervention in the long term in patients undergoing endovascular repair. There is reduced patency after reintervention in the long term in patients with longer lesions and with fewer runoff vessels in the endovascular group.

Correct Answer   D 80%–95%

Reference

Leake, A. E., Segal, M. A., Chaer, R. A., et al. (2017). Meta-analysis of open and endovascular repair of popliteal artery aneurysms. *J Vasc Surg, 65*(1), 246–256.e242. PMID: 28010863

18. RATIONALE

Much of the literature on endovascular management of popliteal aneurysms recommends the use of a center line measurement with higher-resolution CTA imaging in order to determine the true diameter of the target vessel as well as the use of IVUS to guide diameter measurements along with identification of a normal uniform vessel. The instructions for use for the Viabahn endoprostheses suggest a 5%–20% diameter oversizing along with a 10-mm graft-to-vessel overlap without a 1-mm or greater difference between the stent graft diameters. All patients should be imaged with the knee extended and flexed to 90 degrees. Patients should not be imaged with voluntary knee flexion past 90 degrees in the postoperative period to avoid graft-to-graft separation or graft kinking which may lead to occlusion.

Correct Answer　**D** Insufficient overlap in the proximal and distal seal zone, undersizing of the stent, and due to repetitive knee flexion

Reference
Tielliu, I. F., Verhoeven, E. L., Zeebregts, C. J., et al. (2005). Endovascular treatment of popliteal artery aneurysms: results of a prospective cohort study. *J Vasc Surg, 41*(4), 561–567. PMID: 15874916

19. RATIONALE

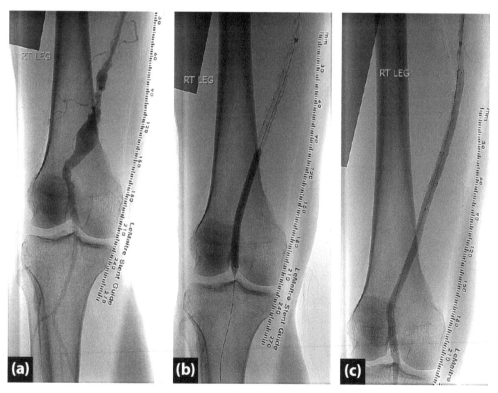

Successful stent graft repair of popliteal aneurysm.

In order to prevent thrombotic complications, careful selection of stent graft length and diameter is important. Data suggests that the use of longer stents or multiple stents is an independent predictor of stent graft thrombosis. It is preferable to cover all aneurysmal and ectatic segments with proximal and distal landing zones of 2 cm with the use of one covered stent, if feasible.

The patient should be started on dual antiplatelet therapy preoperatively and continued for 4–6 weeks after the procedure. Either ipsilateral/antegrade or contralateral/retrograde femoral access using percutaneous access or femoral cutdown is undertaken, depending on the diameter of the endograft and the diameter of the sheath required. Deployment should be done under fluoroscope visualization of the radiopaque markers, using gentle continuous traction on the PTFE suture to minimize device deflection. Aggressive tension on the PTFE suture can bow the tip of the delivery system resulting in deployment within the aneurysmal segment (bowstring phenomenon). If multiple endografts are used, there should be no more than a 1-mm size differential between overlapping devices – the smaller diameter device is placed first, and an overlap of 2–3 cm is maintained.

Correct Answer   **D** Use of multiple and longer stents

Reference
Garg, K., Rockman, C. B., Kim, B. J., et al. (2012). Outcome of endovascular repair of popliteal artery aneurysm using the Viabahn endoprosthesis. *J Vasc Surg*, *55*(6), 1647–1653. PMID: 22608040

20. RATIONALE

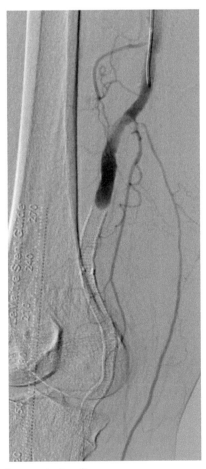

Arteriogram of thrombosis of popliteal artery stent graft.

Most studies have found no significant difference between open and endovascular repair at 1 year with primary patency of over 80%. Long-term follow-up up to 3 years yielded a primary patency of less than 70% with endovascular repair, which is significantly lower than the long-term success of open repair. Many studies have suggested higher rates of perioperative thrombosis with endovascular repair. There has been no evidence of an increased rate of amputation with endovascular repair. Most studies suggest an absence of a definable endoleak upon completion arteriogram. Despite initial success, 5%–10% of these patients were found to have evidence of endoleak on follow-up imaging modalities. With regard to graft-related complications, a single study revealed almost 10% incidence of graft infolding, and all cases had graft occlusion at long-term follow-up.

Correct Answer   **C** At long-term follow-up (3 years) the primary patency of open repair is superior

Reference

Eslami, M. H., Rybin, D., Doros, G., & Farber, A. (2015). Open repair of asymptomatic popliteal artery aneurysm is associated with better outcomes than endovascular repair. *J Vasc Surg, 61*(3), 663–669. PMID: 25454212

21. **RATIONALE**

The Supera stent (Abbott Vascular, Santa Clara, CA) was developed to provide superior radial strength, fracture resistance, and flexibility compared to laser-cut nitinol stents. Due to high mobility of the knee joint, laser-cut nitinol stents in the popliteal artery have the potential for external stent compression fractures resulting in occlusion. A study of 305 Supera stents in 147 patients revealed primary patency, primary assisted patency, and secondary assisted patency of 89.8%, 91.2%, and 93.2% by duplex ultrasound imaging at 12 months, respectively, with mean lesion length of 184.5 +/– 131.8 mm. Knee radiography in 47 patients did not show any stent fracture.

Correct Answer   **C** Deployment of Supera stent

Reference

Montero-Baker, M., Ziomek, G. J., Leon, L., et al. (2016). Analysis of endovascular therapy for femoro-popliteal disease with the Supera stent. *J Vasc Surg, 64*(4), 1002–1008. PMID: 27444365

22. **RATIONALE**

Retrograde tibial/pedal access is an additional option for access if the ipsilateral or contralateral femoral approach is ineffective in crossing the diseased segment. Antegrade recanalization can fail in up to 20% of patients with critical limb ischemia. Access to an artery distal to the occlusion can be obtained with a micropuncture kit under ultrasound guidance. The foot should be placed in plantar flexion when accessing the dorsalis pedis artery or distal anterior tibial artery. Patients are heparinized following sheath insertion. The lesion is crossed with a 0.018 wire, and once the lesion is crossed, the guide wire is snared with a micro-snare from the antegrade approach and brought through the sheath in the groin. Intervention then can be performed in an antegrade fashion.

Correct Answer   **C** 20%

Reference

Bazan, H. A., Le, L., Donovan, M., et al. (2014). Retrograde pedal access for patients with critical limb ischemia. *J Vasc Surg, 60*(2), 375–381. PMID: 24650744

23. RATIONALE

The incidence of surgical site infection following the infrainguinal bypass procedure has been reported to be 4.8%–18%. Preoperative chlorhexidine shower, use of transverse groin incision (avoiding longitudinal incisions), and skip incisions (leaving skin bridges) decrease the incidence of surgical site infection. Use of vacuum-assisted closure dressing in the groin with a single-use negative pressure wound therapy has shown to decrease the incidence of surgical site infection. Other independent risk factors for surgical site infection include ABI <0.35, transfusion of more than two units of packed red blood cells, and operative time of more than 220 minutes. Analysis of NSQIP data (2005–2012) showed 2.1% incidence of surgical site infection during the hospital stay and 6.9% after discharge. In contrast to occurrence of SSI within the perioperative period, late infections can develop months to years after the initial operation with a prosthetic graft. *Staphylococcus aureus* is the most common pathogen and accounts for 25%–50% of infections. In recent years, infections with *Staphylococcus epidermiditis* or Gram-negative bacteria such as *Escherichia coli, Pseudomonas, Klebsiella, Enterobacter serratia*, and *Proteus* have increased in frequency causing surgical site infections.

Correct Answer   B 5%–18%

Reference
Hekman, K. E., Michel, E., Blay, E., et al. (2019). Evidence-based bundled quality improvement intervention for reducing surgical site infection in lower extremity vascular bypass procedures. *J Am Coll Surg, 228*(1), 44–53. PMID: 30359836

24. RATIONALE

The great saphenous vein is the conduit of choice for femoral infrageniculate bypass because of its length, size, compatibility, and durability. The ipsilateral great saphenous vein is inadequate in 20% of patients. The best alternative conduit for lower extremity revascularization in such circumstances remains an issue of ongoing debate. Prosthetic grafts are clearly inferior to autologous conduit for infragenicular arterial reconstructions and should rarely be used. Chew et al. reported 226 infragenicular reconstructions using an autologous vein with use of the contralateral great saphenous vein 31%, single-segment lesser saphenous vein 5%, single-segment arm vein 19%, and autologous composite vein 45% in the absence of an ipsilateral great saphenous vein. These results showed that a 5-year patency rate was significantly better for the contralateral great saphenous vein in patients with an inadequate ipsilateral great saphenous vein.

Correct Answer   D 15%–20% patients

Reference
Chew, D. K., Owens, C. D., Belkin, M., et al. (2002). Bypass in the absence of ipsilateral greater saphenous vein: safety and superiority of the contralateral greater saphenous vein. *J Vasc Surg, 35*(6), 1085–1092. PMID: 12042718

25. RATIONALE

In femoropopliteal bypass surgery, the use of the saphenous vein as an arterial conduit is preferable, but synthetic grafts are often used above the knee. In a meta-analysis of 73 articles from 1986–2004, the pooled primary graft patency was 57.4% for above the knee, polytetrafluoroethylene (PTFE) 77.2% for above the knee vein and 64.8% for below the knee vein at 5 years. The corresponding pooled secondary graft patency was 54% for PTFE, 71.9% above the knee for saphenous vein, and 77.8% below the knee bypass. The prosthetic graft below the knee has a uniformly poor patency, with 3 years; patency of the PTFE graft below the knee is 54%. To improve patency, PTFE grafts covalently bonded to heparin were introduced. An additional way to improve the patency of below the knee prosthetic bypasses involve the use of Miler vein cuff and Taylor vein patches. Randomized trials have shown that the addition of vein cuffs significantly improved the patency of prosthetic grafts for infrageniculate bypass (52%) patency at 2 years for PTFE with vein cuff versus 29% for PTFE without cuff, with the addition of warfarin. Primary patency of femoral-popliteal bypass using an arm vein is 50%–60%.

Correct Answer   **C** 75% above the knee, 65% below the knee

Reference

Pereira, C. E., Albers, M., Romiti, M., et al. (2006). Meta-analysis of femoropopliteal bypass grafts for lower extremity arterial insufficiency. *J Vasc Surg*, *44*(3), 510–517. PMID: 16950427

26. RATIONALE

In patients undergoing bypass to infrapopliteal arteries with circumferential calcification, vascular clamp application may result in dissection and difficulty in obtaining occlusion of the target artery. Tourniquet occlusion in the thigh prior to construction of a distal anastomosis will aid in better visualization of the operative field with less dissection of the target runoff arteries in the calf or paramalleolar region. Since clamp application to small, calcified arteries is avoided, the early failure of the arterial reconstruction may be improved. Tourniquet time of less than 1 hour has not shown any adverse effect in the muscle biopsy specimens. Better primary or secondary patency using tourniquet occlusion has not been demonstrated.

Correct Answer   **B** Improves visualization and avoids clamping of small, calcified target arteries

Reference

Ciervo, A., Dardik, H., Qin, F., et al. (2000). The tourniquet revisited as an adjunct to lower limb revascularization. *J Vasc Surg*, *31*(3), 436–442. PMID: 10709054

27. RATIONALE

Early graft thrombosis has significant prognostic implications in that a failed reconstruction is associated with poor clinical outcome in patients undergoing reconstruction for limb salvage. Despite improvements in revascularization techniques, 5%–10% grafts will fail within 30 days of their placement, with technical error accounting for approximately 25% of the early graft failures. Other factors that contribute to early graft failures include inadequacy of the conduit as well as poor inflow and poor distal runoff. Treatment options for early graft failure include surgical thrombectomy and thrombolysis for PTFE graft. In general, thrombolytic therapy is contraindicated for 2 weeks following major surgical operation.

Correct Answer   **B** 5%–10%

Reference

Conte, M. S., Bandyk, D. F., Clowes, A. W., et al. (2006). Results of PREVENT III: a multicenter, randomized trial of edifoligide for the prevention of vein graft failure in lower extremity bypass surgery. *J Vasc Surg*, *43*(4), 742–751; discussion 751. PMID: 16616230

28. RATIONALE

Selection of specific treatment modalities for managing lower extremity graft infections are based on extent of the graft involvement and its microbiology along with clinical findings. Important adjuncts to attain wound sterilization and graft sterilization include the use of multiple-stage debridements/"old washout" operative procedures to minimize residual bacterial counts, aggressive excision of involved arterial wall and perigraft tissues to healthy tissue planes, wound irrigation, soft tissue coverage with muscle flaps such as sartorius, negative pressure wound therapy, and prolonged culture-specific antibiotics. Infections involving prosthetic grafts require partial or complete graft material excision to eradicate the local septic process. Graft preservation is possible for most arterial infections caused by Gram-positive organisms with autologous tissue reconstruction. Invasive infections caused by *Pseudomonas, Klebsiella, Proteus, E. coli,* and MRSA require graft removal; ex situ revascularization is recommended in this scenario. Acceptable management of infected lower extremity bypass grafts can range from ligation and excision alone to ligation with selective revascularization.

Correct Answer   **C** Complete removal of the graft with ex situ revascularization, excisional debridement, and antipseudomonal antibiotics

Reference

Armstrong, P. A., Back, M. R., Bandyk, D. F., et al. (2007). Selective application of sartorius muscle flaps and aggressive staged surgical debridement can influence long-term outcomes of complex prosthetic graft infections. *J Vasc Surg, 46*(1), 71–78. PMID: 17606124

29. RATIONALE

Late graft occlusion is usually caused by neointimal fibroplasia at the anastomotic site of the graft, usually at the distal anastomosis (vein or prosthetic), structural abnormalities, and progressive atherosclerosis. Late graft occlusion should be treated only if the symptoms are severe enough to warrant intervention based on Rutherford limb ischemia criteria. The longer the graft has been in place, the greater the likelihood that thrombolytic therapy will confer graft patency. If thrombolysis is pursued after systemic heparinization, the initial diagnostic test is arteriography. A hydrophilic 0.035-inch wire can then be used to select the stump of the proximal anastomosis and is manipulated into the body of the graft. Percutaneous mechanical thrombectomy with a pulse spray of tissue plasminogen activator is laced throughout the extent of the thrombosis. If a significant amount of thrombosis persists despite thrombectomy, an infusion catheter with administration of tPA 0.5-1 mg/hour along with heparin 500 units/hour is continued for 24 hours. After restoration of graft patency, further endovascular, or surgical therapy may be required in up to 85% of cases to correct the underlying lesion and to sustain graft patency. Thrombolytic therapy is less effective for thrombosis of the autologous vein grafts.

Correct Answer   **C** Arteriography and thrombolytic therapy

Reference

Schwierz, T., Gschwendtner, M., Havlicek, W., et al. (2001). Indications for directed thrombolysis or new bypass in treatment of occlusion of lower extremity arterial bypass reconstruction. *Ann Vasc Surg, 15*(6), 644–652. PMID: 11769145

30. RATIONALE

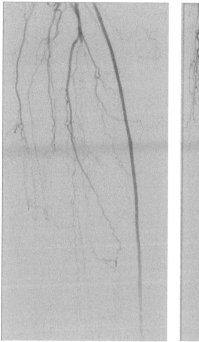
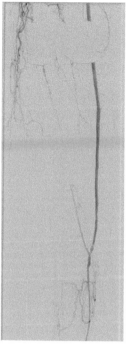
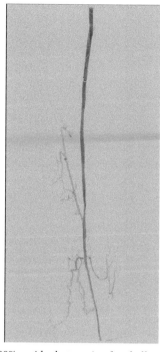

(a) Severe stenosis distal anastomosis RT. (b) Right femoral-PT in situ bypass.

30% residual stenosis after balloon angioplasty.

Carlson et al. reported on 45 percutaneous transluminal angioplasties in 36 patients for failing infrainguinal bypass from 1991 to 2001 due to graft stenosis diagnosed by duplex imaging. Technical success was reported in 91.7% of patients. Stenotic lesions were identified at proximal anastomosis in 3, midgraft in 6, and distal anastomosis in 27 patients. They reported a primary patency of 62.7% at 12 months and 58.4% at 24 months. Cumulative-assisted primary patency was 83.2% at 12 months and 78.9% at 24 months. Stenosis development at the anastomotic site within 10–12 weeks should preferably be treated with open operation for fear of anastomotic disruption during angioplasty. Although initial reports failed to demonstrate an improvement in primary patency with the use of cutting balloon angioplasty for recurrent stenosis following treatment of hyperplastic vein graft lesions, recent reports have shown markedly improved stenosis-free patency with the use of cutting balloon angioplasty versus conventional angioplasty (62% vs. 34% at 4 years).

Correct Answer **B** Percutaneous angioplasty

Reference
Carlson, G. A., Hoballah, J. J., Sharp, W. J., et al. (2004). Balloon angioplasty as a treatment of failing infrainguinal autologous vein bypass grafts. *J Vasc Surg, 39*(2), 421–426. PMID: 14743147

31. RATIONALE

Retained valve leaflets may result in early thrombosis of in situ vein bypass of the lower extremity. In a large-diameter vein, the in situ bypass may not thrombose, but an intimal hyperplastic lesion may threaten the patency of a smaller-diameter vein during follow-up.

The use of intraoperative Doppler ultrasound may produce a continuous high flow signal. Digital compression of the bypass immediately distal to the site of high velocity will result in persistence of flow only if the cause is patency of the side branch AV fistula. After ligation of the fistula, if the continuous localized high-velocity signal persists with flow and disappears with digital compression of the conduit, this is diagnostic of an intraluminal stenosis most likely due to retained valve leaflet. Bergamini et al. reported on 361 consecutive in situ saphenous vein bypasses and observed a 6-year primary patency of 63% and a secondary patency of 87%. They revised 86 (24%) of venous conduits because of a technical failure or inadequate vein segment. In the follow-up period, 95 (26%) bypasses were revised because of thrombus or hemodynamic failure. Operation for retained valve leaflet (n6) and fistula ligation (n4) were required using careful duplex ultrasound assessment during the operation as well as in the follow-up period.

Correct Answer   **A** Retained valve leaflets

Reference
Bergamini, T. M., Towne, J. B., Bandyk, D. F., et al. (1991). Experience within situ saphenous vein bypasses during 1981 to 1989: determinant factors of long-term patency. *J Vasc Surg, 13*(1), 137–147; discussion 148–139. PMID: 1987385

32. **RATIONALE**

Due to the close proximity of lymph vessels and lymph nodes to the corresponding artery and veins, lymphatic complications following infrainguinal bypass procedures are common. Intraoperative dissection contributes to lymphatic injury and/or transection. Fortunately, lymphatic channels often spontaneously heal. However, interruption of lymphatic vessels can lead to lower extremity edema, lymphatic fistula, or lymphocele. Lower extremity edema occurs in 50%–100% of patients undergoing infrainguinal arterial reconstruction for chronic limb ischemia. Significant edema can result in impairment in ambulation and local wound complications. The number of patent lymph nodes were markedly reduced after infrainguinal bypass as proven by lymphography. The lymphatics should be carefully preserved; if they must be divided, they should be ligated or cauterized to avoid leakage of lymph. Prospective randomized studies have demonstrated that endoscopic vein harvesting versus open vein harvesting results in a reduced rate of lymphatic and infectious wound complications. Edema usually becomes worse with ambulation and resolves within 2–3 months following arterial reconstruction.

Correct Answer   **D** 50%–100% of patients

33. **RATIONALE**

Important contributing factors for the development of lymphatic fistula (incidence approximately in 1.1%) include failure to ligate or cauterize lymphatic tissue, inadequate closure of the layers of the incision, and patient factors such as diabetes mellitus or concurrent infection. The diagnosis of a lymphatic fistula is made clinically as persistent leakage of clear or yellow fluid from the groin incision. Conservative management with antibiotics, local wound care, bed rest, and elevation reduce lymph flow. Conservative management does not have a role when a prosthetic graft is present due to risk of infection. Vacuum-assisted closure therapy has been used for an average of 16 days without recurrence of lymphatic complications. If wound VAC therapy fails, isosulfan blue dye is injected into the first and third interdigital space of the foot and a compression pump is placed over the affected leg to increase lymphatic and venous drainage. The groin incision is then reexplored in order to identify the site of lymphatic injury. The area is oversewn, and the wound is closed and dressed.

Correct Answer   C 1.1%

Reference

Hamed, O., Muck, P. E., Smith, J. M., et al. (2008). Use of vacuum-assisted closure (VAC) therapy in treating lymphatic complications after vascular procedures: new approach for lymphoceles. *J Vasc Surg, 48*(6), 1520–1523.e1521–1524. PMID: 19118737

34. RATIONALE

In contrast to a seroma, a lymphocele usually has a well-localized connection with one or more of lymphatic channels. Lymphocele is a localized collection of lymph that develops between two planes of tissue and fails to be reabsorbed. Lymphoscintigraphy can demonstrate a lymphocele. Large lymphoceles can cause local discomfort, pain, and leg swelling. Hematoma, seroma, and wound infection should be considered in the differential diagnosis. The presence of a soft, liquid-filled cyst and intermittent drainage of clear lymph through a fistula confirms the diagnosis of lymphocele. Ultrasonography is helpful in distinguishing a solid, dense hematoma from a cystic lymphocele. CT scan is the imaging modality of choice. When a lymphocele develops several weeks to months after the operative procedure, CT is helpful in excluding graft infection or underlying retroperitoneal lymphocele extending to the groin. Small lymphoceles self-absorb; however, large lymphoceles within the vicinity of the prosthetic graft should undergo exploration to reduce the risk of graft infection. The lymphocele is excised and its pedicle is suture ligated.

Correct Answer   C CT scan

Reference

Uhl, C., Götzke, H., Woronowicz, S., et al. (2020). Treatment of lymphatic complications after common femoral artery endarterectomy. *Ann Vasc Surg, 62*, 382–386. PMID: 31449944

35. RATIONALE

Common femoral endarterectomy in this scenario will correct in-flow stenosis, which may progress during the follow-up period. In addition, it will bring the transected great saphenous vein to be safely anastomosed to the distal portion of the common femoral and proximal superficial femoral artery by performing the proximal anastomosis over the patch grafting in the distal common femoral artery following endarterectomy. The addition of common femoral endarterectomy may further increase the incidence of surgical site infection, which occurs in approximately 11% of patients undergoing lower extremity bypass.

Similarly, during the paramalleolar bypass using in situ technique, if there is difficulty in closing the skin over the distal anastomosis because of swelling secondary to reperfusion in a chronically ischemic lower extremity, a separate release incision (vertical) a few centimeters lateral to the distal arterial anastomotic site should be performed. The release skin incision site is left open, and primary closure over the distal anastomotic site is performed. A split skin graft is applied at the site where the release incision was made approximately 5–7 days later.

Correct Answer   C Common femoral endarterectomy with patch grafting and placement of the proximal anastomosis of the in situ bypass over the distal portion of the patch

Reference
Elbadawy, A., Ali, H., & Saleh, M. (2020). Midterm outcomes of common femoral endarterectomy combined with inflow and outflow endovascular treatment for chronic limb threatening ischaemia. *Eur J Vasc Endovasc Surg, 59*(6), 947–955. PMID: 32224037

36. RATIONALE
Obturator bypass should be considered in patients with unilateral graft limb infection following AFB. CT scan should not reveal any evidence of perigraft fluid and gas in the main body or contralateral limb. At the time of intraabdominal or retroperitoneal exposure, the main body of the graft should be well incorporated. The affected limb is transected, and an opening is made in the anteromedial aspect of the obturator membrane by palpating the pubis and moving the finger laterally until the edge of the firm obturator membrane is exposed and incised with scissors. A tunneler is passed from the obturator fossa into the medial thigh for passage of the graft with subsequent distal anastomosis for arterial reconstruction.

Correct Answer   D Reconstruction with a new graft flush from the origin of the left limb of the AFB with distal anastomosis to the mid-SFA via the obturator canal.

Reference
Bath, J., Rahimi, M., Long, B., et al. (2017). Clinical outcomes of obturator canal bypass. *J Vasc Surg, 66*(1), 160–166. PMID: 28216364

37. RATIONALE
The graft through the obturator foramen is tunneled through the obturator fossa into the medial thigh after proximal anastomosis has been completed. The graft is brought anterior to the adductor longus muscle. The superficial femoral artery is exposed under the sartorius muscle, and the distal anastomosis of an 8-mm PTFE graft (originating flush from the old left limb of the aortobifemoral graft) is performed to the left mid-superficial femoral artery. In patients with an occluded superficial femoral artery, anastomosis may have to be performed to the popliteal artery. After proximal and distal anastomoses are completed, the patient is redraped and the retroperitoneal incision and the incision in the middle/distal thigh are isolated; the groin incision is opened, the infected graft is removed, and excisional debridement is performed.

Correct Answer   C Anterior to adductor longus

Reference
Bath, J., Rahimi, M., Long, B., et al. (2017). Clinical outcomes of obturator canal bypass. *J Vasc Surg, 66*(1), 160–166. PMID: 28216364

38. RATIONALE

Approximately 75% of myxomas occur in women with a mean age of 56 years, whereas the mean age is 25 years for familial cases. The tumor is mostly asymptomatic but fragments as it enlarges. They are gelatinous, polypoid, round, or oval and are usually white, yellowish, or brown in color. The most common site of atrial myxoma is the left atrial cavity. Familial cases are more frequently located in the ventricle. If there is anything atypical about the material removed during embolectomy and the patient is young with no obvious cause to explain embolic occlusion, the specimen should be carefully evaluated and histopathology performed. If histopathology is suggestive of atrial myxoma, the patient should have 2D and transesophageal echocardiography and consultation with a cardiothoracic surgeon for removal of atrial myxoma.

Correct Answer   **B** Embolus from atrial myxoma

Reference

Ha, J. W., Kang, W. C., Chung, N., et al. (1999). Echocardiographic and morphologic characteristics of left atrial myxoma and their relation to systemic embolism. *Am J Cardiol, 83*(11), 1579–1582, a1578. PMID: 10363879

39. RATIONALE

Acute limb ischemia can result from in situ arterial thrombosis (85%) or embolic occlusion 15%. Cardiogenic emboli account for 90% of peripheral arterial emboli and are secondary to atrial fibrillation, valvular disease, myocardial infarction, left ventricular aneurysm, or rarely a paradoxical embolus from a patent foramen ovale. Although many cases can be diagnosed by clinical evaluation, preoperative imaging for acute arterial occlusion includes CTA/MRA/catheter-based contrast arteriography and arterial duplex imaging. A study from British National Health Services in 1996 showed that graft and postangioplasty occlusion was responsible for 15% of acute limb ischemia, most often due to thrombosis. Assessment and treatment are similar to that for native arterial ischemia, but treatment is varied, as many options are available including thrombolysis and open thrombectomy with anticoagulation. From a study of 9736 patients who underwent open surgery and 6493 who had endovascular treatment, the results showed that the primary endovascular treatment for acute limb ischemia appeared to reduce mortality as compared with open surgery without any difference in the risk of amputation.

Correct Answer   **C** 15%

Reference

Grip, O., Wanhainen, A., Michaëlsson, K., et al. (2018). Open or endovascular revascularization in the treatment of acute lower limb ischaemia. *Br J Surg, 105*(12), 1598–1606. PMID: 30043994

40. RATIONALE

The optimal duration of delay before surgery in patients who have had SARS-CoV-2 infection was studied by an international, multicenter, prospective cohort study in patients undergoing elective or emergency surgery. Logistic regression models were used to calculate adjusted 30-day mortality rates stratified by time from diagnosis of SARS-CoV-2 infection to surgery. Among 140,231 patients, 3127 (2.2%), had a preoperative SARS-CoV-2 diagnosis. Adjusted 30-day mortality without SARS-CoV-2 infection was 1.5%. In patients with preoperative SARS-CoV-2 diagnosis, mortality was increased in patients having surgery within 0–2 weeks, 3–4 weeks, and 5–6 weeks of diagnosis (odds ratio 4.1, 3.9, and 3.6, respectively). Surgery performed at or later than 7 weeks after SARS-CoV-2 diagnosis was associated with similar mortality risk as to the baseline. Where possible, surgery should be delayed for at least 7 weeks following SARS-CoV-2 infection. Patients with ongoing symptoms after 7 weeks from diagnosis may benefit from further delay.

Correct Answer **D** Postpone the bypass for 7 weeks

Reference
COVIDSurg Collaborative, & GlobalSurg Collaborative. Timing of surgery following SARS-CoV-2 infection: an international prospective cohort study. (2021). *Anaesthesia, 76*(6), 748–758. PMID: 33690889

41. RATIONALE

Classification of acute arterial ischemia based on its severity is helpful in determining the urgency of intervention and has implications for outcome. Categories of ischemia are based on clinical findings and Doppler measurements performed at the bedside. In patients with class I ischemia (viable) or acute onset of claudication, acute intervention is not necessary. Exercise, the best medical therapy, noninvasive vascular Doppler study, segmental pressures, ABI, and risk modification for atherosclerosis may be all that is necessary. Acute onset of claudication may occasionally result from a thrombosed popliteal aneurysm or compression from adventitial cystic disease of the popliteal artery. In class III irreversible ischemia, there is no indication to improve the blood supply which can potentiate rhabdomyolysis, and the patient most likely will need major amputation. Patients with class II ischemia require intervention, and the distinction between IIa (marginally threatened) or IIb (immediately threatened) is very important. Any delay in treating IIb ischemia may result in irreversible muscle necrosis, whereas in patients with IIa ischemia there is time for investigation and semi-elective intervention while keeping the patient on IV heparin and maintaining hydration and general assessment. The three findings that best differentiate IIa from IIb ischemia are pain at rest, sensory loss, and muscle weakness in class IIb ischemia.

Correct Answer **D** Absence of muscle weakness, minimal loss of motor function (toes) with absent sensory loss, and absence of pain at rest in 2a

Reference
Rutherford, R. B., Baker, J. D., Ernst, C., et al. (1997). Recommended standards for reports dealing with lower extremity ischemia: revised version. *J Vasc Surg, 26*(3), 517–538. PMID: 9308598

42. RATIONALE

From a Swedish Nationwide Vascular Database (1994–2014), 715 cases of acute aortic occlusion were identified with a mean age of 60.7 years; 50.5% were women. The causes were in situ thrombosis (64.1%), saddle embolus (21.3%), and occluded graft/stent/stent graft (14.7%). Patients with saddle embolism were older (mean age 74.3 years) and with a preponderance of women (62.1%). The most common method for revascularization was thromboembolectomy (32%), thrombolysis (22.4%), axillary-bifemoral bypass (18.9%) and aortobiiliac/bifemoral bypass (18.2%). In situ thrombosis was mostly treated with bypass surgery, and embolus treated with embolectomy. Endovascular techniques to treat acute aortic occlusion are becoming more frequent. The amputation rate was 8.6% and mortality was 19.9% within 30 days of surgery, with mortality highest in the embolectomy group (30.9%).

Correct Answer   B In situ thrombosis

Reference
Grip, O., Wanhainen, A., & Björck, M. (2019). Acute aortic occlusion. *Circulation, 139*(2), 292–294. PMID: 30615512

43. RATIONALE

Catheter-directed thrombolysis is an established intervention for all forms of acute arterial occlusion except embolic arterial occlusion. Acute arterial embolus is best managed by embolectomy because embolectomy is a straightforward operation and provides both efficient and definitive revascularization than thrombolysis. For most patients with acute embolic arterial occlusion, the procedure can be performed within 6–8 hours of the onset of symptoms. All current thrombolytic agents are plasminogen activators that accelerate the plasmin production with the degradation of fibrin. Thrombolysis lyses the clot in both large and small arteries as well as the arteriolar and capillary bed. In addition to absolute contraindications to thrombolysis, which include major surgery within 2 weeks, a patient with recent gastrointestinal bleeding, recent stroke, or craniotomy within 3 months, relative contraindications include uncontrolled hypertension, any surgery within 1 month, hepatic failure, bacterial endocarditis, pregnancy, diabetic retinopathy, recent eye surgery, and cardiopulmonary resuscitation within 10 days. In all the choices mentioned, uncontrolled hypertension in the modern era of antihypertensive medication can be controlled as the thrombolytics are started.

Correct Answer   D Uncontrolled hypertension

Reference
Plate, G., Oredsson, S., & Lanke, J. (2009). When is thrombolysis for acute lower limb ischemia worthwhile? *Eur J Vasc Endovasc Surg, 37*(2), 206–212. PMID: 19054698

44. RATIONALE

Of the 110,356 patients in the vascular study group of New England (2010–2014), 365 patients were treated for acute limb ischemia and 1808 patients were treated for chronic limb ischemia. Acute limb ischemia patients were less likely to be treated with self-expanding stents and more likely to undergo thrombolysis than patients with critical limb ischemia. Acute limb ischemia patients were treated with peripheral vascular intervention, had a higher burden of atherosclerotic risk factors, and were more likely to have had prior ipsilateral revascularizations. Acute limb ischemia was associated with high technical failure, increased rate of distal embolization, longer length of stay and higher in-hospital mortality. Acute limb ischemia was not associated with risk of major amputation or mortality at 1 year. Acute limb ischemia patients selected for treatment with endovascular techniques experienced greater short-term adverse events but similar long-term outcomes as their critical limb ischemia counterparts.

Correct Answer   D Similar mortality compared with their chronic limb ischemia counterparts

Reference

Inagaki, E., Farber, A., Kalish, J. A., et al. (2018). Outcomes of peripheral vascular interventions in select patients with lower extremity acute limb ischemia. *J Am Heart Assoc, 7*(8):e004782. PMID: 29650705

45. RATIONALE

From a National Inpatient Sample Database (2010–2014) in patients with a primary diagnosis of acute limb ischemia, 10,484 hospitalizations were reported with endovascular revascularization performed in 5008 (47.8%) and surgical revascularization in 5476 (52.2%). In the propensity score matched cohort ($n = 7746$; 3873 per group), patients who underwent endovascular revascularization had a significantly lower in-hospital mortality, myocardial infarction, composite of death/myocardial infarction/stroke, acute kidney injury, fasciotomy, major bleeding, and need for transfusion. The vascular complications were higher in the endovascular group. Rates of any amputation were similar in both groups. Median length of stay was shorter and hospital costs higher in the endovascular group.

Correct Answer   **D** Lower composite of death/myocardial infarction/stroke

Reference

Kolte, D., Kennedy, K. F., Shishehbor, M. H., et al. (2020). Endovascular versus surgical revascularization for acute limb ischemia: a propensity-score matched analysis. *Circ Cardiovasc Interv, 13*(1), e008150. PMID: 31948292

46. RATIONALE

The ability of percutaneous mechanical thrombectomy to rapidly restore arterial perfusion is an attractive addition to PMT. In patients with significant ischemia that precludes the obligatory delay associated with pharmacologic thrombolysis, percutaneous mechanical thrombectomy devices may rapidly clear a channel through the occluded segment. Partial reperfusion of the extremity may provide enough improvement to allow complete removal of the thrombus, with thrombolytic infusions thereafter. An initial decrease in the size of the thrombus may also help in reduction of the dose and duration of thrombolytic agents, with resultant decrease in the risk of hemorrhagic complications. Hemodynamic devices (Angiojet Peripheral Thrombectomy System, Boston Scientific, Boston, MA), rotational devices (Arrow-Trerotola Thrombectomy Device, Castaneda and Cragg Brushes), and other mechanical adjuncts such as mechanical mixing (Trellis) or ultrasound energy (EKOS) are used to accelerate the speed of lysis. Myoglobinuria is not uncommon after treatment of acute limb ischemia. It is rarely a significant problem except in patients with preexisting renal failure or with the use of greater than 150 mL of contrast agent or when combined with hemoglobinuria. Hemoglobinuria is not uncommon after the use of certain PMT devices, especially if used longer than 5 minutes. Alkalinization of urine and maintenance of urine output greater than 100 mL/hour are important in the management of myoglobinuria. Compartment syndrome is most often seen in patients who have undergone open surgical revascularization or those treated with PMT devices owing to the speed of revascularization. Fasciotomy for compartment syndrome is less frequently required in patients undergoing CDT due to the more gradual resolution of acute limb ischemia.

Correct Answer   **D** Fasciotomy for compartment syndrome is less frequently required

Reference

Björck, M., Earnshaw, J. J., Acosta, S., et al. (2020). Editor's choice — European Society for Vascular Surgery (ESVS) 2020 clinical practice guidelines on the management of acute limb ischemia. *European Journal of Vascular and Endovascular Surgery, 59*(2), 173–218. PMID: 31899099

47. RATIONALE

Compartment pressure in the lower extremity is normally 10–12 mmHg. The studies have suggested that 30 mmHg should be used as a threshold for diagnosis of compartment syndrome. The anterior and the deep posterior compartments are most often affected. The most common causes of compartment syndrome are ischemia-reperfusion phenomenon with acute arterial ischemia, arterial and venous trauma, phlegmasia cerulea dolens, and hemorrhage within a compartment syndrome, as a complication of reperfusion for acute lower extremity ischemia has been reported in approximately 20% of patients. Risk factors for compartment syndrome following acute arterial ischemia include greater than 6 hours of ischemia time, younger age, paucity of arterial collaterals, and hypotension. Clinical criteria for fasciotomy include a swollen tense compartment with pain on passive motion. Pain usually becomes excessive with complaints of associated paresthesias. Any neurological symptoms and/or findings should be treated emergently with fasciotomy to prevent nerve injury. The double incision technique for lower leg fasciotomy involves a lateral incision between the anterior and lateral compartments, and these compartments are opened longitudinally. The second incision is placed on the medial aspect of the leg posterior to the tibia for decompression of the posterior two compartments. Fasciotomy wounds can be closed as a delayed primary closure or allowed to heal by secondary intention, gradual dermal apposition, split-thickness skin grafting, and occasionally with a myocutaneous flap coverage.

Correct Answer   D 20%–21%

Reference

Cone, J., & Inaba, K. (2017). Lower extremity compartment syndrome. *Trauma Surg Acute Care Open*, *2*(1), e000094. PMID: 29766095

48. RATIONALE

The thigh contains three compartments: Anterior, Posterior, and Adductor. In most cases a single lateral incision is used to decompress the posterior and abductor compartments. An incision is made along the lateral thigh beginning just distal to the intertrochanteric line and extending distally to the lateral epicondyle. The iliotibial band is exposed and incised longitudinally to decompress the anterior compartment. The vastus lateralis is reflected medially to expose the lateral intermuscular septum. The intermuscular septum is incised along the length of the incision to release the posterior compartment. The adductor compartment syndrome is decompressed by adding a medial incision. Most fasciotomy wounds are closed by delayed primary closure some by split-thickness skin grafts and a small number by primary closure. Diagnosis is based primarily on physical examination with pain out of proportion to the clinical situation. Pain on passive stretch is the most sensitive finding. Most fasciotomy wounds are closed by delayed primary closure with one-quarter-hand split-thickness clamps and a small number by primary closure. Neurological deficits were the most common complications. There is limited data on thigh compartment syndrome with respect to the cause, use of one versus two incision fasciotomies, method of wound closure, and complication rates.

Correct Answer   D All three compartments

Reference

Ojike, N. I., Roberts, C. S., & Giannoudis, P. V. (2010). Compartment syndrome of the thigh: a systematic review. *Injury*, *41*(2), 133–136. PMID: 19555950

49. RATIONALE

Iliofemoral arterial bypass graft/endarterectomy is a suitable option for high-risk patients with symptomatic unilateral iliac artery occlusive disease. The need for this procedure has declined considerably, as endovascular procedures for iliac artery occlusions are being increasingly successfully performed. If there is extension of the disease to the origin of the common iliac artery or there is extensive calcification, iliofemoral bypass or endarterectomy should be avoided, as it could be challenging to apply a proximal vascular clamp. Iliofemoral bypass is most useful for external iliac artery occlusion when endovascular therapy is unsuccessful or there is also involvement of the common femoral artery. In those cases, a common femoral endarterectomy and iliofemoral bypass or endarterectomy should be considered. Five-year patency of up to 93% has been reported with iliofemoral bypass graft procedures. Another series reported a primary and secondary patency rate of iliofemoral bypass as 94% and 100% at 1 year and 76.7% and 95% at 4 years, respectively.

Correct Answer   **D** 93%

Reference

Carsten, C. G., 3rd, Kalbaugh, C. A., Langan, E. M., et al. (2008). Contemporary outcomes of iliofemoral bypass grafting for unilateral aortoiliac occlusive disease: a 10-year experience. *Am Surg, 74*(6), 555–559; discussion 559–560. PMID: 18557000

50. RATIONALE

The results of the BEST-CLI trial determining the best initial strategy of endovascular therapy vs. surgical therapy revascularization among 1830 patients randomized in two parallel cohort trials. Patient who had a single segment of great saphenous vein that could be used for bypass to Cohort 1. Patients who needed an alternative bypass conduit were assigned to Cohort 2. In Cohort 1, after a median follow-up of 2.7 years, a primary outcome event occurred in 302 of 709 patients (42.6%) in the surgical group and in 408 of the 711 patients in (57.4%) in the endovascular group ($P < 0.001$). In Cohort 2, a primary outcome event occurred in 83 of 194 patients (42.8%) in the surgical group and in 95 of 199 patients (47.7%) in the endovascular group ($P = 0.12$) after a median follow-up of 1.6 years, the incidence of adverse events was similar in the two groups. In patients presenting with chronic limb-threatening ischemia who had an inadequate great saphenous vein for surgical revascularization (Cohort 1) the incidence of a major adverse limb event was significantly lower in the surgical group than in the endovascular group. In patients with inadequate saphenous vein conduit (Cohort 2) the outcomes in the two groups were similar.

Correct Answer   **C** Right femoral-popliteal bypass using GSV

Reference

Farber, A., Menard, M. T., Conte, M. S., et al. for BEST-CLI Investigators (2022). Surgery or endovascular therapy for chronic limb-threatening ischemia. *New England Journal of Medicine, 387*(25), 2305–2316. PMID: 36342173.

SECTION 10: RENAL AND MESENTERIC DISEASE

MCQs 1–23

Q1. If left untreated, a superior mesenteric artery aneurysm will rupture in:
A. <10% of patients
B. 10%–20% of patients
C. 21%–35% of patients
D. 36%–50% of patients

Q2. Intervention for splenic artery aneurysm should be recommended once the aneurysm reaches a diameter of:
A. 1.5 cm
B. 2–2.4 cm
C. 2.5 cm or larger
D. Diagnosis of calcified splenic artery aneurysm is an indication for repair

Q3. One week following coil embolization of a splenic artery aneurysm near the hilum of the spleen, a 43-year-old woman presents with fever, pain in the left upper quadrant, elevated WBC count, and C-reactive protein. The most likely diagnosis is:
A. Splenic infarct
B. Post-embolization syndrome
C. Splenic abscess
D. Pseudocyst pancreas

Q4. The rupture rate of hepatic artery aneurysm is:
A. 10%
B. 15%
C. 20%
D. Hepatic artery aneurysm rupture is encountered only in patients with hepatic artery pseudoaneurysms

Q5. The lifetime risk of rupture of a celiac artery aneurysm is in the range of:
A. 0%–5%
B. 6%–20%
C. 21%–24%
D. 25%

Q6. The following statement best reflects the presentation and mortality of gastroepiploic aneurysms:
A. <50% present with rupture with 50% mortality
B. 60% present with rupture with 60% mortality
C. 70% present with rupture with 70% mortality
D. 90% present with rupture with 70% mortality

Q7. The rupture of renal artery aneurysm is associated with a mortality of:
A. <5%
B. 10%
C. 15%
D. 20%

Q8. The conduit of choice for open renal artery aneurysm repair in a 16 year old is:
A. Great saphenous vein (reversed)
B. Great saphenous vein (non-reversed with lysis of the valves)
C. Hypogastric artery
D. PTFE (Polytetraflouroethylene) graft

Q9. Postoperative renal artery patency rates 10 years following open repair of renal artery aneurysm are:
A. 90% or greater
B. 80%
C. 75%
D. 70%

DOI: 10.1201/9781003389897-10

Q10. A 38-year-old woman with underlying connective tissue disorder presents with a spontaneous isolated renal artery dissection with poor perfusion of the right kidney. The next best management option is:
A. IV heparin
B. Open repair of renal artery dissection
C. Steroids
D. Covered stent

Q11. An 85-year-old woman came to the ER with a history of intermittent abdominal pain for the past 3–4 days. She was on warfarin for atrial fibrillation but had discontinued it on her own. Abdominal examination is unremarkable. CBC and serum lactate levels are elevated. The next best option is:
A. Exploratory laparotomy
B. CT scan of the abdomen and pelvis with IV contrast
C. MRA abdomen and pelvis
D. Catheter-based angioplasty

Q12. A 66-year-old woman complains of postprandial abdominal pain, weight loss, and food fear. CTA of the abdomen and pelvis shows 50% stenosis of the celiac artery, occlusion of the first 2 cm of the superior mesenteric artery, and an occluded inferior mesenteric artery with large mesenteric collaterals. Which revascularization procedure will provide the best long-term outcome?
A. Retrograde abdominal aorta to superior mesenteric artery bypass
B. Antegrade supraceliac aorta to superior mesenteric artery bypass
C. Aortic endarterectomy
D. Angioplasty/stenting of the celiac artery with a retrograde superior mesenteric artery bypass

Q13. A 68-year-old woman presents with a history of vague periumbilical abdominal pain for 6 months without food fear and has no history of weight loss. GI endoscopy is negative. Duplex imaging and CTA of the abdomen and pelvis show 50% stenosis of the celiac artery, 60% stenosis of the superior mesenteric

artery, and a patent inferior mesenteric artery. Mesenteric collaterals are not seen on arteriography. Optimal management consists of:
A. SMA stenting
B. Celiac and SMA stenting
C. Medical management and follow-up CTA abdomen and pelvis in 1 year
D. Medical management with surveillance duplex imaging of celiac and superior mesenteric artery

Q14. A 78-year-old woman presents with a history of postprandial abdominal pain and significant weight loss, with imaging studies showing occlusion of the celiac artery, occlusion of proximal 4-cm segment of the superior mesenteric artery, and a patent inferior mesenteric artery with large mesenteric collaterals. Supraceliac aorta shows circumferential calcification. Infrarenal aorta is only 10 mm in diameter with a posterior plaque. Optimal surgical management consists of:
A. Antegrade bypass from supraceliac aorta to superior mesenteric artery
B. Bypass to celiac and superior mesenteric artery from supraceliac aorta using left retroperitoneal flank approach via ninth intercostal space
C. Retrograde bypass using a ringed prosthetic graft from infrarenal aorta or right common iliac artery to superior mesenteric artery
D. Retrograde bypass from infrarenal aorta to superior mesenteric artery using non-reversed great saphenous vein

Q15. A 76-year-old man with a prior history of coronary artery bypass graft presents with symptoms of chronic mesenteric ischemia with occlusion of the proximal 2-cm segment of celiac and superior mesenteric artery with a failed prior percutaneous intervention. Optimal management consists of:
A. Antegrade aortoceliac/hepatic and superior mesenteric artery bypass
B. Retrograde bypass from the infrarenal aorta to the superior mesenteric artery

C. Retrograde stenting of the superior mesenteric artery following aortoceliac bypass

D. Trapdoor aortic endarterectomy

Q16. **A 60-year-old woman presented with ischemic rest pain and postprandial abdominal pain without any weight loss. Abdominal aortogram showed juxtarenal aortic occlusion and occlusion of the proximal 4 cm of the superior mesenteric artery with a patent inferior mesenteric artery (small diameter) and large mesenteric collaterals. The celiac artery showed 50% stenosis at this origin. The superior mesenteric artery could not be catheterized using brachial access. She underwent aortobifemoral graft with proximal anastomosis end-to-end with a 14 × 7-mm knitted Dacron graft. After completion of proximal anastomosis and closure of the distal abdominal aorta above the inferior mesenteric artery, the terminal 6 inches of the small intestine became ischemic with no Doppler flow in its mesentery. Preferable management in the patient is:**

A. Medial visceral rotation and aorto-to-superior mesenteric artery bypass using 8-mm ringed PTFE graft

B. Supraceliac aorta to superior mesenteric artery bypass using great saphenous vein

C. Retrograde stenting of the superior mesenteric artery

D. Retrograde bypass from the right limb of the aortobifemoral graft to the superior mesenteric artery using great saphenous vein harvested from right groin and upper thigh

Q17. **A 77-year-old woman with a history of prior distal pancreatectomy and radiation therapy with adjuvant chemotherapy for carcinoma of the body of the pancreas develops 50% stenosis of the superior mesenteric artery, inferior mesenteric artery occlusion, and 50%** stenosis of the celiac artery with a 3.1-cm infrarenal abdominal aortic aneurysm. Vascular surgery is called in by the general surgeon who has performed a laparotomy, which revealed acute ischemia of the terminal ileum and cecum. The optimal management is:

A. Bowel resection with discontinuity

B. Superior mesenteric artery stenting via left brachial approach

C. Retrograde superior mesenteric artery stenting and bowel resection with bowel in discontinuity

D. Bowel resection with primary anastomosis and closing the abdomen with the patient taken to the IR for superior mesenteric artery stenting

Q18. **In-stent restenosis of the superior mesenteric artery is best treated with:**

A. Open bypass

B. Superior mesenteric artery endarterectomy

C. Stent angioplasty

D. Thrombolysis using PTA followed by angioplasty

Q19. **In order to avoid the complication of embolization during superior mesenteric artery stenting for severe eccentric stenosis in its proximal 2-cm segment:**

A. Predilatation of the lesion should never be performed

B. Inadequate anticoagulation is not an important factor

C. Femoral access is the best option

D. Preprocedure planning with selection of the site of arterial access and availability of filter option

Q20. **Arterial dissection during stenting of visceral arteries for occlusive disease can best be avoided by:**

A. Forceful predilation

B. Heparinization

C. Always use self-expanding stent

D. Ensuring true lumen position of the crossing wire by contrast injection through a low-profile crossing catheter

Q21. An 8-year-old child has infrarenal abdominal aortic coaractation with associated renal artery ostial stenosis. The optimal management is:
A. Medical management
B. Primary angioplasty with PTFE patch and bilateral renal artery reimplantation
C. Percutaneous transluminal angioplasty (PTA)
D. Primary aortal renal bypass with right renal artery reimplantation and left splenorenal anastomosis

Q22. An aortorenal bypass is planned for a 10-year-old male for treatment of distal main renal artery stenosis. The best conduit for bypass is:
A. PTFE graft
B. Dacron graft
C. Saphenous graft
D. Internal iliac artery graft

Q23. Conventional surgical revascularization for pediatric renovascular hypertension results in a cure among:
A. 50% of patients
B. 60% of patients
C. 70% of patients
D. 80% of patients

RATIONALE 1–23

1. RATIONALE

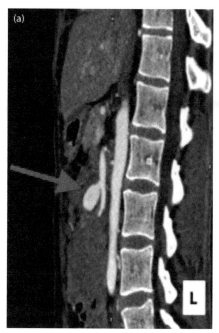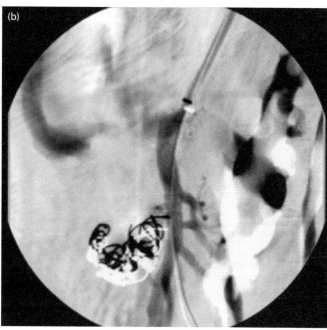

(a) Saccular SMA aneurysm. (b) Stent graft and coils in the SMA and aneurysm sac.

Superior mesenteric artery aneurysms account for 5% of all visceral aneurysms. The most common cause of superior mesenteric artery aneurysm is mycotic (60%) secondary to bacterial endocarditis or intravenous drug abuse. Staphylococcus and streptococcus species are the most common bacteria responsible for aneurysm degeneration. Patients may be asymptomatic or present with symptoms of intestinal ischemia. Due to higher resistance bed of the small intestine vasculature, superior mesenteric artery aneurysms frequently present with thrombosis. Other etiologies of superior mesenteric artery aneurysms include medial degeneration, connective tissue disease, and polyarteritis nodosa. Rupture rates for SMA aneurysms range from 38% to 50% with a mortality of 90% secondary to bleeding and bowel ischemia. Repair is indicated in symptomatic mycotic superior mesenteric artery aneurysms or those measuring greater than 2.5 cm in Ap/Tr. diameter.

Correct Answer   D 36%–50% of patients

Reference
Corey, M. R., Ergul, E. A., Cambria, R. P., et al. (2016). The natural history of splanchnic artery aneurysms and outcomes after operative intervention. *J Vasc Surg*, *63*(4), 949–957. PMID: 26792545

2. RATIONALE

Splenic artery aneurysms account for over 60% of all splanchnic aneurysms with an incidence of 0.8%. They are often detected in multiparous women with a female-to-male ratio of 4 to 1. The majority are located in the distal one-third portion of the splenic artery. The risk of rupture is estimated to be close to 3%. This risk is higher in the setting of pregnancy, portal hypertension, liver transplant, and vasculitis. Intervention is currently recommended for all symptomatic patients as well as those with an aneurysm diameter larger than 2.5 cm. Small calcified splenic artery aneurysms incidentally identified on CT scans of the abdomen do not require repair in most instances.

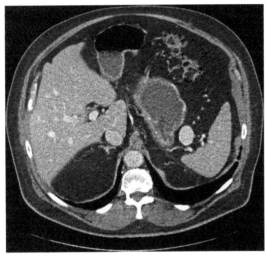

CTA abdomen showing splenic artery aneurysm.

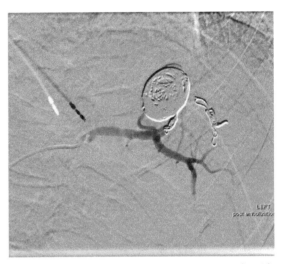

Complete thrombosis of aneurysm sac using coils with preserved flow to the spleen.

Correct Answer   **C** 2.5 cm or larger

Reference
Barrionuevo, P., Malas, M. B., Nejim, B., et al. (2019). A systematic review and meta-analysis of the management of visceral artery aneurysms. *J Vasc Surg*, *70*(5), 1694–1699. PMID: 31126761

3. **RATIONALE**

Post-embolization syndrome is characterized by fever, abdominal pain, and leukocytosis and is more common after embolization of hepatic tumors and is likely caused by an inflammatory response to the necrotic tissue. Splenic infarct following coil embolization does not require any treatment unless splenic abscess develops. Distal splenic artery embolization is associated with greater incidences of splenic infarct and abscess then proximal embolization. Splenic abscess is encountered less frequently but often requires percutaneous drainage or splenectomy following confirmation with non-contrast CT scan of the abdomen.

Correct Answer   **C** Splenic abscess

Reference
Ahuja, C., Farsad, K., & Chadha, M. (2015). An overview of splenic embolization. *AJR Am J Roentgenol*, *205*(4), 720–725. PMID: 26397320

4. RATIONALE

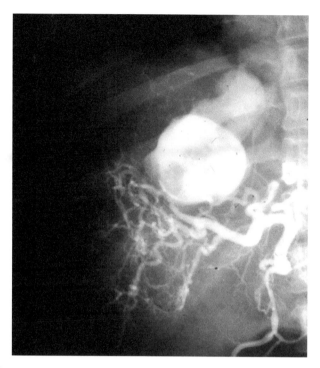

Hepatic artery aneurysm.

Hepatic artery aneurysms are the second most common visceral aneurysms, and the majority are extrahepatic and occur in the common hepatic artery. The most common cause is atherosclerotic degeneration with less common causes such as fibromuscular dysplasia, polyarteritis nodosa, mycotic degeneration, and inflammatory pseudoaneurysms due to acute pancreatitis and cholecystitis. Traumatic pseudoaneurysms account for almost half of the intrahepatic aneurysms encountered. Rupture rate can be as high as 20%, with intrahepatic aneurysms reporting even higher rupture rates. Hepatic artery aneurysms have one of the highest rates of rupture of all visceral artery aneurysms and a high mortality rate of 40% when presenting with rupture. Rupture can also occur into the gastrointestinal or biliary tract. Current management recommendations include treatment for all symptomatic hepatic aneurysms and all true aneurysms >2 cm. Pseudoaneurysms of the hepatic artery should be treated regardless of their size. Because of a high rate of anatomic variations (replaced right or left hepatic arteries originating from the superior mesenteric artery in 18% or from the left gastroduodenal artery in 12%), careful attention to exposure of the hepatic artery must be performed. Surgical exposure can be obtained by right subcostal incision. If the aneurysm is proximal to the gastroduodenal artery, the aneurysm can be ligated with collateral flow precluding the need for in-line reconstruction. If the aneurysm extends into the proper hepatic artery, reconstruction will be required, avoiding branch ligation, which can result in hepatic necrosis if the distal portion of the right hepatic artery is ligated. Cholecystectomy should be considered in this instance. Hepatic artery ligation should be avoided in patients with baseline liver dysfunction or liver cirrhosis. Catheter-based approaches are preferable for intraparenchymal lesions. Embolization does carry the risk of liver necrosis, abscess, and sepsis.

Correct Answer **C** 20%

Reference
Berceli, S. A. (2005). Hepatic and splenic artery aneurysms. *Semin Vasc Surg, 18*(4), 196–201. PMID: 16360576

5. RATIONALE

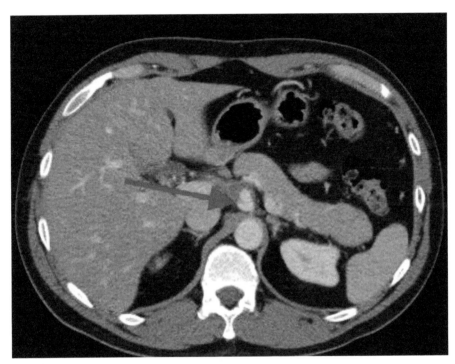

Celiac artery aneurysm.

The lifetime risk of rupture of celiac artery aneurysm is between 6% and 20% with a mortality of 50%. Because of the low incidence of celiac artery aneurysm, it is difficult to reliably identify risk factors for rupture. As with splenic artery aneurysms, a "double-rupture" phenomenon can occur with initial contained lesser sac bleeding followed in variable time intervals by extension into the peritoneal cavity. Several contemporary studies do not report rupture of celiac artery aneurysm smaller than 2.5 cm diameter. Therefore, for asymptomatic patients, a celiac artery aneurysm less than 2.5 cm can be monitored by visceral duplex imaging or CTA of the abdomen. Endovascular technique usually includes embolization and/or exclusion of the celiac artery because of the short length of the celiac trunk. The short length of the celiac trunk limits complete stent graft exclusion of most aneurysms. Successful endovascular repair, therefore, relies on adequate collateral blood supply to the liver. The preferred open surgical treatment of celiac artery aneurysms is aneurysm resection with revascularization. Autologous vein or a prosthetic bypass is used as a conduit for the celiac artery with distal anastomosis to the common hepatic artery or the divided end of the celiac trunk. An aortic punch is useful to create a circular opening in the aorta, and occasionally aortic reimplantation of celiac artery is possible. Aneurysmorrhaphy has been employed in less than 10% of cases for saccular aneurysms involving a small portion of the arterial circumference. However, most patients will require an aortoceliac or aorto-hepatic bypass after resection of the aneurysm.

Correct Answer   **B** 6%–20%

Reference

Stone, W. M., Abbas, M. A., Gloviczki, P., et al. (2002). Celiac arterial aneurysms: a critical reappraisal of a rare entity. *Arch Surg, 137*(6), 670–674. PMID: 12049537

6. RATIONALE

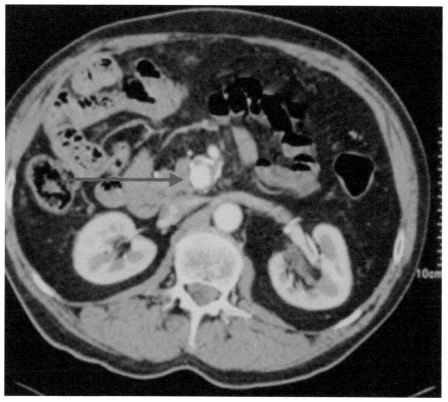

Pancreaticoduodenal artery aneurysm.

Gastric artery aneurysms and gastroepiploic artery aneurysms are rare; in combination they account for 4% of all visceral aneurysms. The etiology includes atherosclerosis (30%), trauma (25%), and inflammation (15%), including pancreatitis, peptic ulcer disease, and vasculitis. More than 90% of gastroepiploic artery aneurysms are ruptured at presentation because they are intraperitoneal. The mortality rate from rupture is 70%. Management generally consists of operative ligation with or without arterial reconstruction. Aneurysm in the distribution of the jejunal, ileal, and colic branches is rare and comprises 2% of all visceral aneurysms. Rupture of jejunal and ileal aneurysms is less common than colic aneurysms. Gastroduodenal aneurysms and pancreaticoduodenal aneurysms are uncommon (1.5%–2% of visceral aneurysms). They are commonly associated with acute pancreatitis resulting in pseudoaneurysm formation from pancreatic inflammation or pseudocyst. When true pancreaticoduodenal aneurysms are associated with celiac artery occlusive disease, both aneurysm and celiac stenosis or occlusion should be treated to minimize the risk of abolishing the collateral supply. Endovascular techniques have changed the approach to gastroduodenal artery aneurysms and pancreaticoduodenal artery aneurysms. Coil embolization has been the most popular option but requires close surveillance, as recanalization causing recurrent bleeding is common. True pancreaticoduodenal artery aneurysms associated with celiac artery stenosis or occlusion are difficult to treat with endovascular means alone, and combined open and endovascular approaches are a better option. Hybrid repair is often required.

Correct Answer   **D** 90% present with rupture, with 70% mortality

Reference
Shanley, C. J., Shah, N. L., & Messina, L. M. (1996). Uncommon splanchnic artery aneurysms: pancreaticoduodenal, gastroduodenal, superior mesenteric, inferior mesenteric, and colic. *Ann Vasc Surg, 10*(5), 506–515. PMID: 8905073

7. RATIONALE

Most renal artery aneurysms are asymptomatic and are usually found incidentally on imaging for unrelated conditions. Of those that develop symptoms, hypertension is the most common. Hypertension may be the result of renin-mediated vasoconstriction in the setting of renal artery stenosis, which can result in formation of post-stenotic fusiform aneurysms. Other symptoms include flank pain and hematuria. The most serious complication is rupture, presenting as flank or abdominal pain with hypotension, with a mortality of about 10%. Among survivors of aneurysm ruptures, 90% have a loss of the kidney. The mortality is significantly greater in the pregnant population, where it is associated with a 50% maternal mortality and a 75% fetal mortality. Traditionally a 2-cm diameter was considered the threshold for repair, but many authorities now advise waiting until the aneurysm reaches 3 cm or larger in light of a benign natural history of renal artery aneurysms. Preoperative imaging with thin-cut high-quality computed tomography angiogram of the abdomen is performed. Three-dimensional reconstruction is imperative to define the aneurysm and branch anatomy preoperatively. Most of these aneurysms are saccular and arise at the bifurcation/branch points, and 75% are bilateral.

Correct Answer   **B** 10%

Reference
Klausner, J. Q., Lawrence, P. F., Harlander-Locke, M. P., et al. (2015). The contemporary management of renal artery aneurysms. *J Vasc Surg, 61*(4), 978–984. PMID: 25537277

8. RATIONALE

The saphenous vein is the most commonly used bypass conduit in about 75% of patients requiring repair of a renal artery aneurysm. However, its risks include aneurysmal dilatation over time. Therefore, the hypogastric artery is favored for children and young adults in order to avoid late degeneration. Autologous tissue is often favored due to its resistance to infection, ease of handling for branched renal artery aneurysm repair, and long-term durability. Primary patency rates with the use of saphenous vein graft and PTFE are comparable. Early graft failures are due to thrombosis or stenosis requiring urgent intervention to avoid renal compromise. An end-to-end anastomosis with generous spatulation of the graft and artery can lessen the risk of stricture. Interposition graft or endovascular techniques (transluminal angioplasty with and without stenting) in a high-risk situation are useful techniques. Over time, saphenous vein grafts may demonstrate dilation, which has been reported to occur in 20%–40% of vein grafts when used for aortorenal bypass. However, progression to a true aneurysm in these vein grafts is less common. Aneurysm at branch points, most commonly the main renal artery bifurcation, is more frequent than main renal artery lesions and requires complex repair. For saccular aneurysms, aneurysmorrhaphy with or without patching can be performed, but salvage of all branches frequently require resection, grafting, and consideration of branch reimplantation. In complex distal branch aneurysms, ex vivo repair and auto-transplantation should be considered.

Correct Answer   **C** Hypogastric artery

Reference
Coleman, D. M., & Stanley, J. C. (2015). Renal artery aneurysms. *J Vasc Surg, 62*(3), 779–785. PMID: 26213273

9. RATIONALE

Postoperative mortality following open aneurysmectomy in most high-volume centers is unusual following renal artery aneurysm repair. However, early complications, including acute thrombosis of the reconstructed renal artery or one of its branches, occurs in 1%–2% of cases. Segmental arterial occlusion usually causes a limited infarction of a small segment of the kidney, resulting in renovascular hypertension. Late stenosis of the reconstructed arteries may affect 2% of cases. Improvement in blood pressures has been observed in more than 50% of patients undergoing surgical treatment of a renal artery aneurysm without coexisting stenotic disease. Most large series document excellent postoperative renal artery patency rates well above 90% at 10 years.

Correct Answer   **A** 90% or greater

Reference
Henke, P. K., Cardneau, J. D., Welling, T. H., et al. (2001). Renal artery aneurysms: a 35-year clinical experience with 252 aneurysms in 168 patients. *Ann Surg, 234*(4), 454–462; discussion 462–453. PMID: 11573039

10. RATIONALE

The most frequent presenting feature of spontaneous renal artery dissection is uncontrolled hypertension and sudden onset of severe flank pain. Definitive diagnosis is made by catheter-based angiography, multidetector CTA, and MRA, which are quite reliable in the diagnosis of spontaneous renal artery dissection. Unilateral spontaneous renal dissection may be a risk factor for the subsequent dissection of the contralateral renal artery. Medical management with pain control and management of hypertension should be immediately started. The role of anticoagulation is controversial. Endovascular options are preferred, and in patients with luminal thrombosis, thrombolytics followed by covered stent are recommended. In this patient, a 6 Fr Ansel sheath was used for support and a 0.018″ wire was maneuvered successfully into the true lumen. Two 6 mm × 2.5 cm overlapping Viabahn (W.L. Gore, Newark, DE) stents were deployed up to the first bifurcation point, favoring the true lumen and restoring flow to the kidney. Surgical repair as a definitive treatment has also been described in the literature but carries a higher morbidity.

Correct Answer   **D** Covered stent

Reference
Afshinnia, F., Sundaram, B., Rao, P., et al. (2013). Evaluation of characteristics, associations and clinical course of isolated spontaneous renal artery dissection. *Nephrol Dial Transplant, 28*(8), 2089–2098. PMID: 23563282

11. RATIONALE

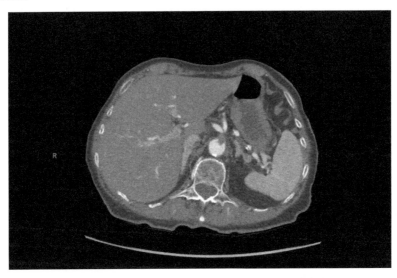

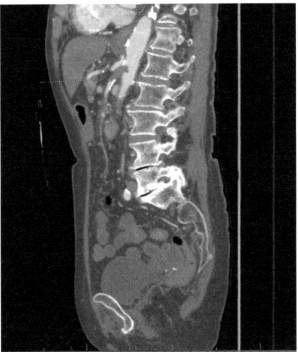

CTA filling defect at the origin of SMA is consistent with embolus.

The patient's history, lack of physical findings with elevated WBC count, and serum lactate level are suggestive of superior mesenteric artery embolus. Fluid resuscitation and an emergency CTA of the abdomen and pelvis with contrast enhancement should be performed. The findings showed a filling defect near the origin of the superior mesenteric artery with some contrast seen in the superior mesenteric artery distal to the filling defect. The patient underwent superior mesenteric artery via midline laparotomy using inframesocolic approach. Acute mesenteric ischemia is the result of superior mesenteric artery embolus in 40% of cases and is usually associated with atrial fibrillation, valvular disease, recent myocardial infarction, and arterial thrombosis in 30% of cases; arterial dissection in <5%; and venous mesenteric infarction in 5%–15% with nonocclusive mesenteric hypoperfusion in 10%–15% of cases. In contrast to thrombotic occlusion, the proximal 10–16 inches of jejunum is usually spared as the embolus lodges beyond the origin of the pancreaticoduodenal arteries near the origin of the middle colic artery. In thrombotic occlusion, the entire small bowel from the ligament of Treitz to the distal transverse colon is involved with ischemia. Emergent treatment is necessary in acute mesenteric ischemia, which has a mortality approaching 50%.

Correct Answer   **B** CT scan of the abdomen and pelvis with IV contrast

Reference
Acosta, S., & Björck, M. (2003). Acute thrombo-embolic occlusion of the superior mesenteric artery: a prospective study in a well defined population. *Eur J Vasc Endovasc Surg, 26*(2), 179–183. PMID: 12917835

12. RATIONALE

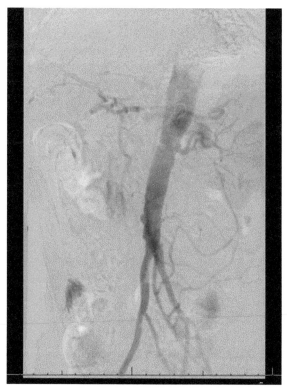

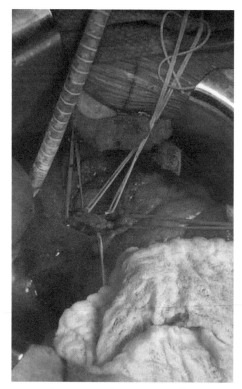

Preoperative arteriography showing occlusion of proximal superior mesenteric artery and enlarged gastroduodenal artery and arc of Rolen.

Intraoperative picture showing opened supramesenteric artery beyond occlusion and prosthetic graft to be sutured to the artery for distal anastomosis.

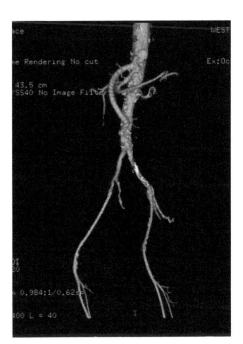

Postoperative CTA showing patent antegrade supraceliac aorta to superior mesenteric artery bypass.

The diagnosis of chronic mesenteric artery ischemia remains a challenge and results in considerable morbidity and high mortality in patients affected with this condition. One of the most devastating complications of chronic mesenteric ischemia is mesenteric arterial thrombosis resulting in infarction of the bowel. Acute arterial thrombosis superimposed on preexisting atherosclerotic disease represents the second most common cause of acute mesenteric ischemia, as up to 20% of patients with acute mesenteric ischemia have a demonstrated history of chronic mesenteric ischemia. The diagnosis can be confirmed by readily available celiac and mesenteric duplex imaging. The optimal method of treatment and type of revascularization (open versus endovascular) and type of open reconstruction (transaortic endarterectomy versus antegrade aortomesenteric versus retrograde aortomesenteric bypass) remains controversial. In most reported series long-term patency using objective means is lacking. Endovascular therapy is less invasive, but its success depends on the type of occlusion (stenosis versus total long segment occlusion). Jimenez et al. reported on 47 patients with antegrade aortomesenteric bypass using a prosthetic graft with satisfactory functional outcome, with in-hospital mortality of 11%, primary patency of 69%, primary assisted patency 94%, and secondary patency of 100% at 5 years.

Correct Answer   B Antegrade supraceliac aorta to superior mesenteric artery bypass

Reference
Jimenez, J. G., Huber, T. S., Ozaki, C. K., et al. (2002). Durability of antegrade synthetic aortomesenteric bypass for chronic mesenteric ischemia. *J Vasc Surg, 35*(6), 1078–1084. PMID: 12042717

13. RATIONALE

Diagnosis of chronic mesenteric ischemia can be challenging. Classic symptoms include "food fear" (sitophobia), abdominal pain, and weight loss. Abdominal pain is postprandial. In some patients, the clinical presentation of chronic mesenteric ischemia can be less specific with vague abdominal pain, nausea, and vomiting with or without change in bowel habits. In the past, high-grade stenosis or occlusion of at least two arteries (celiac, SMA, or IMA) had to be demonstrated before diagnosing mesenteric ischemia. Since the superior mesenteric artery supplies the major portion of the GI tract, severe stenosis or occlusion of the superior mesenteric artery in isolation can present with symptoms of chronic mesenteric ischemia. The old concept that mesenteric ischemia is due to limited blood supply to the small intestine during digestion has been challenged. The latest concept is that ischemia of the small bowel is due to preferential blood supply to the stomach upon food ingestion. Absence of collaterals (gastroduodenal, arc of Riolan or marginal artery) indicates that celiac/mesenteric arterial occlusive disease is unlikely to be hemodynamically significant.

Correct Answer   D Medical management with surveillance duplex imaging of celiac and superior mesenteric artery

Reference
Chang, R. W., Chang, J. B., & Longo, W. E. (2006). Update in management of mesenteric ischemia. *World J Gastroenterol, 12*(20), 3243–3247. PMID: 16718846

14. RATIONALE

A retrograde bypass originating from the distal abdominal aorta or from the right common iliac artery to the superior mesenteric artery in selected high-risk patients for whom an endo-vascular option does not exist can be used. This operation is performed using a transperitoneal approach. An 8-mm externally supported PTFE graft is selected. The superior mesenteric artery is exposed in the root of the mesentery to the right of the superior mesenteric vein and is dis-sected up to the level of the left renal vein. The distal aorta and right common iliac artery are mobilized. The inflow anastomosis is performed first in an end-to-side fashion. The superior mesenteric artery anastomosis is performed in an end-to-side antegrade manner. It is impera-tive to allow a gentle curve (C shape) for the graft to avoid kinking as the bowel returns to its normal anatomic position in the abdomen. The graft is covered with the retroperitoneum and greater omentum depending on the anatomical situation. An autologous conduit (femoral-pop-liteal vein) is preferred in patients with bowel infarction requiring resection.

Correct Answer   C Retrograde bypass using a ringed prosthetic graft from infrarenal aorta or right common iliac artery to superior mesenteric artery

Reference
Cho, J. S., Carr, J. A., Jacobsen, G., et al. (2002). Long-term outcome after mesenteric artery reconstruc-tion: a 37-year experience. *J Vasc Surg, 35*(3), 453–460. PMID: 11877692

15. RATIONALE

Trapdoor aortic endarterectomy is best indicated in the setting of chronic mesenteric ischemia with significant perivisceral aortic disease. It is most useful when the occlusion of the celiac and superior mesenteric artery is confined to the proximal 2–3 cm. This operation should not be used for acute mesenteric ischemia. The aorta is exposed using a left flank retroperitoneal approach with the incision extending to the ninth intercostal space. The left kidney is mobilized anteriorly, and the lumbar vein of the left renal vein is identified, ligated, and divided. Left crus of the diaphragm is divided, and the supraceliac aorta with the origin of celiac and superior mesenteric artery is exposed. The supraceliac aorta is dissected circumferentially. Following heparinization, the aorta is clamped 2–3 cm above the celiac axis and 2–3 cm below the superior mesenteric artery. The distal clamp may have to be placed below the left renal artery. The celiac axis and superior mesenteric artery are controlled with double silastic vessel loops. Intravenous mannitol (25–50 gm) is administered by the anesthesia team. The aortotomy is performed around the orifices of the celiac and superior mesenteric artery. The plane of endarterectomy is developed, and the visceral vessel orifices and extraction of the plaque is carried out with a smooth feathered end. The aortotomy is closed with 4-0 cardiovascular polypropylene suture.

Correct Answer   **D** Trapdoor aortic endarterectomy

Reference

Cho, J. S., Carr, J. A., Jacobsen, G., et al. (2002). Long-term outcome after mesenteric artery reconstruction: a 37-year experience. *J Vasc Surg, 35*(3), 453–460. PMID: 11877692

16. **RATIONALE**

In the presence of bowel ischemia, one should strongly consider using autologous vein reconstruction. Although more time consuming and with the potential risks of kinking, redundancy, and twisting, autologous grafts are more resistant to infection. One should be cognizant of the anatomic position of the anastomosed bypass to the superior mesenteric artery, as the bypass may assume a slightly different course when the bowel is returned to its proper anatomical position.

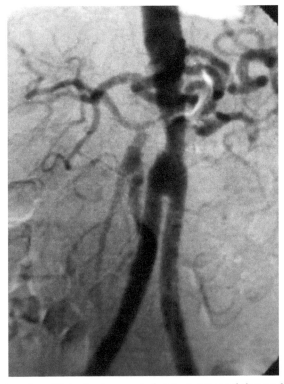

During ABF graft distal 16 inches of small intestine became ischemic. A retrograde bypass from the right limb of the graft to SMA using reversed GSV–postoperative DSA.

Correct Answer **D** Retrograde bypass from the right limb of the aortobifemoral graft to the superior mesenteric artery using great saphenous vein harvested from the groin and upper thigh

Reference

Hans, S. S. (2020). Mesenteric revascularization in a patient with acute on chronic bowel ischemia. In S. S. Hans (Ed.), *Challenging arterial reconstructions: 100 clinical cases* (pp. 229–233). Cham, Switzerland: Springer Nature Switzerland AG.

17. RATIONALE

Retrograde open superior mesenteric artery stenting is an attractive alternative to open bypass or percutaneous stenting in patients with acute mesenteric ischemia who require abdominal exploration and in those with flush mesenteric occlusion who have failed to respond to conservative treatment and are unsuitable for stenting using percutaneous access. During abdominal exploration, the transverse mesocolon is retracted cranially. The rest of the mesentery is retracted to the right and opened longitudinally anterior to the superior mesenteric artery. The superior mesenteric artery and its branches are dissected free and controlled with silastic vessel loops. Following systemic heparinization the superior mesenteric artery is accessed in a retrograde manner using a 0.018-inch micropuncture kit, which is subsequently exchanged for a 0.035-inch guide wire, and a 6 Fr sheath is inserted. Limited angiography is performed. A 5 Fr catheter angled 0.035″, 180 cm glide wire (Terumo Interventional System, Sommerset, NJ) is used to cross the superior mesenteric artery lesion into the abdominal aorta. The wire is then exchanged for a stiff Amplatz guide wire (Cook Medical, Bloomington, IN). Primary stenting with a balloon-expandable stent is performed. If retrograde access could not be obtained, antegrade access via a left brachial access approach may be used.

Correct Answer **C** Retrograde superior mesenteric artery stenting and bowel resection with bowel in discontinuity

Reference

Oderich, G. S., Macedo, R., Stone, D. H., et al. (2018). Multicenter study of retrograde open mesenteric artery stenting through laparotomy for treatment of acute and chronic mesenteric ischemia. *J Vasc Surg, 68*(2), 470–480.e471. PMID: 29548812

18. RATIONALE

Superior mesenteric artery stenting is less durable than open bypass, with a lower primary patency and significant incidence of in-stent restenosis (20%–66%). Treatment with stent angioplasty is recommended in patients who develop recurrent symptoms of chronic mesenteric ischemia or those with preocclusive in-stent restenosis. Tallarita et al. reported on 30 patients with reintervention for mesenteric artery in-stent restenosis, with 24 patients presenting with recurrent symptoms (21 chronic, 3 acute), and 6 had asymptomatic preocclusive lesions. Twenty-six patients underwent repeat endovascular treatment with stent placement in 17 and stent angioplasty in 9. The remaining four patients had open bypass, and one was performed for acute ischemia. Mesenteric reinterventions were associated with low mortality (3%), high complication rate (27%), and excellent symptom improvement (92%).

Correct Answer **C** Stent angioplasty

Reference
Tallarita, T., Oderich, G. S., Macedo, T. A., et al. (2011). Reinterventions for stent restenosis in patients treated for atherosclerotic mesenteric artery disease. *J Vasc Surg*, 54(5), 1422–1429.e1421. PMID: 21963821

19. RATIONALE

Embolization is a dreaded complication that can be identified following a technically successful angioplasty and stenting. Some inherent risks arise from the "shaggy aorta." These irregularities can include soft plaque, calcific lesions, and ectatic segment that are crossed with the balloon or stent delivery system. To reduce the risk of distal embolization in these high-risk patients, it is paramount to have adequate preprocedure planning so that the approach allows for the least catheter manipulation within the diseased aorta. In patients with severe acute angle of a superior mesenteric artery in a diseased aortic segment, the femoral approach has an increased risk of distal embolization. On the contrary, if the descending thoracic aorta has severe disease, a retrograde femoral approach may be safer. Filter options should be considered in patients with a high risk of embolization. Predilatation of the target lesion should not be overly aggressive and should be performed to allow a safe passage of the stent. Inadequate anticoagulation can result in thrombus formation in the sheath or catheter. If embolization does occur, aspiration embolectomy catheters can be used to clear the debris by advancing the large-bore sheath close to the embolic debris and performing strong aspiration. If the sheath cannot be advanced to the area of embolization, a 5 Fr diagnostic catheter or an aspiration embolectomy catheter such as Export catheter (Medtronic Corp., Santa Ana, CA) can be used to aspirate the debris. If aspiration is not successful, inflating the balloon may break the emboli into smaller pieces, resulting in occlusion of very small branches of the mesenteric arteries and resulting in minimal ischemic damage.

Correct Answer   D Preprocedure planning with selection of arterial access and availability of filter options

Reference
Molnar, R. G., & Gandillion, C. (2021). Complications of endovascular therapy for occlusive disease of splanchnic arteries including renal arteries. In S. S. Hans & M. J. Conrad (Eds.), *Vascular and endovascular complications: a practical approach* (pp. 35–40). Boca Raton, FL: CRC Press.

20. RATIONALE

A meticulous technique ensuring true luminal positioning of the crossing wire is fundamental in treating occlusive lesions of the visceral vessels. Once the crossing catheter is confirmed to be in the true lumen, a 0.014″ support wire and the use of balloon-expandable stents should be used in small-diameter vessels with eccentric high-grade stenotic plaques. Balloon-expandable stents are necessary for these ostial lesions to provide strong radial force. For severely diseased segments, predilation with a standard balloon to approximately greater than 5% of the reference vessel diameter will allow for safe placement of the stent at the target lesion. If this is not performed, the balloon-mounted stent may not be able to cross the lesion without resistance and with the possibility of stent becoming dislodged from the balloon. The stent size should be one-to-one with the reference vessel diameter to avoid vessel perforation; distal dissection and undersizing can lead to malposition of the stent. Should the crossing wire not be within the true lumen, the stent will be deployed in a subintimal plane and will likely lead to vessel occlusion.

Correct Answer **D** Ensuring true lumen position of the crossing wire by contrast injection through a low-profile crossing catheter

Reference
Molnar, R. G., & Gandillion, C. (2021). Complications of endovascular therapy for occlusive disease of splanchnic arteries including renal arteries. In S. S. Hans & M. J. Conrad (Eds.), *Vascular and endovascular complications: a practical approach* (pp. 35–40). Boca Raton, FL: CRC Press.

21. RATIONALE

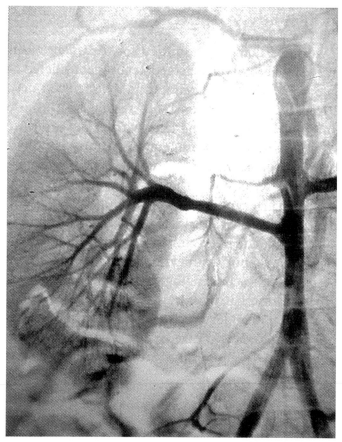

Aortorenal bypass with an internal iliac artery graft. (Reproduced with permission from Stanley JC, Zelenock GB, Messina LM, et al. (1995). Pediatric renovascular hypertension: a thirty-year experience of operative treatment. *J Vasc Surg*, 21,219.)

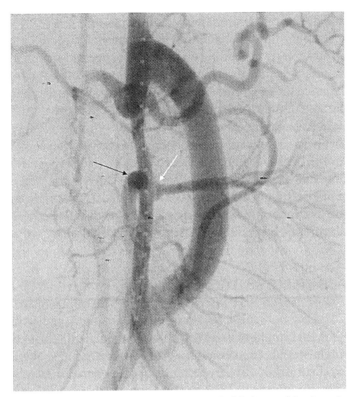

Renal artery-aortic (white arrow) and superior mesenteric artery-aortic (black arrow) implantation in conjunction with a thoracoabdominal bypass for a suprarenal abdominal aortic coarctation and severe ostial stenoses of the implanted arteries. (Reproduced with permission from Stanley JC, Criado E, Upchurch GR Jr., et al. (2006). Pediatric renovascular hypertension: 132 primary and 30 secondary operations in 97 children. *J Vasc Surg*, 44:1219–1228. p. 1225.)

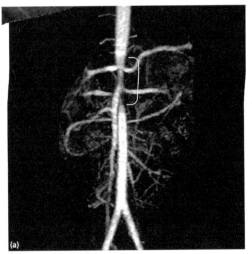 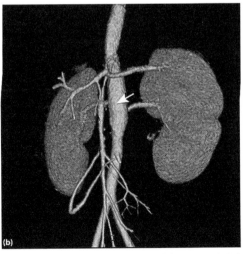

Intrarenal abdominal aortic coarctation (bracket), (a) associated with renal artery ostial stenoses. (b) Proximal abdominal patch aortoplasty (arrow) and bilateral renal artery aortic implantations. (Reproduced with permission from Stanley JC, Criado E, Eliason JL, et al. (2008). Abdominal aortic coarctation: surgical treatment of 53 patients with a thoracoabdominal bypass, patch aortoplasty, or interposition aortoaortic graft. *J Vasc Surg*, 44:1073–1082. p. 1077.)

Patients with TA should undergo vascular reconstruction when the disease is in remission. Renal artery-aortic reimplantation with abdominal aortic patch angioplasty using a PTFE patch is preferred, as the Dacron patch may undergo late aneurysmal deterioration. Patches are made large enough so as not to be constrictive as the child grows into adulthood. In certain instances, a primary thoracoabdominal bypass is favored over aortoplasty because of the patient's age and the risk of anastomotic disease affecting the renal or splanchnic arteries. PTFE prostheses are preferable over a Dacron graft. Extraperitoneal reflection of the abdominal viscera provides excellent access to the upper abdominal aorta, which is the site of bypass origin. Grafts originating in the chest are easily tunneled through the posterior diaphragm, behind the left kidney though the distal aorta. Critical ostial stenosis of the celiac and superior mesenteric artery should be reconstructed at the time of treatment of developmental aortic and renal artery narrowing. However, many children are often critically ill, which will add to the complexity of the procedure. Recurrent stenosis or technical failures affect nearly 15% of these.

Correct Answer **B** Primary angioplasty with PTFE patch and bilateral renal artery reimplantation

Reference
Stanley, J. C., Criado, E., Eliason, J. L., et al. (2008). Abdominal aortic coarctation: surgical treatment of 53 patients with a thoracoabdominal bypass, patch aortoplasty, or interposition aortoaortic graft. *J Vasc Surg*, *48*(5), 1073–1082. PMID: 18692352

22. RATIONALE

Exposure of aortorenal bypass procedures in children is like that undertaken in adults undergoing similar bypass procedures. The internal iliac artery is the preferred conduit when treating mid-stenosis or distal main renal artery stenosis in children. In children, stenosis involving the origin of the main renal artery, small-diameter renal artery branches, or accessory renal arteries beyond a stenotic segment can be implanted into aorta. In the case of branches, an accessory renal artery can be implanted into the non-diseased adjacent main or segmental renal artery. Anastomoses are spatulated and completed with interrupted sutures in very young children with small arteries. Stenosis of multiple small renal arteries may require approximation of these vessels to form a large common orifice to which an aortorenal graft can be anastomosed. Synthetic prosthetic grafts are rarely used for pediatric renal artery reconstruction because of the risk of infection, technical difficulties, and unpredictable long-term durability. Vein grafts are not favored because of their propensity to undergo late aneurysmal dilation. When other, more acceptable reconstructive procedures prove impossible and a vein is the only conduit available, it should be covered with a synthetic mesh to decrease the chance of aneurysmal dilation.

Correct Answer **D** Internal iliac artery graft

Reference
Stanley, J. C., Criado, E., Eliason, J. L., et al. (2008). Abdominal aortic coarctation: surgical treatment of 53 patients with a thoracoabdominal bypass, patch aortoplasty, or interposition aortoaortic graft. *J Vasc Surg*, *48*(5), 1073–1082. PMID: 18692352

23. RATIONALE

Direct renal artery implantation and single-staged concomitant aortic reconstruction offer excellent results with a cure of hypertension in 70%, improved in 25%, and unchanged in 5%, with a negligible operative mortality. Impaired renal function before and after the operative procedure occurs in <1% of these patients. Recurrent stenosis or technical failure affects nearly 15% of these young children and will require later secondary intervention. These children have very complex disease, and optimal care demands careful planning of open arterial reconstruction.

Correct Answer   **C** 70% of patients

Reference
Stanley, J. C., Criado, E., Eliason, J. L., et al. (2008). Abdominal aortic coarctation: surgical treatment of 53 patients with a thoracoabdominal bypass, patch aortoplasty, or interposition aortoaortic graft. *J Vasc Surg, 48*(5), 1073–1082. PMID: 18692352

SECTION 11: UPPER EXTREMITY ARTERIAL DISEASE

MCQs 1–10

Q1. The most common reason for repair of a subclavian artery aneurysm is:
A. To prevent thromboembolic complications
B. Brachial plexopathy
C. Subclavian vein compression
D. To prevent rupture

Q2. The most common nerve injured during open repair of a subclavian artery aneurysm in its second portion is:
A. Vagus
B. Recurrent laryngeal
C. Phrenic
D. Lower cord of brachial plexus

Q3. The incidence of axillary and brachial artery aneurysms among peripheral artery aneurysms is:
A. <1%
B. 1%–3%
C. 3.1%–4%
D. 4.1%–5%

Q4. Repair of axillary and brachial artery aneurysm is recommended for an aneurysm size of:
A. 0.5–1 cm
B. 1.1–1.5 cm
C. 1.6–1.9 cm
D. >2 cm

Q5. For distal ulnar arterial bypass, the conduit of choice is:
A. Great saphenous vein
B. Basilic vein/cephalic vein from ipsilateral arm

C. Basilic vein/cephalic vein from contralateral arm
D. Contralateral radial artery

Q6. Patients with critical hand ischemia resulting from arterial occlusive disease secondary to diabetes mellitus and associated end-stage renal disease have a 2-year survival of:
A. 60%
B. 50%
C. 45%
D. 30%

Q7. Hypothenar hammer syndrome is caused by:
A. Occlusion of the radial artery
B. Trauma to the distal ulnar artery as it passes through Guyon canal
C. Post-stenotic dilatation/aneurysm from arterial thoracic outlet syndrome
D. Scleroderma

Q8. Upper extremity compartment syndrome most often involves:
A. Extensor compartment
B. Superficial flexor compartment
C. Deep flexor compartment
D. Superficial and deep flexor compartments

Q9. The risks of upper extremity ischemia in patients with occlusion of an axillofemoral graft is:
A. <1%
B. 1%–2%
C. 2.5%
D. 3%

DOI: 10.1201/9781003389897-11

Q10. **Anastomotic disruption and pseudoaneu-rysm following axillofemoral bypass graft at proximal anastomosis is due to:**

A. Technical error

B. Infection

C. Failure to leave redundancy in the graft

D. Infection, technical error, and failure to leave redundancy in the graft

RATIONALE 1–10

1. RATIONALE

The majority of subclavian artery aneurysms (SAAs) are located in the proximal segment (39%). The middle segment accounts for 25% and distal segment 24% with associated involvement of the proximal axillary artery. Indications for subclavian artery aneurysm repair include size >2 cm, symptoms, or size >1.5 cm and concurrent operation for other aortic pathology. Proximal aneurysms are mostly caused by atherosclerotic disease, collagen disorders, trauma, and infection. The middle segment SAAs are mainly caused by collagen disorders and trauma. Distal SAAs are mostly described in relation to thoracic outlet syndrome or as a consequence of blunt or penetrating trauma. Most patients present with a pulsating mass and shoulder pain. Other symptoms include pain from distal embolization and symptoms from local compression, thrombosis, and rupture. Duplex ultrasound scanning for distal SCCA, CTA, and catheter-based angiography are often necessary prior to open repair. Despite the increasing interest in endovascular repair of the aneurysm, open repair of the subclavian artery is preferable and requires thoracotomy. For repair of proximal SAAs, sternotomy without supraclavicular and transclavicular/infraclavicular incision with partial resection of the clavicle may be necessary. The majority of subclavian artery aneurysm and nearly all aberrant subclavian artery aneurysms can now be repaired using a TEVAR-based approach without the need for sternotomy or thoracotomy.

Correct Answer   **A** To prevent thromboembolic complications

Reference
Andersen, N. D., Barfield, M. E., Hanna, J. M., et al. (2013). Intrathoracic subclavian artery aneurysm repair in the thoracic endovascular aortic repair era. *J Vasc Surg, 57*(4), 915–925. PMID: 23375432

2. RATIONALE

The recurrent laryngeal nerve injury is the most common nerve to be injured during open repair of a subclavian artery aneurysm resulting in hoarseness. Stent graft repair is being increasingly utilized, but these options are dependent on the anatomical characteristics of the aneurysm and vascular access. Traumatic subclavian artery aneurysm and iatrogenic subclavian artery aneurysm are best repaired using endovascular techniques. Patency of the reconstruction following endovascular repair may further improve with the development of better stent grafts, as in-stent stenosis and thrombosis were reported in an earlier series.

Correct Answer   **B** Recurrent laryngeal

Reference
Vierhout, B. P., Zeebregts, C. J., van den Dungen, J. J., & Reijnen, M. M. (2010). Changing profiles of diagnostic and treatment options in subclavian artery aneurysms. *Eur J Vasc Endovasc Surg, 40*(1), 27–34. PMID: 20399124

3. RATIONALE

Most aneurysms involving the upper extremity arteries are posttraumatic or secondary to connective tissue disorders or congenital in origin. These aneurysms are relatively uncommon and account for <1% of all peripheral artery aneurysms. Chronic repetitive trauma from the use of crutches can cause aneurysmal degeneration in the proximity arteries (axillary and high brachial) in the upper extremity. All symptomatic true and all pseudoaneurysms in the axillary and brachial artery distribution should be repaired. Brachial and radial artery pseudoaneurysms may be secondary to vascular access for coronary or peripheral arteriography with or without associated intervention. Mycotic pseudoaneurysms have also been reported in patients with a history of intravenous drug abuse. During repair of axillary and brachial artery aneurysms, the median nerve needs to be protected, as the median nerve courses lateral to the brachial artery in the upper arm. However, the nerve crosses the artery from the lateral to medial side as it descends. Just before it enters the forearm, the medial nerve passes between the tendons of the biceps brachii and brachialis.

Correct Answer   **A** <1%

Reference
Gray, R. J., Stone, W. M., Fowl, R. J., et al. (1998). Management of true aneurysms distal to the axillary artery. *J Vasc Surg, 28*(4), 606–610. PMID: 9786253

4. RATIONALE

All symptomatic true or pseudoaneurysms involving the axillary and brachial artery should be repaired. The most common presentation of axillary and brachial artery aneurysms is distal embolization resulting in hand ischemia. Patients may also present with neurological symptoms associated with brachial plexus (axillary artery) or median nerve (brachial artery) compression. Pseudoaneurysm due to infection can be safely ligated due to abundant collaterals. Asymptomatic true aneurysms should be repaired if equal to or greater than 2 cm in transverse/AP diameter. Primary repair, resection with end-to-end anastomosis, patch angioplasty and interposition graft are many options for repair depending upon the anatomy and local findings at the time of repair.

Correct Answer   **D** >2 cm

Reference
Gray, R. J., Stone, W. M., Fowl, R. J., et al. (1998). Management of true aneurysms distal to the axillary artery. *J Vasc Surg, 28*(4), 606–610. PMID: 9786253

5. RATIONALE

For distal ulnar artery bypass, the conduit of choice is the contralateral radial artery because of a better size match and superior long-term performance. Continuity of the palmar arch is evaluated by the Allen test and duplex imaging before the radial artery is harvested. Either end-to-side or end-to-end anastomosis is performed with an interrupted or running 7-0 polypropylene suture under optical magnification.

Correct Answer   **D** Contralateral radial artery

Reference
Bassiouny, H. S. (2017). Upper extremity arterial bypass. In S. S. Hans, A. D. Shepard, H. R. Weaver, P. G. Bove, & G. W. Long (Eds.), *Endovascular and open vascular reconstructions: a practical approach* (pp. 191–196). Boca Raton, FL: CRC Press.

6. RATIONALE

Hemodialysis and complications of hemodialysis access such as steal syndrome are risk factors for chronic hand ischemia. This is usually the result of progressive atherosclerosis involving arteries of the palmar arch and digital arteries. As the number of patients on hemodialysis are living longer, it is conceivable that patients with chronic hand ischemia will increase. The role of endovascular therapy, except for balloon angioplasty, in forearm arteries is limited except in patients with associated proximal stenotic lesions in the subclavian/axillary/brachial artery. The prognosis of patients with chronic hand ischemia is poor, with 44% survival at a mean follow-up of 26.8 months.

Correct Answer   **C** 45%

Reference
Tomoi, Y., Soga, Y., Fujihara, M., et al. (2016). Outcomes of endovascular therapy for upper extremity peripheral artery disease with critical hand ischemia. *J Endovasc Ther, 23*(5), 717–722. PMID: 27421289

7. RATIONALE

Hypothenar hammer syndrome results from repetitive trauma to the ulnar artery at the hypothenar eminence as it exits Guyon canal and branches into superficial and deep palmar arches. The ring (fourth) finger is most frequently symptomatic, whereas the thumb is spared due to its radial artery blood supply. A pulsatile mass secondary to ulnar artery aneurysm may be present. In many patients, the aneurysm is thrombosed and there is associated embolization with significant ischemia of the hand and fingers. Duplex imaging and upper extremity catheter-based arteriography or CT angiography is diagnostic. Treatment is initially conservative depending on the severity of symptoms and digital ischemia. Conservative therapy consists of avoidance of initiating trauma, palmar padding, cessation of smoking, and antiplatelet medications. Surgical treatment is indicated when conservative management fails, aneurysm formation is present, or digital ischemia is severe. Interventions include sympathectomy and surgical excision of the aneurysm with end-to-end anastomosis, as there is associated tortuosity of the artery. However, an interposition graft using an autologous vein or contralateral radial/ulnar artery may be necessary. Long-term graft patency is variable, with up to 75% occlusion of vein grafts at 10 years.

Correct Answer   **B** Trauma to the distal ulnar artery as it passes through Guyon canal

Reference
Ravari, H., Johari, H. G., & Rajabnejad, A. (2018). Hypothenar hammer syndrome: surgical approach in patients presenting with ulnar artery aneurysm. *Ann Vasc Surg, 50*, 284–287. PMID: 29477685

8. RATIONALE

The compartment syndrome of the forearm is associated with high-energy injuries to the upper extremity with or without brachial artery occlusion. The decompression of the upper extremity compartment syndrome involves the volar approach using a curvilinear incision that begins proximal to the antecubital fossa and medial to the biceps tendon, where it crosses the antecubital crease and extends to the radial side of the forearm, where it extends distally along the medial border of brachioradialis muscle. The incision from the distal forearm extends across the carpal tunnel along the thenar crease. The fascia overlying the superficial compartment is incised along the entire length of the skin incision. The radial nerve and the brachioradialis muscle are retracted to the radial side of the forearm, and the flexor carpi radialis and the radial artery are retracted to the ulnar side. The fascia covering the muscles of the deep flexor compartment is incised to complete the superficial and deep flexor compartment fasciotomy. Fasciotomy of the hand depends on the symptoms of pain with passive stretch or extension of the fingers associated with swelling of the hand. All patients require careful carpal tunnel release.

Correct Answer **D** Superficial and deep flexor compartment

Reference
Friedrich, J. B., & Shin, A. Y. (2007). Management of forearm compartment syndrome. *Hand Clin, 23*(2), 245–254, vii. PMID: 17548015

9. RATIONALE

Upper extremity ischemia following axillofemoral bypass graft occlusions has been reported in 2.5% of cases. Arterial steal syndrome has also been described after axillofemoral graft reconstruction. Axillary artery thrombosis may occur as a result of sharp angulation, or "pulling down," of the artery from graft due to tension. The residual stump of the proximal anastomosis of a nonfunctioning axillofemoral bypass graft may also be a source of arterial emboli to the distal ipsilateral upper extremity. If this occurs, in addition to performing thrombo-embolectomy of the upper extremity, the axillary anastomosis should be taken down and patch angioplasty at the site of anastomosis performed to prevent future embolic events.

Correct Answer **C** 2.5%

Reference
Rashleigh-Belcher, H. J., & Newcombe, J. F. (1987). Axillary artery thrombosis: a complication of axillofemoral bypass grafts. *Surgery, 101*(3), 373–375. PMID: 3824166

10. RATIONALE

Anastomotic disruption in the early postoperative period is likely to occur as a result of a technical error. Late disruptions are highly concerning for infection. Failure to leave some redundancy on the graft can cause excessive tension, which may lead to disruption even after a minor trauma or shoulder movement. Proximal anastomosis should be constructed at the first portion of the axillary artery (medial to pectoralis minor), as the axillary artery does not have significant variation in its length during arm movement in its first portion. Proximal anastomotic disruption may be associated with forceful movement of the ipsilateral upper extremity such as arm abduction or shoulder elevation. Patients often present with pain, swelling, and pulsatile mass. Duplex ultrasound and CT angiography are confirmatory. Surgical repair usually includes the need for supraclavicular exposure of the subclavian artery for proximal control. Balloon occlusion of the subclavian artery is another option for obtaining proximal control, following which the axillary artery is repaired with patch angioplasty or a short interposition graft, making certain that there is no tension in the graft.

Correct Answer **D** Infection, technical error, and failure to leave redundancy in the graft

Reference
Piazza, D., Ameli, F. M., von Schroeder, H. P., & Lossing, A. (1993). Nonanastomotic pseudoaneurysm of expanded polytetrafluoroethylene axillofemoral bypass graft. *J Vasc Surg, 17*(4), 777–779. PMID: 8464101

SECTION 12: VASCULAR TRAUMA

MCQs 1–16

Q1. The hard signs of cervical penetrating vascular injury are all of the following except:
- **A.** Pulsatile bleeding
- **B.** Audible bruit/palpable thrill
- **C.** Expanding hematoma
- **D.** Diminished pulse

Q2. A 30-year-old man presented with a large stab wound to zone II of his neck. There was clear violation of the platysma muscle and partial transection of the sternocleidomastoid muscle. The patient is hemodynamically stable. The next best option is:

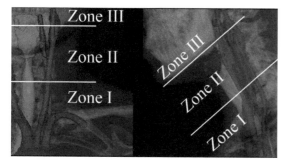

- **A.** Diagnostic neck exploration
- **B.** CTA
- **C.** Catheter-based arteriography
- **D.** Observation in the ICU

Q3. Following a zone II penetrating neck injury, a 21-year-old man presents with a pulsatile mass in the middle of the right neck with unstable cervical spine fracture. CTA of the neck shows a carotid pseudoaneurysm. The best management option is:

- **A.** Open repair first followed by neck fixation
- **B.** Fixation of neck fracture first followed by open repair
- **C.** Stent graft repair
- **D.** Carotid ligation

Q4. A 38-year-old man is involved in an MVA and sustained greater than 25% intimal injury to the right common carotid artery. There is no associated neurological deficit. There is no other head or torso injury. Optimal management consists of:
- **A.** Observation
- **B.** Antiplatelet medication
- **C.** Heparin
- **D.** Stenting

Q5. A 45-year-old man presents with 25% left vertebral artery intimal injury with a Glasgow Coma Scale score of 12. Optimal management consists of:
- **A.** Antiplatelet medications
- **B.** Observation
- **C.** Heparin
- **D.** Stenting

Q6. A 36-year-old man sustained a grade II intramural hematoma of the thoracic aorta at the isthmus with no other significant injuries. Optimal management consists of:
- **A.** Thoracic stent graft
- **B.** Observation
- **C.** Open repair
- **D.** Thoracic stent graft with left subclavian to carotid bypass

DOI: 10.1201/9781003389897-12

Q7. Greater than 25% oversizing of the thoracic stent graft for blunt thoracic aortic injury may result in:
A. Pseudoaneurysm
B. Rupture
C. Distal aortic dissection
D. Stent graft collapse

Q8. A 36-year-old woman sustained a traumatic aortic injury involving 30% of the circumference of the abdominal aorta and concomitant inferior vena cava injury with small bowel laceration. The optimal management following resuscitation includes laparotomy, antibiotics, and:
A. Primary repair of the aorta and interposition of a 12-mm PTFE graft for inferior vena cava reconstruction
B. Primary repair of the aorta and replacement of the inferior vena cava with a rifampin-soaked Dacron graft
C. Repair of the aorta with bovine pericardial patch angioplasty and interposition with 12-mm PTFE graft for IVC reconstruction
D. Repair of the aorta with bovine pericardial patch angioplasty and interposition bovine carotid graft for inferior vena cava injury

Q9. A 54-year-old woman undergoes right total knee replacement for degenerative arthritis. She had a prior history of tibial osteotomy. In the recovery room the right foot is slightly cooler than the left; ABI on the right is 0.9 and on the left is 1.0. The next best option is:
A. Explore the right popliteal artery via a medial approach
B. Obtain catheter-based arteriogram of the right lower extremity
C. CTA of the lower extremity
D. IV heparinization and close monitoring in the ICU

Q10. A 78-year-old woman complains of pain and swelling in the right calf for the past 2 months following right total knee arthroplasty. Duplex venous study is negative for deep venous thrombosis, but there is suggestion of right popliteal pseudoaneurysm behind the knee. The best management option is:
A. Thrombin injection into the pseudoaneurysm
B. Ultrasonic compression
C. Covered stent via contralateral femoral approach
D. Open repair

Q11. A 68-year-old man underwent coronary stenting using right radial artery access. Two months later the patient presented with a 2 cm × 2 cm pulsatile mass on the right radial aspect of the front of the wrist joint. The next best management option is:
A. Open exploration of the volar aspect of the wrist, including duplex imaging with Allen test
B. CTA of the right upper extremity
C. Duplex imaging of the ulnar artery with Allen test
D. Catheter-based arteriography of right upper extremity

Q12. A 21-year-old man sustained a gunshot wound to the left groin 3 inches below the groin crease and 1 cm lateral to the midinguinal point. On examination he has a non-expansile, moderate-size hematoma in the left groin. The right groin appears to be normal. The next best management option is:
A. Real-time duplex ultrasonography of the left groin
B. Catheter-based arteriography
C. CTA
D. Measurements of ankle-brachial index

Q13. The peak incidence of tracheoinnominate fistula occurs after how many days following tracheostomy:
A. 0–6 days
B. 7–14 days
C. 15–20 days
D. 21–30 days

Q14. **Open surgical repair of tracheoinnominate artery fistula is associated with:**
- **A.** 20% mortality
- **B.** 30% mortality
- **C.** 40% mortality
- **D.** 50% mortality

Q15. **Following knee arthroscopy and meniscectomy, a 48-year-old woman develops popliteal venous pseudoaneurysm and popliteal arterial venous fistula. The best management option is:**
- **A.** Thrombin injection in the neck of the pseudoaneurysm
- **B.** Covered stent deployment in the popliteal vein
- **C.** Coil embolization of the neck of pseudoaneurysm and covered stent in the popliteal artery at the site of fistula
- **D.** Direct open repair

Q16. **Ten years following stapling of the biceps tendon at the left shoulder a 49-year-old man presented with acquired arterial venous fistula arising from the branches of axillary artery. The best management strategy is:**
- **A.** Sclerotherapy
- **B.** Covered stent placement excluding the feeding branches of the axillary artery
- **C.** Surgical excision
- **D.** Coil embolization with coaxial microcatheter using access from the brachial artery, basilic vein, and cephalic vein and placement of a covered stent at the origin of the feeding branches of the axillary artery

RATIONALE 1–16

1. RATIONALE

Penetrating neck trauma represents 1% of all traumatic injuries in the United States, resulting in up to 3%–6% of all mortalities from great vessel injury. The initial decision to operate is based on the hard signs of vascular trauma which includes (a) pulsatile bleeding, (b) palpable thrill/audible bruit, and (c) expanding hematoma. Further diagnostic imaging (soft signs) is warranted in patients with a history of moderate hemorrhage, diminished pulse, and stable size of the hematoma. Surgical exploration is also warranted in patients with evidence of cerebral ischemia (neurological deficit) or altered mental status and evidence of tracheobronchial injury (esophageal disruption manifested as palpable crepitus, air bubbling from the penetrating injury, and respiratory distress).

Correct Answer   **D** Diminished pulse

Reference

Brywczynski, J. J., Barrett, T. W., Lyon, J. A., & Cotton, B. A. (2008). Management of penetrating neck injury in the emergency department: a structured literature review. *Emerg Med J, 25*(11), 711–715. PMID: 18955599

2. RATIONALE

Zone II injuries with platysma violation were traditionally managed with mandatory diagnostic neck exploration. However, this approach resulted in historically high rates of negative findings ranging from 30% to 89%. Cervical computed tomographic angiography is becoming the initial modality of choice for all stable patients because of its scanning speed, widespread availability, and technical ease of performance. The sensitivity of CTA for detecting vascular injury approaches 100%, making it a suitable replacement for catheter-based arteriography, with the added benefit of identifying aerodigestive injuries.

Correct Answer   **B** CTA

Reference

Demetriades, D., Asensio, J. A., Velmahos, G., & Thal, E. (1996). Complex problems in penetrating neck trauma. *Surg Clin North Am, 76*(4), 661–683. PMID: 8782468

3. RATIONALE

In patients with unstable neck fractures, open repair of vascular injury may result in cervical spinal cord ischemia during intubation and neck positioning. Carotid ligation is a morbid procedure, with a stroke rate of 30%, and is usually recommended for gunshot wounds involving the neck, face, and oropharynx with brisk back bleeding from a large circumferential defect in the distal internal carotid artery (zone III) in an unstable patient who is otherwise comatose. The procedural mortality rate is reported to be 45%. Open repair of CCA/ICA in a patient without neurological deficit has a 1% rate of permanent deficit. Patients with a neurological deficit have a 50% chance of improvement with revascularization. Carotid stent has an overall primary patency of 80% at 2 years, mortality <1%, and a stroke rate of 3.5%. A stent graft repair for carotid pseudoaneurysm would be considered the best mode of treatment in this patient.

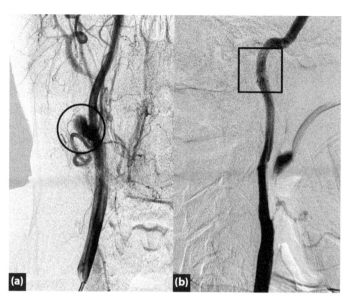

(a) Unstable neck fractures and carotid artery pseudoaneurysm (circled). (b) Treatment with stent graft-embolic protection device (squared).

Correct Answer **C** Stent graft repair

Reference
du Toit, D. F., van Schalkwyk, G. D., Wadee, S. A., & Warren, B. L. (2003). Neurologic outcome after penetrating extracranial arterial trauma. *J Vasc Surg*, *38*(2), 257–262. PMID: 12891106

4. RATIONALE

Blunt carotid artery injury is present in 0.1% of all trauma patients and 0.67% of motor vehicle accidents. The mortality is high, and a large proportion of patients have a permanent neurological deficit (58%). Screening for these injuries is based on the Denver or Memphis Criteria, and intervention is based on the grade of the injury on the Denver scale, with grade I intimal irregularity or hematoma <25% stenosis of the vessel diameter, grade II with intimal disruption or hematoma >25% stenosis of the vessel diameter, grade III pseudoaneurysm, grade IV occlusion, and grade V transection. Generally, a greater grade of injury or greater wound size warrants endovascular or open repair. In-stent thrombosis is a highly feared complication, and dual antiplatelet therapy is often employed following stent placement. Either aspirin or heparin anticoagulation is the recommended treatment in patients who have only medical management for a blunt carotid injury. In patients with contraindications to heparin, anticoagulation antiplatelet therapy should be considered. Biffl et al. reported a stroke risk of 3% in grade I patients, 11% in grade II, 33% in grade III, and 44% in grade IV if anticoagulation/antiplatelet therapy was not started. When it can be used (in the absence of head injury or intraabdominal bleeding), anticoagulation has also demonstrated trends toward improved neurological recovery in this group of patients.

Correct Answer **C** Heparin

Reference
Biffl, W. L., Moore, E. E., Offner, P. J., et al. (1999). Blunt carotid arterial injuries: implications of a new grading scale. *J Trauma*, *47*(5), 845–853. PMID: 10568710

5. RATIONALE

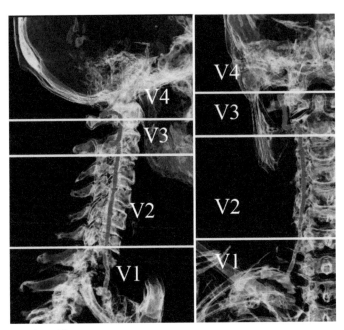

Segments of the vertebral artery (V1–V4).

Penetrating vertebral artery injury is relatively uncommon outside of the iatrogenic setting due to the vertebral arteries' relatively protected position as they course through the vertebral bodies. Blunt vertebral artery injury is relatively more common. In the absence of a cervical spine injury, vertebral artery contusion or dissection may go undiagnosed. Missed vertebral artery injury can result in vessel thrombosis and embolization causing cerebellar brainstem, mid-brain, thalamic, and areas of temporal and occipital lobe infarction (posterior circulation which may occur days to weeks after missed injury). Grading of the vertebral artery is similar to carotid artery injury on the Denver scale. Many vertebral artery injuries require only anti-coagulation or antiplatelet administration and neurological monitoring. Higher-grade injuries may require endovascular or open repair. Exposure of the vertebral artery may be beneficial for injuries to the V1 or V3 segments of the vertebral artery. The V2 and V4 segments are within the bony confines and require an endovascular approach. Open exposure of the proximal verte-bral artery requires attention to the thoracic duct, phrenic nerve, and sympathetic ganglion. Due to its proximity to the cervical transverse foramina and the skull base, the vertebral artery can be difficult to control proximally and distally, especially in the setting of laceration and hemorrhage. Proximal ligation is unlikely to result in complete resolution of bleeding due to retrograde flow from the opposite vertebral artery. Ligation of the dominant proximal vertebral artery may result in thrombosis of the basilar artery and stroke in the distribution of cerebellum and brainstem with a very high mortality.

Correct Answer   **A** Antiplatelet medications

Reference
Mwipatayi, B. P., Jeffery, P., Beningfield, S. J., et al. (2004). Management of extra-cranial vertebral artery injuries. *Eur J Vasc Endovasc Surg, 27*(2), 157–162. PMID: 14718897

6. RATIONALE

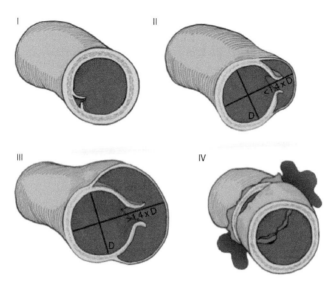

Proposed grades of blunt traumatic aortic injury.

Proposed grades of blunt traumatic injury are grade I intimal injury, grade II small pseudoaneurysm <50% circumference and injury diameter of <1.4 × normal diameter, grade III large pseudoaneurysm >50% circumference or injury diameter >1.4 normal diameter, and grade IV frank rupture. Grade I and II injuries are monitored. Grade III and IV injuries are most commonly managed with thoracic endovascular aortic aneurysm repair (TEVAR). Patients without secondary signs of injury (pseudocoarctation, mechanical hematoma, or large left hemithorax) are generally safe for waiting and a delayed repair. A novel BTAI (blunt trauma aortic injury) score was recently developed to predict early rupture in high-grade injuries more accurately than clinical assessment. This score is based on the size of the pseudoaneurysm to aortic diameter ratio (>1.4), the presence of descending thoracic aortic hematoma (>10 mm), and lactate (>4 mmol/l). There is high risk for rupture when two or more of these three risk factors are present, suggesting the need for immediate repair in these groups of patients.

Correct Answer   B Observation

Reference
Harris, D. G., Rabin, J., Kufera, J. A., et al. (2015). A new aortic injury score predicts early rupture more accurately than clinical assessment. *J Vasc Surg, 61*(2), 332–338. PMID: 25195146

7. RATIONALE

Oversizing of a thoracic stent graft for trauma in thoracic aortic injury by 20%–30% may lead to degeneration of the aortic wall over time. One study reported that a 10% increase in oversizing leads to a 3.4% increase in proximal aortic diameter. Most concerning is oversizing of 25%–30% is associated with stent graft collapse, predominately occurring in the first 2–4 weeks following placement but can also occur at a later time. Oversized TEVAR in the setting of thoracic aortic injury results in poor apposition of the lesser curve of the aortic arch, resulting in a bird-beak configuration and has been reported in 65% of patients. Some patients with bird-beak configuration go on to develop type I endoleak and stent graft collapse. In situ thrombosis due to angulation of the proximal portion of the graft may also occur along with stent graft collapse.

Correct Answer **D** Stent graft collapse

Reference

Gennai, S., Leone, N., Andreoli, F., et al. (2020). Influence of thoracic endovascular repair on aortic morphology in patients treated for blunt traumatic aortic injuries: long-term outcomes in a multicentre study. *Eur J Vasc Endovasc Surg, 59*(3), 428–436. PMID: 31911139

8. RATIONALE

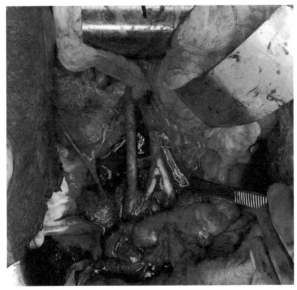

Traumatic aortic injury with concomitant IVC injury following MVA. Aorta repaired with bovine pericardial patch angioplasty. IVC repaired with bovine carotid graft due to contaminated field.

Management of abdominal vascular trauma is determined by the mechanism of injury and zone of injury. There are three zones within the abdomen and pelvis; zone I is the center portion of the abdomen and contains the aorta, mesenteric vasculature, and the inferior vena cava; zone II involves bilateral flanks and contains renal vasculature; and zone III involves the pelvis with iliac arteries and veins. Blunt abdominal trauma in the absence of instability and/or expanding hematoma does not necessitate operative intervention, while all penetrating trauma warrants operative exploration. Zone I injury is managed by laparotomy for aortic repair or replacement. Primary repair with or without patch angioplasty should be performed if the tear in the vessel in question involves <50% diameter and the quality of the edges of the vessel are satisfactory. Replacement should be performed if the diameter of the injury is >50% or the length of injury mitigates against primary repair. Gunshot wounds require debridement prior to repair. If replacement is necessary in a contaminated field, use of a synthetic conduit for repair is not a desirable option. Small-diameter blood vessels can be replaced by the great saphenous vein as a conduit. For aorta and inferior vena cava, femoral and popliteal veins (deep veins) harvest may be necessary. However, this procedure is time consuming, and if there is concomitant arterial or venous injury in the extremity, the deep vein harvest should not be performed. Other options include a rifampin-soaked Dacron graft or cryopreserved aortic homograft. The patient may need lifelong antibiotics in this type of clinical scenario.

Correct Answer **D** Repair of aorta with bovine pericardial patch angioplasty and interposition bovine carotid graft for inferior vena cava injury

Reference
Chapellier, X., Sockeel, P., & Baranger, B. (2010). Management of penetrating abdominal vessel injuries. *J Vasc Surg, 147*(2), e1–12. PMID: 20638931

9. RATIONALE

Iatrogenic arterial injury occurs in less than 1% of patients following total knee arthroplasty. The mechanism of injury involves direct trauma (heat injury or instrumental injury) or indirect (arterial stretching during retraction). Diagnostic testing should be done with CT angiography if the patient is outside the operating room or arteriogram from the contralateral femoral artery in patients who are still in the operating room undergoing knee arthroplasty. Most patients have thrombosis or a laceration of the popliteal artery, and open repair is required. If the injury is suspected in the operating room, the patient should be kept supine and the popliteal artery exposed via the medial approach. The drawback of this approach is the relative inaccessibility of the middle portion of the popliteal artery, which is directly behind the knee, and the potential risk of skin incision breakdown, as the medial incision is quite near the anterior incision for the knee arthroplasty. If the injury is discovered after the patient has left the operating room, an emergent operation should consider using the posterior approach. Direct repair, patch angioplasty, or interposition graft may be necessary depending on the extent of involvement of the popliteal artery. In patients with prolonged ischemia, a lower-extremity four-compartment fasciotomy is often required.

Correct Answer   C CTA lower extremity

Reference
Hans, S. S., Shepard, A. D., Reddy, P., et al. (2011). Iatrogenic arterial injuries of spine and orthopedic operations. *J Vasc Surg, 53*(2), 407–413. PMID: 21055898

10. RATIONALE

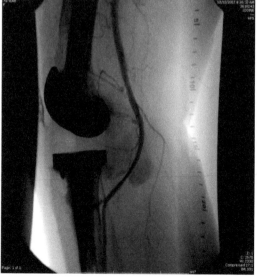

Right popliteal pseudoaneurysm following right knee arthroplasty.

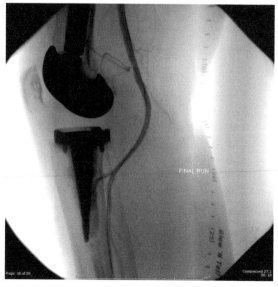

Covered stent placement for repair of right popliteal pseudoaneurysm.

The pseudoaneurysm involving the popliteal artery without arteriovenous fistula is best managed by a covered stent, preferably using contralateral femoral access. Pseudoaneurysm is probably the result of a partial laceration of the popliteal artery. Excessive bleeding following tourniquet release should be suspicious for arterial injury. Complete transection of the popliteal artery is relatively uncommon. Patients at increased risk of arterial injury are those with peripheral arterial disease with or without prior arterial bypass and patients who are undergoing redo joint arthroplasty.

Correct Answer   **C** Covered stent via contralateral femoral approach

Reference
Hans, S. S., Shepard, A. D., Reddy, P., et al. (2011). Iatrogenic arterial injuries of spine and orthopedic operations. *J Vasc Surg*, *53*(2), 407–413. PMID: 21055898

11. RATIONALE

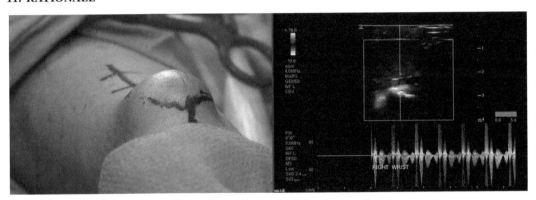

Left: Radial artery pseudoaneurysm. *Right*: Duplex ultrasound radial artery pseudoaneurysm.

This presentation is highly suggestive of radial artery pseudoaneurysm, which can be easily confirmed by duplex imaging. The Allen test will help in evaluation of the integrity of the palmar arch and the patency of the ulnar artery. If the ulnar artery and palmar arch are not patent, repair of the right radial artery pseudoaneurysm, if complicated by postoperative radial artery thrombosis, will result in severe ischemia in the hand. Catheter-based arteriography and CTA are usually not necessary unless arteriovenous fistula or other vascular injury is suspected. Diminished radial artery flow or thrombosis associated with radial artery line placement (arterial line) has been reported in 25%–33% of patients after decannulation, but hand ischemia occurs in <1% of patients. Treatment of distal thromboembolism from atherosclerosis or catheter-related debris with a patent radial artery would require catheter removal, anticoagulation/antiplatelet medications, or both if clinically appropriate. For patients who present with thrombotic radial artery occlusion, they may undergo radial artery exploration or thromboembolectomy followed by patch angioplasty. Pseudoaneurysm is the most common nonischemic complication. The patient may undergo primary repair, vein patch angioplasty, or ligation in the setting of a ruptured pseudoaneurysm. Mycotic pseudoaneurysms should be treated with antibiotics, excision, and wide debridement of infected tissues.

Correct Answer   **C** Duplex imaging of the ulnar artery with Allen test

Reference
Garg, K., Howell, B. W., Saltzberg, S. S., et al. (2013). Open surgical management of complications from indwelling radial artery catheters. *J Vasc Surg*, *58*(5), 1325–1330. PMID: 23810262

12. RATIONALE

The patient has a hematoma in close proximity to the left femoral vessels. Ankle-brachial index is very useful when the physical signs are not definitive (hard signs) of arterial injury. An ankle brachial index of >0.9 approaches 100% predictive value for home discharge, and an ABI of <0.9 has a sensitivity of 95% and a specificity of 97% for the diagnosis of arterial trauma. Patients with an ABI of <0.9 should undergo CT angiography or catheter-based arteriography.

Correct Answer **D** Measurements of ankle-brachial index

Reference

Fox, N., Rajani, R. R., Bokhari, F., et al. (2012). Evaluation and management of penetrating lower extremity arterial trauma: an Eastern Association for the Surgery of Trauma practice management guideline. *J Trauma Acute Care Surg*, *73*(5 Suppl 4), S315–S320. PMID: 23114487

13. RATIONALE

Tracheoinnominate artery fistula is a potentially life-threating iatrogenic complication that is typically associated with percutaneous or surgical placement of a tracheostomy tube. It has also been described in cases of tracheal resection and tracheal stenting. The incidence after surgical tracheostomy has been reported to be 0.1%–1%, with a peak incidence typically seen 7–14 days after the procedure, but it can be seen as early as 3 days and as late as 6 weeks after the procedure. Risk factors for fistula development include high cuff pressure, necrosis, mucosal trauma from a malpositioned cannula, low tracheal incision, excessive neck motion, or radiation therapy. Most patients manifest minor bleeding episodes prior to a massive hemorrhage. For the successful management of tracheoinnominate fistula, treatment should be initiated immediately for control of bleeding before contemplating definitive surgical management. The tracheostomy cuff should be overinflated to help tamponade the bleeding from the fistula; flexible bronchoscopy should be performed through the tracheostomy tube to clear and secure the airway. Digital compression should be applied around or through the tracheostomy incision. No attempt should be made to manipulate the tracheostomy tube. Once the bleeding can be controlled locally, operative intervention is the treatment of choice. A medial sternotomy is performed to gain access to the innominate artery. Ligation and resection of the fistulous segment of the innominate artery without vascular reconstruction is the recommended treatment. The condition is fatal if not immediately recognized.

Correct Answer **B** 7–14 days

Reference

Grant, C. A., Dempsey, G., Harrison, J., & Jones, T. (2006). Tracheo-innominate artery fistula after percutaneous tracheostomy: three case reports and a clinical review. *Br J Anaesth*, *96*(1), 127–131. PMID: 16299043

14. RATIONALE

If tracheoinnominate artery fistula (TIF) is suspected, placement of a finger in the stoma to compress the innominate artery should be the first maneuver. Temporizing measures can be useful for patients who present with tracheoinnominate artery fistula until definitive repair is performed. Manual pressure or a pressure dressing in the neck may be helpful. Suction via bronchoscopy may be necessary to prevent aspiration of the blood. In a few reported cases the endovascular approach has afforded a faster hemorrhage control than thoracotomy or median sternotomy, but there is potential for stent graft infection. Stent graft deployment can be performed using the brachial artery, axillary artery, or femoral artery access with placement of a covered stent at the site of the fistula. Open surgical repair is associated with a mortality rate of approximately 50%. Operative management includes a median sternotomy to expose the aortic arch vessels and trachea with repair sutured over pericardial pledgets. Innominate artery exclusion and extra-anatomic graft such as carotid-carotid, axillo-axillary, or femoral-axillary artery bypass may offer a less morbid option than direct revascularization.

Correct Answer   **D** 50% mortality

Reference
Hamaguchi, S., & Nakajima, Y. (2012). Two cases of tracheoinnominate artery fistula following tracheostomy treated successfully by endovascular embolization of the innominate artery. *J Vasc Surg*, *55*(2), 545–547. PMID: 21958569

15. RATIONALE

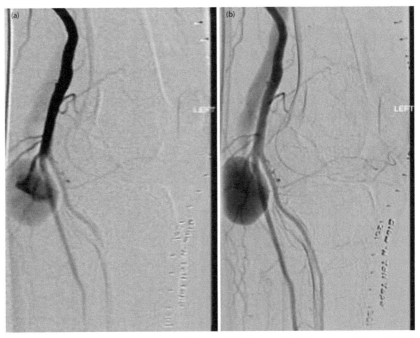

(a) An angiographic image demonstrating AP views in the arterial phase and with two vessel opacification and delayed filling of the pseudoaneurysm. (b) Lateral projections demonstrate the arteriovenous fistula communication to the venous pseudoaneurysm.

Bleeding, infection, and deep venous thrombosis have been reported following knee arthroscopy. Uncommon complications include arterial nerve injury and injury to articular cartilage. During knee arthroscopy, laceration of a genicular artery and vein may result in the formation of a fistula with high pressure in a dilated (aneurysmal) popliteal vein. During meniscectomy with manipulation and external rotation of the knee, the neurovascular bundle in close approximation to the posterior horn of the meniscus may get injured, which may result in the formation of an arterial venous fistula. Vascular injury should be considered in the differential diagnosis in a patient with new onset of pain with fullness or mass in the popliteal fossa following knee arthroscopy or surgery. It is important to obtain a lateral view during arteriography to confirm the site of fistula and location of the pseudoaneurysm before undertaking repair. In low-risk patients open repair via the posterior approach is preferable; if the site of the fistula is distal to the knee joint line, the medial approach is also a satisfactory option. Endovascular options are reserved for high-risk patients.

Correct Answer   **D** Direct open repair

Reference

Hans, S. S. (2020). Popliteal venous pseudoaneurysm and associated arteriovenous fistula following knee arthroscopy in challenging arterial reconstructions. In S. S. Hans (Ed.), *Challenging arterial reconstructions: 100 clinical cases* (pp. 265–267). Cham, Switzerland: Springer Nature Switzerland AG.

16. RATIONALE

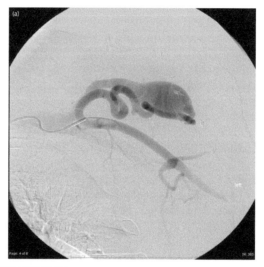

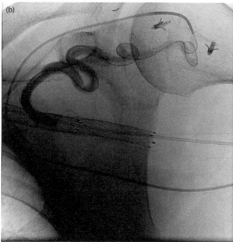
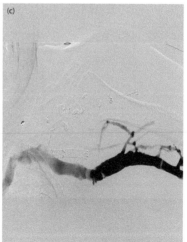

Coil embolization with coaxial microcatheter using access from the brachial artery, basilic vein, and cephalic vein and placement of a covered stent at the origin of the feeding branches of the axillary artery (femoral access).

Iatrogenic injuries to the branches of the axillary artery may result from orthopedic operations on the shoulder joint, pacemaker wire manipulation, lead extraction, or insertion of a large-bore catheter (hemodialysis). Duplex imaging is readily available for confirming the diagnosis, and CT angiography is extremely helpful in identification of inflow and outflow vessels; 3D rendering is useful in selecting treatment options and preplanning for obliteration of traumatic arteriovenous fistulas. Most traumatic fistulas require open repair, as spontaneous resolution occurs in less than 2% of patients. Depending on the location of the fistula, many patients with arteriovenous fistula have minimal symptoms or may be completely asymptomatic. Surgical closure may be the only option available for closure of traumatic fistulas involving axial vessels in younger patients. Other treatment options are now available that include covered stents, coil embolization, glue, alcohol ablation, etc. An endovascular solution provides a less invasive choice with less morbidity and is especially suitable in hemodynamically unstable patients. Long-standing fistulas may have multiple smaller draining channels that would be difficult to visualize if a power injector is not used. To satisfactorily achieve endovascular repair, coil embolization of the draining vein using a coaxial microcatheter system by puncture of the cephalic and basilic vein should be performed. Any small branches of the axillary artery should also be coil embolized using percutaneous brachial access. For covered stent placement to obliterate large circumflex humeral branches at their origin, femoral artery access may be preferable, as a large-size sheath is necessary to deploy a large-diameter covered stent (6 mm or 8 mm). Coverage of the axillary artery in isolation at the site of the main arterial inflow to the fistula is not effective in obliteration of the traumatic arterial venous fistula.

Correct Answer D Coil embolization with coaxial microcatheter using access from brachial artery, basilic vein, and cephalic vein and placement of a covered stent at the origin of the feeding branches of the axillary artery

Reference
Hans, S. S., Shepard, A. D., Reddy, P., et al. (2011). Iatrogenic arterial injuries of spine and orthopedic operations. *J Vasc Surg, 53*(2), 407–413. PMID: 21055898

SECTION 13: VENOUS DISEASE

MCQs 1–52

Q1. The most common nerve injured during endovenous ablation of the lesser saphenous vein is:
- **A.** Saphenous nerve
- **B.** Sural nerve
- **C.** Posterior tibial nerve
- **D.** Common peroneal nerve

Q2. The incidence of superficial burns following endovenous ablation is:
- **A.** <0.2%
- **B.** 0.2%–3.7%
- **C.** 3.8%–4.5%
- **D.** 4.6%–5%

Q3. Following endovenous ablation of the great saphenous vein, a 28-year-old woman presents with class IV endothermal heat-induced thrombosis (EHIT). The optimal treatment is:
- **A.** Heparin
- **B.** Warfarin
- **C.** Apixaban
- **D.** Lovenox

Q4. Arteriovenous fistula following endovenous thermal ablation occurs in:
- **A.** <0.2%
- **B.** 0.2%–0.4%
- **C.** 0.5%–0.8%
- **D.** 0.9%–1.0%

Q5. Recanalization following endovenous thermal ablation occurs in:
- **A.** <2% of patients
- **B.** <4% of patients
- **C.** 4%–6% of patients
- **D.** 7%–8% of patients

Q6. A 44-year-old woman with a BMI of 44 undergoes laparoscopic Roux-en-Y gastric bypass. On postoperative day 3, she has a swollen, mottled, slightly cooler left lower extremity. Duplex venous study shows a left femoral-popliteal venous thrombosis with probable extension into the left external iliac vein. CT venography shows thrombosis of the left common and external iliac vein. The next best step in management besides intravenous heparinization is:
- **A.** Continue heparin for 2 weeks followed by warfarin
- **B.** Apixaban
- **C.** Retrievable inferior vena cava filter
- **D.** Catheter-based mechanical pharmacologic venous thrombectomy

Q7. The incidence of arterial puncture during access of the internal jugular vein in the neck during insertion of a central venous catheter is:
- **A.** <4.0%
- **B.** 4.2%–9.3%
- **C.** 9.4%–10%
- **D.** 11%–12%

Q8. Which of the following statements is true regarding central line–associated bloodstream infection (CLABSI)?
- **A.** Peripherally inserted central catheters (PICC-line) are associated with increased catheter-associated thromboembolism in the upper extremity
- **B.** The adherence to an insertion checklist or bundles has no effect on central line associated–bloodstream infection rates
- **C.** The infection rate in the outpatient setting is higher with a PICC-line than with central venous catheters
- **D.** The PICC-line is associated with a lower in-hospital infection rate as compared with central venous catheters

DOI: 10.1201/9781003389897-13

Q9. A 22-year-old woman who is 18 weeks pregnant presents 8 days after an uncomplicated laparoscopic ovarian cystectomy with a markedly swollen left lower extremity without any pain. Clinical examination and duplex venous study reveal left femoropopliteal acute deep venous thrombosis with extension into the left external iliac vein. The optimal management for acute deep venous thrombosis is:
A. IVC filter via right IJ vein placed at suprarenal level
B. Catheter-directed mechanical-pharmacological thrombolysis
C. Subcutaneous low molecular weight heparin during the entire pregnancy
D. Unfractionated heparin intravenously followed by oral warfarin

Q10. The incidence of stent thrombosis following stent placement for acute iliac vein thrombosis is:
A. <5%
B. 6%–7%
C. 8%–9%
D. >10%

Q11. The incidence of stent thrombosis following venous stenting for post-thrombotic syndrome is:
A. 1%–3%
B. 4%–5%
C. 6%–7%
D. 8%–10%

Q12. The incidence of pulmonary embolism following iliofemoral venous stent placement is:
A. <1%
B. 1%–2%
C. >2% but <3%
D. Pulmonary embolism is not a known complication of venous stenting

Q13. The incidence of clinically significant bleeding following endovascular iliocaval procedures is:
A. 0.3%–1.1%
B. 1.2%–1.5%
C. 1.6%–1.8%
D. 2%

Q14. During resection of a pancreatic adenocarcinoma with involvement of the portal vein, the most satisfactory conduit for reconstruction of the portal vein is:
A. PTFE graft
B. Femoral vein
C. External iliac vein
D. Internal jugular vein

Q15. Resection of a retroperitoneal sarcoma with inferior vena cava includes en-bloc resection and inferior vena cava reconstruction. The most satisfactory conduit for inferior vena cava reconstruction is:
A. Aortic homograft
B. Cryopreserved inferior vena cava
C. Superficial femoral vein (femoral vein)
D. Externally reinforced PTFE graft

Q16. Tilt of the IVC filter (defined as greater than 15 degrees angulation from the long axis of IVC) is least common with:
A. Gunther-Tulip filter
B. Trapease
C. Vena tech
D. Bird nest

Q17. The venogram shown in this figure is diagnostic of:

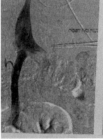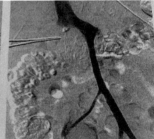

A. Left-sided inferior vena cava
B. Duplicated inferior vena cava
C. Normal vena cava with large left gonadal vein
D. Nutcracker syndrome

Q18. Filter fracture after 1 year of implantation of an IVC filter occurs in:
A. <2%
B. <5%
C. 5.9%–27%
D. 28%–30%

Q19. Symptomatic perforation of the IVC after filter placement occurs in approximately:
A. <5% of patients
B. 5%–7% of patients
C. 8%–9% of patients
D. >10% of patients

Q20. The reported incidence of IVC thrombosis after IVC filter placement is:
A. <2%
B. 2%–30%
C. 31%–35%
D. 36%–40%

Q21. The reported incidence of recurrent pulmonary embolism following IVC filter placement is:
A. <3%
B. <6%
C. 6%–9%
D. 10%–12%

Q22. The incidence of deep venous thrombosis as a late complication of an indwelling IVC filter is as high as:
A. 12%
B. 22%
C. 33%
D. 43%

Q23. A 74-year-old man is scheduled for removal of a retrievable IVC filter for deep venous thrombosis of the common femoral vein and pulmonary embolism with a prior history of craniotomy. Venacavogram at the time of retrieval showed a significant amount of thrombus within the filter. The best management option is:
A. Remove the filter and place the patient on low molecular weight heparin
B. Remove the filter and start the patient on apixaban
C. Cancel the retrieval, continue anticoagulation, and reevaluate for clearance of the thrombus in 4–6 weeks
D. Cancel the retrieval, anticoagulation for 2 weeks, followed by removal of the filter

Q24. Retrieval rates for retrievable IVC filters has been reported as:
A. 10%
B. 20%–23%
C. 24%–30%
D. 31%–40%

Q25. All are known complications of IVC filter retrieval except:
A. Device fracture
B. Caval intussusception
C. Dissection and hemorrhage
D. Perforation of duodenum

Q26. An advanced strategy to facilitate retrieval of a removable IVC filter by snaring the retrieval hook of the filter is not successful. The next best option is:
A. Use of a CloverSnare
B. Division of struts by biopsy forceps followed by removal
C. Benson wire and a snare catheter are maneuvered so that the wire passes through the opposite interstices of the filter then snaring the wire with EN Snare™ (Merit Med, South Jordan, UT) with a "lasso" pulled below the filter collar
D. Photothermal tissue ablation with an excimer laser

Q27. The incidence of post-thrombotic syndrome following deep venous thrombosis of the lower extremity occurs in:
A. 20% of patients
B. 30% of patients
C. 40% of patients
D. 50% of patients

Q28. The normal luminal diameters of the common iliac, external iliac, and common femoral veins are:
A. Common iliac vein 18 mm, external iliac vein 16 mm, common femoral vein 14 mm
B. Common iliac vein 16 mm, external iliac vein 14 mm, common femoral vein 12 mm
C. Common iliac vein 14 mm, external iliac vein 12 mm, common femoral vein 10 mm
D. Common iliac vein 12 mm, external iliac vein 10 mm, common femoral vein 10 mm

Q29. Patients selected for endovascular treatment of chronic venous insufficiency (CVI) should undergo the procedure:

A. Under local anesthesia with intravenous sedation and using access to the ipsilateral popliteal vein in prone position

B. Under general anesthesia with the patient supine and puncture of the ipsilateral proximal femoral vein

C. Under general anesthesia with puncture of the ipsilateral left femoral vein in the midthigh

D. Under local anesthesia and intravenous sedation with puncture of the contralateral common femoral vein

Q30. Which of the following statements best reflects the results of stenting for chronic, nonmalignant, post-thrombotic lesions of the femoro-ilio-caval segment with a 6-year follow-up?

A. Primary patency 65%, primary assisted patency 75%, and secondary patency 90%

B. Primary patency 57%, primary assisted patency 80%, and secondary patency 86%

C. Primary patency 50%, primary assisted patency 70%, and secondary patency 80%

D. Primary patency 45%, primary assisted patency 65%, and secondary patency 70%

Q31. A 67-year-old woman presents with a longstanding history of chronic venous insufficiency of the bilateral lower extremities associated with pain and swelling, more marked on the left side; the workup (venous duplex ultrasound, air plethysmography, and CTV) confirmed luminal compromise of the femoro-ilio-caval segment, most likely post-thrombotic in nature, with compromise of the left calf muscle function. The optimal management consists of:

A. Venous angioplasty of the left common femoral vein, external iliac vein, and common iliac vein

B. Venous angioplasty and stenting of the left common femoral vein, external iliac vein, and common iliac vein

C. Venous angioplasty and stenting with wall stent endoprosthesis

D. Venous angioplasty and stenting with wall stent endoprosthesis and Gianturco Z stent only after trial of conservative therapy

Q32. The incidence of stent compression/in-stent restenosis following common iliac, external iliac, and common femoral vein stenting for chronic venous insufficiency is:

A. 15%–20%

B. 21%–25%

C. 26%–30%

D. 31%–35%

Q33. The indications for operative venous thrombectomy in patients with massive iliofemoral deep venous thrombosis include those with:

A. Multiple trauma with bleeding

B. Intracranial bleeding

C. Pregnant patient or patient refusing catheter-directed thrombolysis

D. Multiple traumas, intracranial bleeding, and in pregnancy

Q34. The long-term iliac vein patency following iliofemoral venous thrombectomy with arteriovenous fistula has been reported in:

A. 60% of patients

B. 70% of patients

C. 80% of patients

D. 90% of patients

Q35. After open iliofemoral venous thrombectomy, a patient is fitted with below the knee compression stockings with a 30–40 mm pressure gradient. This will reduce the morbidity of post-thrombotic syndrome by:

A. 20%

B. 30%

C. 40%

D. 50%

Q36. The best indication for saphenopopliteal vein bypass is to treat:

A. Unilateral occlusion of the femoral vein with a patent contralateral femoral vein

B. Unilateral occlusion of the femoral vein with ipsilateral iliac vein occlusion

C. Unilateral occlusion of the femoral vein with a patent iliac venous system and occlusion of the profunda femoris vein

D. Unilateral occlusion of the femoral vein and occlusion of the popliteal vein (ipsilateral)

Q37. A 32-year-old woman presents with back pain and bilateral lower extremity fatigue for 6 days prior to coming to the emergency room. Duplex ultrasound demonstrated bilateral deep venous thrombosis up to the iliac veins. An MRV demonstrated absence of contrast in the intrahepatic inferior vena cava, bilateral common iliac veins, and external iliac veins with large paracaval collaterals suggestive of chronic inferior vena cava thrombosis or inferior vena cava atresia. The optimal management consists of:

A. Venography with thrombolysis, suction thrombectomy, and balloon angioplasty from above the knee popliteal veins to external iliac vein followed by bilateral iliofemoral vein recanalization and stenting/angioplasty

B. Venography with thrombolysis, balloon angioplasty, suction thrombectomy from above the knee popliteal veins to external iliac veins followed by bilateral iliofemoral recanalization with bilateral overlapping wall stents from common iliac vein, external iliac vein, and rostral femoral vein 6 months later

C. Hybrid repair with interposition of 14-mm ringed PTFE graft from infrarenal inferior vena cava to bilateral common iliac veins and bilateral stenting of external iliac vein, femoral vein, and rostral femoral veins 6 months later

D. Open thrombectomy of bilateral popliteal, femoral, and common femoral veins followed by simultaneous interposition of 14-mm ringed PTFE graft from infrarenal inferior vena cava to common iliac bifurcation

Q38. A 28-year-old woman presented with a chronically occluded right common iliac vein stent despite multiple attempts at recanalization and thrombolysis.

She presents with heaviness and swelling of the right lower extremity. A crossover femoro-femoral venous bypass using the left great saphenous vein as a conduit and tunneled into the right groin (Palma procedure) was carried out, where an end-to-side anastomosis was performed to the right common femoral vein. There is concern for poor inflow. What is the next best option?

A. Anticoagulation with low molecular weight heparin

B. Anticoagulation with apixaban

C. Low molecular weight heparin

D. Creation of arteriovenous fistula

Q39. The repair of a popliteal venous aneurysm is recommended:

A. To prevent rupture

B. To prevent thrombosis

C. To prevent pulmonary embolism

D. To prevent local compression symptoms

Q40. The reported incidence of early thrombosis following popliteal venous aneurysm repair is:

A. 10%

B. 15%

C. 20%

D. 25%

Q41. The most common symptom associated with nutcracker syndrome (left renal vein compression) is:

A. Hematuria

B. Flank pain

C. Orthostatic proteinuria

D. Fatigue

Q42. The positive predictive value as a cut-off diameter of the left ovarian vein by transvaginal ultrasound for diagnosis of pelvis venous congestion syndrome is reported to be:

A. 60% at 5 mm, 70% at 6 mm, 72% at 7 mm, and 75% at 8 mm

B. 71.2% at 5 mm, 83.3% at 6 mm, 81.1% at 7 mm, and 75.8% at 8 mm

C. 55% at 5 mm, 65% at 6 mm, 70% at 7 mm, and 72% at 8 mm

D. 50% at 5 mm, 60% at 6 mm, 65% at 7 mm, and 68% at 8 mm

Q43. The incidence of post-embolization syndrome following embolization for pelvic congestion syndrome is:

A. 10%
B. 20%
C. 25%
D. 30%

Q44. The lowest incidence of major bleeding as a complication of an anticoagulation regimen is with:

A. Oral apixaban
B. Parenteral unfractionated heparin followed by warfarin
C. Low molecular weight heparin
D. Low molecular weight heparin combined with dabigatran

Q45. A 46-year-old woman presents with painful swelling of the left lower extremity with purplish discoloration extending up to the left groin. She has a history of large uterine myoma and oral contraceptive use. The most plausible diagnosis is:

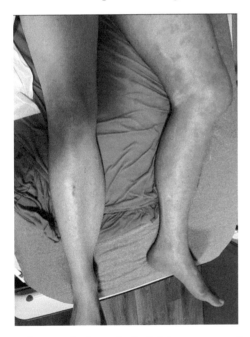

A. Lymphedema in the left lower extremity
B. Acute arterial occlusion in the left lower extremity
C. Phlegmasia cerulea dolens
D. Livedo reticularis

Q46. May–Thurner syndrome is the cause of DVT in:

A. 1%–2% of cases
B. 2%–5% of cases
C. 5%–7% of cases
D. 7%–10% of cases

Q47. In the assessment of congenital vascular malformation, the most helpful imaging modality is:

A. Duplex ultrasound
B. CTA
C. Dynamic contrast-enhanced MRI
D. Catheter-based arteriography

Q48. For low-flow vascular malformations, the optimal management strategy consists of:

A. Conservative management
B. Foam sclerotherapy
C. Surgical resection
D. All of the above

Q49. A 62-year-old man had significant pelvic bleeding during robotic prostatectomy, which was controlled by clips and suture repair. In the recovery room the left leg was found to be purplish up to the midthigh with significant swelling. The most likely diagnosis is:

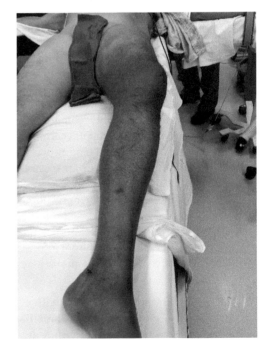

A. Acute arterial occlusion of the left lower extremity

B. Left iliac vein occlusion

C. Hematoma in pelvis causing extrinsic compression of the left iliac vein

D. Livedo reticularis

Q50. A 50-year-old man with known cirrhosis of the liver presents with vague abdominal pain. CT scan of the abdomen shows thrombus in the portal vein and superior mesenteric vein near the junction with the portal vein. The optimal management for this condition is:

A. Distal splenorenal shunt

B. Liver transplant

C. Anticoagulation

D. Endovenous thrombectomy

Q51. Which condition is associated with the greatest risk of venous thromboembolism?

A. Morbid obesity (BMI greater than 32)

B. Age greater than 70 years

C. Prolonged bed rest

D. Acute spinal cord injury

Q52. A 56-year-old man presents with a superficial ulcer above the ankle on the medial side with surrounding pigmentation, induration, and dermatitis of 2 months' duration. The most effective initial treatment for healing of the venous ulcer is:

A. PICC-line with administration of intravenous antibiotics for 6 weeks

B. Silver-impregnated local dressings

C. Graduated compression stockings with local wound care and management of dermatitis

D. Open ligation of feeding perforators at the ankle

RATIONALE 1–52

1. RATIONALE

Reasons for neve injury during endovenous thermal ablation (EVTA) include needle stick injury during vein cannulation or during administration of tumescent anesthesia or heat transfer during EVTA. Nerve injury is a common complication of endovenous thermal ablation, as paresthesia is seen in 19.6% of patients after varicose vein surgery versus 9.7% after radiofrequency ablation and 4.8% after endovenous laser ablation. The risk of nerve injury during EVTA is directly related to the relative proximity of several nerves to the most commonly ablated veins. The sural nerve travels along the lesser saphenous vein from the mid-posterior calf to the posterior aspect of the lateral malleolus. Damage to the sural nerve due to thermal ablation can result in paresthesia to the heel and lateral aspect of the foot. The common peroneal nerve may also get injured during EVTA of the lesser saphenous vein and may result in partial or complete foot drop. Most nerve injuries are self-limiting and usually spontaneously resolve within 2–3 weeks.

Correct Answer **B** Sural nerve

Reference

Atkin, G. K., Round, T., Vattipally, V. R., & Das, S. K. (2007). Common peroneal nerve injury as a complication of short saphenous vein surgery. *Phlebology, 22*(1), 3–7. PMID: 18265547

2. RATIONALE

During endovenous thermal ablation (EVTA) there can be a significant amount of heat dispersed around the vein intended for treatment. Most of the heat generated remains within the venous lumen. When the vein becomes epifascial or close to the skin surface, the patient can suffer a full-thickness skin burn. The reported incidence of superficial burns following EVTA is 0.2%–3.7%. Cutaneous burns can be painful and unsightly but are usually self-limiting. Local wound care and frequent evaluation for possible infection should be undertaken. If the burn is apparent at the time of ablation, it can be excised and a primary closure performed. Most skin burns can be prevented by appropriate tumescent anesthesia. Correct energy doses, stopping laser activation at the entry site, and caution at the extrafascial site will decrease the incidence of skin burns.

Correct Answer **B** 0.2%–3.7%

Reference

Kheirelseid, E. A. H., Crowe, G., Sehgal, R., et al. (2018). Systematic review and meta-analysis of randomized controlled trials evaluating long-term outcomes of endovenous management of lower extremity varicose veins. *J Vasc Surg Venous Lymphat Disord, 6*(2), 256–270. PMID: 29292115

3. RATIONALE

Endothermal heat-induced thrombosis (EHIT) is defined as the propagation of thrombosis from the superficial vein into a deep vein. The incidence of EHIT was 1.4% after EVTA of the great saphenous vein, with potential for pulmonary embolism in up to 5.7% being reported. Risk factors include a large diameter of the great saphenous vein at the saphenofemoral or lesser saphenous vein at the saphenopopliteal junction, presence of reflux at the junction, tobacco use, advanced body mass index, prior intervention, prior DVT, hypercoagulable state, clinical classification greater than C3, male gender, and increased Caprini risk assessment score model. EHITs are more echogenic as compared to de novo DVTs and are more stable with complete regression. Based on classification EHITs are divided into four classes; a treatment algorithm is suggested. For class 1, serial duplex ultrasound monthly until clot regresses. For class 2, low molecular weight heparin is advised for 2 weeks but continued if the clot does not regress on duplex imaging. For class 3 and class 4, it should be treated like any other provoked deep venous thrombosis as per guidelines with full dose anticoagulation. In a study, patients presenting with EHIT level more than or equal to 2 or deep venous thrombus after EVTA, therapeutic anticoagulation with rivaroxaban or fondaparinux was initiated until complete recanalization on ultrasound imaging was documented. They observed that rivaroxaban offered an oral medication approach showing no difference in preventing EHIT and DVT compared with fondaparinux without increased bleeding risk.

Correct Answer **C** Apixaban

Reference
Lawrence, P. F., Chandra, A., Wu, M., et al. (2010). Classification of proximal endovenous closure levels and treatment algorithm. *J Vasc Surg*, *52*(2), 388–393. PMID: 20646894

4. RATIONALE

Concomitant venous and arterial injuries during administration of tumescent anesthesia as well as transmission of thermal energy across the venous wall into the adjacent artery can lead to later vascular degeneration and formation of an arteriovenous fistula. Arteriovenous fistula occurrence during venous ablation is quite uncommon with an incidence of 0.15%. Potential anatomical pitfalls include the external pudendal artery as it courses posterior to the great saphenous vein and sural artery branches close to the lesser saphenous veins or perforators. Potential serous sequelae of post-ablation arterial venous fistulas include severe limb edema, steal syndrome with claudication, and distal ischemia. Some fistulas will close spontaneously, and some may remain but are usually asymptomatic. Open repair, embolization, or endovascular treatment is reserved for symptomatic patients.

Correct Answer **A** <0.2%

Reference
Rudarakanchana, N., Berland, T. L., Chasin, C., et al. (2012). Arteriovenous fistula after endovenous ablation for varicose veins. *J Vasc Surg*, *55*(5), 1492–1494. PMID: 22119247

5. RATIONALE

Residue varicosities that persist after EVTA should be differentiated from recurrent varicose veins. The extent of residual varicosities depends on the pretreatment anatomical distribution of varicosities and their hemodynamic relationship with the incompetent axial vein. Recanalization occurs in up to 4% of axial veins after EVLA, although most are not associated with recurrent varicose veins, unless it occurs within 6 weeks of treatment (primary treatment failure due to thrombus dissolution). It is thought to occur during treatment with low energy less than or equal to 60 J/cm.

Correct Answer **B** <4% of patients

Reference

Theivacumar, N. S., Dellagrammaticas, D., Darwood, R. J., et al. (2008). Fate of the great saphenous vein following endovenous laser ablation: does re-canalisation mean recurrence? *Eur J Vasc Endovasc Surg*, *36*(2), 211–215. PMID: 18474444

6. RATIONALE

Anticoagulants alone do not dissolve the occluding thrombus, decrease the venous outflow obstruction, or have any significant impact on the inflammatory reaction caused by persistent thrombus, venous reflux, and post-thrombotic syndrome. The results of a randomized multi-center trial in 692 patients assigned to either anticoagulation alone (control group) or antico-agulation plus pharmaco-mechanical thrombolysis (catheter-mediated or device-mediated tPA with thrombus aspiration or maceration with or without stenting) did not result in a lower risk of post-thrombotic syndrome but was associated with a higher risk of bleeding. The severity score for PTS was lower in the pharmaco-mechanical thrombolysis group than in the control group (anticoagulation alone) at 6, 12, 18, and 24 months of follow-up. The risk of bleeding complications in the early postoperative period must be balanced against the benefits of thrombolysis and clot clearance in a patient with findings suggestive of phlegmasia cerulea dolens. However, the patient presented here is likely to benefit from mechanical-pharmacological thrombectomy.

Correct Answer   D Catheter-based mechanical-pharmacologic venous thrombectomy

Reference

Vedantham, S., Goldhaber, S. Z., Julian, J. A., et al. (2017). Pharmacomechanical catheter-directed thrombolysis for deep-vein thrombosis. *N Engl J Med*, *377*(23), 2240–2252. PMID: 29211671

7. RATIONALE

The most serious complication with central venous puncture is pericardial tamponade, which can result in mortality if not immediately recognized and treated. The incidence of arterial puncture ranges from 4.2% to 9.3% during central venous catheterization using internal jugular vein access. Inadvertent arterial puncture in the neck with a smaller gauge needle (micropunc-ture needle size 21) should prompt withdrawal and light pressure for 5–10 minutes. Arterial puncture with a larger-bore catheter (>7 Fr) can lead to hematoma, pseudoaneurysm, arterio-venous fistula, dissection, bleeding, stroke, and death. Risk factors for iatrogenic arterial injury include obesity, previous radiation to the neck, multiple attempts, and operator inexperience. Vascular surgery consult should be promptly obtained and open neck exploration with control of bleeding from the artery using 5-0 or 6-0 cardiovascular polypropylene suture to obtain satis-factory hemostasis is often necessary.

Correct Answer   B 4.2%–9.3%

Reference

Yoon, D. Y., Annambhotla, S., Resnick, S. A., et al. (2015). Inadvertent arterial placement of central venous catheters: diagnostic and therapeutic strategies. *Ann Vasc Surg*, *29*(8), 1567–1574. PMID: 26256713

8. RATIONALE

Many efforts have been spent to decrease CLABSI (central line–associated bloodstream infection). In the inpatient population, the rate of CLABSI by number of catheter days is similar between

PICC-line and central venous catheters without any difference in rates of infection in these two groups. In the outpatient population, patients with a PICC-line have lower rates of infection. There is increased incidence of catheter-associated venous thromboembolism with PICC-lines, (presumably due to their longer length) and in patients with an associated diagnosis of malignancy.

Correct Answer A Peripherally inserted central catheters (PICC-line) are associated with increased catheter-associated thromboembolism in the upper extremity

Reference

Chopra, V., Anand, S., Hickner, A., et al. (2013). Risk of venous thromboembolism associated with peripherally inserted central catheters: a systematic review and meta-analysis. *Lancet, 382*(9889), 311–325. PMID: 23697825

9. RATIONALE

Women are at increased risk of both venous and arterial thrombosis during pregnancy. Compared to nonpregnant women, the risk of arterial thromboembolism (stroke and heart attacks) is increased three- to fourfold and the risk of venous thromboembolism is increased four- to fivefold. In the postpartum period the risk is even higher (20-fold). Approximately 20% of thromboembolic events are arterial and the other 80% are venous. Approximately 80% of venous thromboembolic events during pregnancy are deep venous thrombosis and 20% are pulmonary embolism. Approximately one-third of pregnancy-related DVT and half of pregnancy-related pulmonary embolisms occur after delivery. Deep venous thrombosis during pregnancy is more likely to be proximal, massive, and more common in the left lower extremity due to relative stenosis of the left common iliac vein where it lies between the right common iliac artery and body of the lumbar vertebra. Ten percent of DVT during pregnancy and the postpartum period involve the pelvic veins. The most important reason for increased risk of venous thromboembolism during pregnancy is hypercoagulability, and the most important risk factor for VTE in pregnancy is a prior history of thrombosis. The preferred agent for anticoagulation in pregnancy is heparin compounds. Neither unfractionated or low molecular weight heparin crosses the placenta and are safe in pregnancy. Higher doses are necessary, as unfractionated heparin and low molecular weight heparin have shorter half-lives. Low molecular weight heparin is preferable in deep venous thrombosis and pulmonary embolism, as administration is easier as an outpatient. Pregnant women may be converted from low molecular weight heparin to unfractionated heparin in the last month of pregnancy or sooner if delivery appears imminent. Unfractionated heparin is short acting; therefore, if epidural anesthesia is to be administered, unfractionated heparin with a shorter half-life as compared to 12–24 hours for the half-life of low molecular weight heparin makes it preferrable.

Correct Answer C Subcutaneous low molecular weight heparin during the entire pregnancy

Reference

James, A. H. (2009). Venous thromboembolism in pregnancy. *Arterioscler Thromb Vasc Biol, 29*(3), 326–331. PMID: 19228606

10. RATIONALE

Occlusion or in-stent thrombosis in the deep venous system is usually related to thrombosis rather than a cellular hyperplastic reaction such as seen in the arteries. As such, the conditions that predispose to thrombosis are the main risk factors for early occlusion of stents.

From a meta-analysis, stent thrombosis has been reported to occur in 6.5% of patients with acute thrombotic conditions. It has been postulated that poor-quality inflow and/or outflow predisposes patients to early thrombosis. A suboptimal anticoagulation regimen or patient non-compliance may also predispose to early stent thrombosis. Unexplained early stent thrombosis is usually a poor prognostic sign. The incidence of rethrombosis in such patients is high after attempts at reintervention.

Correct Answer **B** 6%–7%

Reference
Razavi, M. K., Black, S., Gagne, P., et al. (2019). Pivotal study of endovenous stent placement for symptomatic iliofemoral venous obstruction. *Circ Cardiovasc Interv, 12*(12), e008268. PMID: 31833414

11. RATIONALE

The incidence of early (within 30 days) stent thrombosis is 6.8% in patients with chronic post-thrombotic lesions. The risk of DVT after stent placement in patients with non-thrombotic venous obstructive lesions (VOLs) has been reported to be 1.5% at 30 days. Poor quality of inflow such as a chronically occluded external iliac and common femoral vein with subacute thrombosis of the profunda femoris vein with chronic DVT in the femoral vein, even in the presence of satisfactory outflow (common iliac vein), stenting of the external iliac vein, and common femoral vein, will, in all probability, lead to stent thrombosis. In such cases consideration should be given to open femoral and external iliac vein exploration with removal of the fibrous scar, subacute thrombus, and patch grafting. Placement of a stent in a difficult-to-dilate lesion will lead to suboptimal stent expansion. In such cases cutting balloon or serial high-pressure balloon dilation is often necessary prior to stent placement. Risk factors for late loss of patency depend on the etiology of the disease, with chronic post-thrombotic occlusions posing the highest risk followed by stenting after thrombolysis in acute thrombotic conditions. Non-thrombotic obstruction is associated with a 12-month patency >96% in the PIVOTAL trial for venous stent placement. The presence of residual thrombus inflow channels is another risk factor for late loss of stent patency. Lesion length and stent extension into the common femoral vein also increase the incidence of stent thrombosis.

Correct Answer **C** 6%–7%

Reference
Neglén, P., Hollis, K. C., Olivier, J., & Raju, S. (2007). Stenting of the venous outflow in chronic venous disease: long-term stent-related outcome, clinical, and hemodynamic result. *J Vasc Surg, 46*(5), 979–990. PMID:17980284

12. RATIONALE

Death and pulmonary embolism are rare but the most serious complications of deep venous intervention. The 30-day mortality after iliofemoral venous stent placement ranges from 0.1% to 0.7%. This mortality rate is comparable to that of an age-matched population with deep venous disease and, hence, is unlikely to be directly related to the procedure of venous stenting by itself. Pulmonary embolism is reported in 0.2%–0.9% of patients within 30 days of the procedure. Given the low rate of clinically significant pulmonary embolism, prophylactic IVC filter placement during venous recanalization procedures, even in the setting of acute iliofemoral deep venous thrombosis, is not necessary in most instances. Following outcome research from

37 studies reporting 45 treatment effects (non-thrombotic 8; acute thrombotic 19; and chronic post-thrombotic 18) from 2869 patients (non-thrombotic 1122; acute thrombotic 629; and chronic post-thrombotic 1118), technical success rates were comparable among groups ranging from 94% to 96%. Complication rates ranged from 0.3% to 1.1% among groups for major bleeding, from 0.2% to 0.9% for pulmonary embolism, from 0.1% to 0.7% for periprocedure mortality, and from 1.0% to 6.8% for early thrombosis. At 1 year, primary and secondary patency were 96% and 99% from non-thrombotic, 87% and 89% for acute thrombotic, and 79% and 94% for chronic post-thrombotic. From this meta-analysis it was concluded that stent placement for iliofemoral outflow obstruction results in high-technical success and acceptable complication rates regardless of the cause of obstruction.

Correct Answer   A <1%

Reference

Razavi, M. K., Jaff, M. R., & Miller, L. E. (2015). Safety and effectiveness of stent placement for iliofemoral venous outflow obstruction: systematic review and meta-analysis. *Circ Cardiovasc Interv*, *8*(10), e002772. PMID: 26438686

13. RATIONALE

Clinically significant bleeding or venous rupture are rare complications of iliofemoral vein interventions. The reported rates of 0.3%–1.1% are mostly related to either the use of thrombolytic or anticoagulant drugs used during the procedure, with majority of the bleeding being at the site of puncture. Vascular injury with hematoma and AV fistula formation have also been reported. Concomitant thrombolytic therapy increases the risk of access site bleeding complications. Rupture of a chronically occluded venous channel or balloon dilatation of inadvertently crossed venous collaterals may occur. Venous perforation in patients undergoing recanalization of chronic occlusion of iliofemoral veins requiring blood transfusion have been reported. Prolonged balloon inflation at the site of injury or use of covered stents will help control bleeding and obtain hemostasis. A potentially disastrous bleeding may occur as the result of inadvertent passage of a wire or catheter into the epidural space via the epidural venous plexus. Frequent venography in orthogonal projections can avoid this rare but devastating complication that may result in serious neurological injury.

Correct Answer   A 0.3%–1.1%

Reference

Kölbel, T., Lindh, M., Akesson, M., et al. (2009). Chronic iliac vein occlusion: midterm results of endovascular recanalization. *J Endovasc Ther*, *16*(4), 483–491. PMID: 19702343

14. RATIONALE

Several methods of portal vein reconstruction are possible if tumor invasion is present. Primary venorrhaphy is acceptable if there is not any risk of luminal narrowing >30%. An autologous vein conduit is preferable. The internal jugular vein is the most suitable conduit as compared to the great saphenous vein because of its better size match. Other graft options include femoral vein, left renal vein, external iliac vein, or prosthetic graft (PTFE or Dacron).

Correct Answer   D Internal jugular vein

Reference
Etkin, Y., Foley, P. J., Wang, G. J., et al. (2016). Successful venous repair and reconstruction for oncologic resections. *J Vasc Surg Venous Lymphat Disord*, *4*(1), 57–63. PMID: 26946897

15. RATIONALE

If following en-bloc resection, less than 50% circumference of the inferior vena cava has been removed due to its involvement, primary repair with a fine cardiovascular polypropylene suture can be performed with minimal narrowing of the inferior vena cava. En-bloc resection with complete iliocaval venous excision and reconstruction with externally reinforced PTFE interposition graft is most commonly used. Though other conduits like Dacron, cryopreserved inferior vena cava, aorta, and femoral vein have all been used. The advantage of using externally reinforced PTFE is the avoidance of kinking and compression of the neo-IVC by the abdominal viscera. In some cases, primary IVC ligation has been reported. However, patients often develop massive lower extremity edema, renal dysfunction, and ascites; therefore, ligation of the inferior vena cava should be avoided.

Correct Answer   D Externally reinforced PTFE graft

Reference
Etkin, Y., Foley, P. J., Wang, et al. (2016). Successful venous repair and reconstruction for oncologic resections. *J Vasc Surg Venous Lymphat Disord*, *4*(1), 57–63. PMID: 26946897

16. RATIONALE

Filter tilt is defined as greater than 15 degrees angulation of the filter from the long axis of the vena cava, which is encountered with all types of filter designs except bird nest filter (Cook Medical, Bloomington, IN), due to its inherent design. An increased tilt angle may increase the risk of pulmonary embolism, but it does not increase the risk of thrombosis. Attempts to adjust the filter to correct the tilt is not generally recommended. The ideal positioning of an IVC filter is with the apex just inferior to the renal veins and the base superior to the caval bifurcation. Misplacement or migration of the device above the renal veins may lead to renal vein thrombosis, while positioning in a unilateral iliac vein leaves the contralateral side patent for thrombi from the lower extremities to reach the pulmonary circulation. There have been rare reported cases of inadvertent placement into the infrarenal aorta and spinal canal.

Correct Answer   D Bird nest

Reference
Nguyen, N. T., Barshes, N. R., Bechara, C. F., & Pisimisis, G. T. (2014). Natural history of an intra-aortic permanent inferior vena cava filter. *J Vasc Surg*, *60*(3), 784. PMID: 25154964

17. RATIONALE

The incidence of duplicated inferior vena cava varies from 0.39% to 3%. A duplicated inferior vena cava results from failure of regression of the left subcardinal vein. The left and right inferior vena cava joins at the level of the renal arteries to the suprarenal inferior vena cava. During inferior vena cava placement, a duplicated inferior vena cava should be suspected if the inferior vena cava appears unusually small on the ipsilateral side as imaged on initial venogram. The venogram may also uncover an interiliac communication with filling of the contralateral inferior vena cava. In patients with bilateral deep venous thrombosis or in the presence of a large interiliac communicating branch, filter deployment should be considered in both the right and left inferior vena cava. Duplicate inferior vena cava should be considered in the event of a recurrent pulmonary embolism after placement of the inferior vena cava filter.

Correct Answer   **B** Duplicated inferior vena cava

Reference
Siddiqui, R. A., & Hans, S. (2008). Double inferior vena cava filter implantation in a patient with a duplicate inferior vena cava. *J Invasive Cardiol*, *20*(2), 91–92. PMID: 18252974

18. **RATIONALE**

In review of the FDA manufacturer guidelines and user facility device experience (MAUDE) database from 2014, the most common later complication after IVC filter placement was fracture, accounting for 5.9%–27% of all complications. Filter fracture occurs due to structural integrity failure of the material, most commonly seen 1 year following placement, and may lead to fragment embolization. Fracture is more common with retrievable filters. This can result in alterations in flow dynamics within the IVC, with higher risk of thrombosis, and decrease the effectiveness of the prevention of pulmonary embolism. Fragment embolization has been reported within the pulmonary vasculature, renal veins, and heart. Filter and fragment retrieval is recommended for patients upon discovery of the fracture. Endovascular retrieval is successful in most cases. Most fragments in the cardiopulmonary system remain asymptomatic. Surgical removal is rarely necessary.

Correct Answer   **C** 5.9%–27%

Reference
Sella, D. M., & Oldenburg, W. A. (2013). Complications of inferior vena cava filters. *Semin Vasc Surg*, *26*(1), 23–28. PMID: 23932558

19. **RATIONALE**

IVC filter perforation is defined as a filter strut >3 mm outside the vessel wall and entering the retroperitoneum or surrounding anatomic structures. The majority are asymptomatic. In a literature review of 9002 cases, caval perforation was reported in 19% of cases. However, only 8% were symptomatic, with pain being the most common symptom; 5% had major complications requiring implant intervention, which included surgical removal of the filter (n63), endovascular stent graft placement for aortic pseudoaneurysm (n8), endovascular retrieval (n4), arterial embolization for bleeding (n2), percutaneous nephrostomy (n1), and ureteral stent (n1). Perforated struts involved other organs like the duodenum, lumbar vertebra, and aorta. The mechanism of IVC penetration is not well understood. The conical-shaped filters with free struts have a higher frequency of penetration. Filters without free struts may increase the risk of caval thrombosis. Other mechanisms include increase in filter span, sharpness of barbs, decreased strength of the caval wall, significant tilt, and small-caliber inferior vena cava. For symptomatic filter perforation, retrieval should be considered. Most perforations into the duodenum necessitate laparotomy and caval exploration. For filters unable to be removed, the offending struts are trimmed with wire cutters.

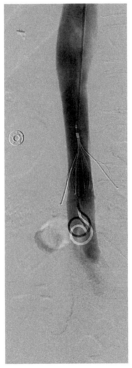

Struts of the filter outside of the wall of the IVC.

Correct Answer   **C** 8%–9% of patients

Reference
Jia, Z., Wu, A., Tam, M., Spain, J., et al. (2015). Caval penetration by inferior vena cava filters: a systematic literature review of clinical significance and management. *Circulation*, *132*(10), 944–952. PMID: 26169756

20. RATIONALE

IVC thrombosis after filter placement is reported in 2%–30% of patients with symptoms of bilateral lower extremity pain and swelling; renal failure may occur if the thrombus extends above the level of the renal veins. The incidence of recurrent pulmonary embolism is 1%–7% if the thrombus extends above the filter. The cause of thrombus of the filter is often due to the patient's initial risk factors or the presence of a foreign body with accumulation of thrombus in the struts. There is also the possibility of entrapped mobile thrombus within the filter. There is no statistical difference in the rate of IVC thrombosis between patients with or without malignancy, although patients with metastatic disease have an increased risk of recurrent pulmonary embolism despite filter placement. Rates of recurrent pulmonary embolism in patients with metastatic disease are reported at 10.4% compared to 2.3% in those with nonmetastatic malignancy. Once caval thrombosis is diagnosed, current practice guidelines recommend anticoagulation with the majority managed without additional intervention. Catheter-directed thrombolysis for symptomatic patients is usually not successful, as the thrombus is often subacute or chronic. Prophylactic anticoagulation with an indwelling filter does not seem to improve the rate of IVC thrombosis. Pharmaco-mechanical thrombolysis using Angio-jet device (Boston Scientific, Marlborough, MA) or with Inari clot Treiver system (Inari Med, Irvine, CA) are options. Angio-jet uses tPA and represents rheolytic thrombectomy. Angiovac-system (Angiodynamics, Latham, NY) and Inari clot Treiver system do not use tPA.

Correct Answer   B 2%–30%

Reference
Golowa, Y., Warhit, M., Matsunaga, F., & Cynamon, J. (2016). Catheter directed interventions for inferior vena cava thrombosis. *Cardiovasc Diagn Ther, 6*(6), 612–622. PMID: 28123981

21. RATIONALE

The reported incidence of recurrent pulmonary embolism after IVC filter placement is between 0.5% and 6%, although the true incidence is difficult to document due to the number of unreported events. The PREPIC study randomized 400 patients with deep venous thrombosis at higher risk for pulmonary embolism to either filter or nonfilter group and then further randomized them to receive low molecular weight heparin or unfractionated heparin. An 8-year follow-up demonstrated a pulmonary embolism rate of 6.2% in the filter group compared to 15.1% in the nonfiltered group, but there was a significant increased rate of DVT in those with IVC filter (35.7% versus 27.5%). Current recommendation for IVC filter patients with recurrent pulmonary embolism is that systemic anticoagulation should be used unless contraindicated. The presence of a filter should not alter the duration or intensity of anticoagulation.

Correct Answer   B <6%

Reference
Herve Decousus (Chairman), Fabrice-Guy Barral, Andrea Buchmuller-Cordier, Bernard Charbonnier, Phillippe Girard, Christian Lamer, Silvy Laporte, Alain Leizorovicz, Patrick Mismetti, Florence Parent, Sara Quenet, Karine Rivron-Guillot, Bernard Tardy. (2005). Eight-year follow-up of patients with permanent vena cava filters in the prevention of pulmonary embolism: the PREPIC (Prevention du Risque d'Embolie Pulmonaire par Interruption Cave) randomized study. *Circulation, 112*(3), 416–422. PMID: 16009794

22. RATIONALE

Deep venous thrombosis is a common late complication of an indwelling IVC filter, with an incidence as high as 43%. In the PREPIC study, at 8 years, vena cava filters reduced the risk of pulmonary embolism but increased that of deep vein thrombosis and had no effect on survival. At 2 years, the risk of DVT in patients with IVC filter was doubled than those without and is probably related to alterations in venous blood flow and the underlying coagulopathy of patients requiring an IVC filter. This risk may be mitigated by a retrievable filter, but only if they are removed. The incidence of DVT with an indwelling retrievable filter is comparable to permanent filters (11.3% vs. 12.6%).

Correct Answer   D 43%

Reference

Kim, H. S., Young, M. J., Narayan, A. K., et al. (2008). A comparison of clinical outcomes with retrievable and permanent inferior vena cava filters. *J Vasc Interv Radiol, 19*(3), 393–399. PMID: 18295699

23. RATIONALE

Prior to removal of the IVC filter, venacavogram should be obtained via injection through the catheter (OmniFlush-Pigtail). If there is occlusion of the filter by the thrombus or if there is a large amount of thrombus in the filter, retrieval should be abandoned. The patient should be continued on anticoagulation and reevaluated in 4–6 weeks by CT venography. Removal of the filter in the presence of thrombus poses undue risk to the patient for pulmonary embolism even if the thrombus is subacute/chronic.

Correct Answer   C Cancel the retrieval, continue anticoagulation, and reevaluate for clearance of thrombus in 4–6 weeks

Reference

Major, M. T., Bove, P. G., & Long, G. W. (2021). Complications of IVC filters in Vascular and endovascular complications. In *Vascular and endovascular complications: a practical approach* (pp. 96–103). Boca Raton, FL: CRC Press.

24. RATIONALE

In a retrospective review of 605 patients with retrievable IVC filters, a retrieval rate of 23% was demonstrated with an overall technical success of 93%. The most common reason for technical failure was a large amount of thrombus in the filter. Average indwelling filter time was 111 days. Predictive risk factors for non-retrievable filters included age >80 years, acute bleed, current malignancy, post-filter anticoagulation, and history of venous thromboembolism.

Correct Answer   B 20%–23%

Reference

Siracuse, J. J., Al Bazroon, A., Gill, H. L., et al. (2015). Risk factors of nonretrieval of retrievable inferior vena cava filters. *Ann Vasc Surg, 29*(2), 318–321. PMID: 25308241

25. RATIONALE

Complications associated with filter retrieval include device fracture, caval intussusception, dissection, and hemorrhage. Factors that increase the rate of complications include longer indwelling times, increased tilt angle, and hook embedded in the vena cava wall. Complications for retrieval performed within 30 days of filter placement are rare, and there are increasing numbers of reports demonstrating safe retrieval with increasing dwell times. In patients with much longer dwell times, a subapical guide wire loop is used to dissect the tissue and allow the release of the filter. Once released, the apex was snared and a 16 Fr sheath was advanced in an attempt to collapse the struts of the filter. A CloverSnare (Cook Med, Inc., Bloomington, IN) kit consisting of a 10 Fr outer and 8 Fr inner sheath is inserted through the 16 Fr sheath, with gradual telescopic advance of the sheaths over the struts to allow the release of the struts from the fibrous tissue.

Correct Answer   **D** Perforation of duodenum

Reference
Grewal, S., Chamarthy, M. R., & Kalva, S. P. (2016). Complications of inferior vena cava filters. *Cardiovasc Diagn Ther, 6*(6), 632–641. PMID: 28123983

26. RATIONALE

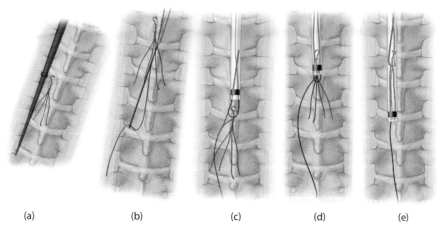

     (a)   (b)   (c)   (d)   (e)

Lasso technique for IVC filter retrieval.

A "fallback" technique for difficult IVC filter retrieval in cases where the hook cannot be snared by standard technique involves an 18 Fr sheath 85 cm long inserted over a stiff wire under fluoroscopic guidance to the level of the filter. A Benson wire (0.035) (Cook Medical, Bloomington, IN) and a snare catheter are maneuvered so that they pass through the interstices in the opposite side of the device. The wire is snared with an EN Snare (Merit Medical Systems, South Jordan, UT) below the filter, and the resulting "lasso" is pulled up below the filter collar. The 18 Fr sheath is then advanced over the filter to collapse the filter legs and the filter is removed. The 18 Fr sheath is removed from the neck with the patient in Trendelenburg position, and a purse-string suture is used to ensure hemostasis. In a series of 34 patients, a success rate of 100% was reported without any morbidity. An emerging strategy to facilitate retrieval of long-standing filters is photothermal tissue ablation with an excimer laser. Laser-assisted retrieval is successful 99.2% with a complication rate of 1.6%.

Correct Answer   **C** Benson wire and a snare catheter are maneuvered so that the wire passes through the opposite interstices of the filter. Snaring the wire with EN Snare (Merit Med, South Jordan, UT) with a "lasso" pulled below the filter collar

Reference
Foley, P. J., Nathan, D. P., Wang, G. J., et al. (2012). A "fall-back" technique for difficult inferior vena cava filter retrieval. *J Vasc Surg, 56*(6), 1629–1633. PMID: 22607712

27. RATIONALE

Chronic venous insufficiency (CVI) can be primary (non-thrombotic) or secondary (post-thrombotic). Post-thrombotic syndrome can develop in up to 50% of patients with a prior history of deep venous thrombosis. Non-thrombotic conditions include May–Thurner syndrome, which is the most common form of primary chronic venous insufficiency. Clinical manifestations of chronic venous insufficiency include pain, claudication, swelling, skin changes (eczema, lipodermatoscle-rosis, dermatitis), and ulceration of the involved limb, usually near the ankle. Diagnostic testing should focus on determining the etiology of CVI in addition to determining the inflow and outflow of the affected segment. The pertinent tests include venous duplex ultrasound, air plethysmography, computed tomographic venography, MRV, and ascending venography.

Correct Answer   **D** 50% of patients

Reference

Kahn, S. R., Comerota, A. J., Cushman, M., et al. (2014). The postthrombotic syndrome: evidence-based prevention, diagnosis, and treatment strategies: a scientific statement from the American Heart Association. *Circulation, 130*(18), 1636–1661. PMID: 25246013

28. RATIONALE

These diameters help in determination of the extent of femoro-ilio-caval narrowing. CTV and MRV elucidate anatomy and status of the vein in regard to compression or occlusion and collateral circulation. In addition, any unexpected abdominal and pelvic pathology, including malignancy, can also be evaluated if present. Most patients with chronic venous insufficiency can be managed by conservative management with elevation of the extremity, graduated compression stockings, and local wound care for ulceration and antibiotics if the ulcer shows evidence of infection. Endovascular treatment should be reserved for patients who do not tolerate or fail conservative treatment.

Correct Answer   **B** Common iliac vein 16 mm, external iliac vein 14 mm, common femoral vein 12 mm

Reference

Kahn, S. R., Comerota, A. J., Cushman, M., et al. (2014). The postthrombotic syndrome: evidence-based prevention, diagnosis, and treatment strategies: a scientific statement from the American Heart Association. *Circulation, 130*(18), 1636–1661. PMID: 25246013

29. RATIONALE

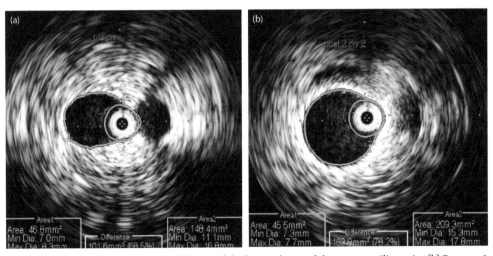

(a) Intravascular ultrasound planimetry. Predilation of the luminal area of the common iliac vein. (b) Post-angioplasty and stenting of the luminal area of the common iliac vein.

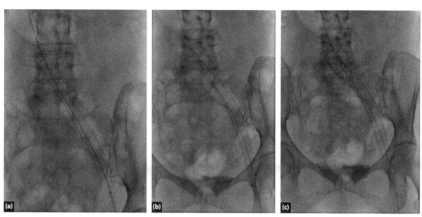

Stenting of the left distal femoroal-ilio-caval tract. (a) Intitial stent placement across iliocaval confluence. (b) Stent extension distally. (c) Stent stack postdeployement of Gianturco Z™ stent across the confluence.

Stenting of the femoro-ilio-caval segment is the most common modality of treatment for patients who fail conservative treatment for chronic venous insufficiency. Stenting is preferably performed under general anesthesia, as there is significant pain during venous angioplasty. With the patient in a supine position, the left (more commonly involved) femoral vein is punctured under ultrasound guidance. Either a micropuncture needle or an 18-gauge needle is used for puncture and a 0.035-inch glide wire (Terumo Medical Corporation, Sommerset, NJ) is used to enter the inferior vena cava in its proximal segment. An 11 Fr 10-cm-long sheath is advanced. Ascending venogram is performed if renal function is not compromised. Intravascular ultrasound (IVUS) is then performed with a 0.035-inch probe (Volcano Corporation, San Diego, CA). Using planimetry, luminal areas of the common femoral vein (CFV), external iliac vein (EIV), and common iliac vein (CIV) are assessed (normal cutoffs of 125 mm², 150 mm², and 200 mm² are used as normal cutoffs for CFV, EIV, and CIV, respectively). Any decrease in the luminal area in a symptomatic patient is considered abnormal thereby meriting angioplasty and stenting. Pre-dilation is performed with an 18 × 60 mm Atlas PTA dilation catheter (Bard Vascular, Inc., Tempe, AZ) proceeding from the CFV to the distal IVC. Stenting is then carried out with 20-mm WALLSTENT™ Endoprosthesis (Boston Scientific Corporation, Hallborough MA). The proximal landing zone is typically 1–2 cm above the iliac confluence, while the distal landing zone is in the CFV. Given the decreased radial strength of the WALLSTENT™ endoprosthesis, a Gianturco Z stent (Cook Medical, Bloomington, IN) is used to provide additional strength across the confluence of common iliac veins. The Gianturco stent should extend 5 mm beyond the wall stent proximally into the inferior vena cava. An overlap of 3 cm between the wall stent is required to compensate for shortening during angioplasty. Post-dilatation is performed with an 18 × 60 Atlas PTA dilatation catheter (Bard Peripheral Vascular, Inc., Murray Hill, New Providence, NJ). Any residual narrowing on IVUS interrogation is overcome with repeat dilatation with a larger balloon (20 mm). Completion venography is then performed. The 11 Fr sheath is subsequently withdrawn to just outside the vein and a surgical fibrillar absorbable hemostat (Ethicon US, LLC, Sommerville, NJ) is introduced via the sheath to aid in local hemostasis. Manual pressure is then held to complete the hemostasis, and a pressure dressing is applied.

Correct Answer   **C** Under general anesthesia with puncture of the ipsilateral left femoral vein in the midthigh

Reference
Neglén, P., Hollis, K. C., Olivier, J., & Raju, S. (2007). Stenting of the venous outflow in chronic venous disease: long-term stent-related outcome, clinical, and hemodynamic result. *J Vasc Surg, 46*(5), 979–990. PMID: 17980284

30. RATIONALE

Results following deployment of 982 stents for chronic, nonmalignant, obstructive lesions of the femoro-ilio-caval venous segment with a 6-year follow-up demonstrated primary patency, primary assisted, and secondary patency rates of 79%, 100%, and 100% for non-thrombotic lesions and 57%, 80%, and 86% for post-thrombotic lesions, respectively. The main risk factor for restenosis/stent occlusion after venous stenting was the presence and severity of post-thrombotic disease; thrombophilia by itself was not a risk factor. In-stent restenosis/stent compression is reported in 25% and is the result of a buildup of robust neointimal hyperplastic tissue and fibrotic tissue causing extrinsic compression of the stent. Hyperdilation is used to treat this complication.

Correct Answer **B** Primary patency 57%, primary assisted patency 80%, and secondary patency 86%

Reference

Neglén, P., Hollis, K. C., Olivier, J., & Raju, S. (2007). Stenting of the venous outflow in chronic venous disease: long-term stent-related outcome, clinical, and hemodynamic result. *J Vasc Surg, 46*(5), 979–990. PMID: 17980284

31. RATIONALE

It is important to confirm the lumen of the common femoral vein, external iliac vein, and common iliac vein following angioplasty and stenting by IVUS and by venography. Layering of the thrombus within the stent occurs because of poor inflow and outflow. Contributing factors include stent undersizing, understenting, and lack of perioperative use of anticoagulation/antiplatelet medications. Restenting after fracture of a previously undersized stent with a large-caliber angioplasty balloon or extending the stent stack proximally and distally is required for undersized stents and understenting, respectively. Contralateral iliac vein thrombosis can occur from jailing of the contralateral common iliac via an ipsilateral stent. It can be overcome with a wall stent and Gianturco Z stent.

Correct Answer **D** Venous angioplasty and stenting with wall stent endoprosthesis and Gianturco Z stent only after trial of conservative therapy

Reference

Neglén, P., Hollis, K. C., Olivier, J., & Raju, S. (2007). Stenting of the venous outflow in chronic venous disease: long-term stent-related outcome, clinical, and hemodynamic result. *J Vasc Surg, 46*(5), 979–990. PMID: 17980284

32. RATIONALE

The development of stent compression/in-stent restenosis is from extrinsic compression of the stent because of fibrotic tissue or a significant buildup of neohyperplastic tissue. The incidence of 21%–25% has been reported. Hyperdilatation may result in stent compression/in-stent restenosis. The fracture of stents in the arterial system has been well studied, and its incidences, predisposing factors, and sequelae are much better understood. None of these have been studied in depth or reported in the iliofemoral venous segments. Studies on stent fractures in the arterial system reveal a direct correlation between fracture rate and biomechanical forces exerted on the stents. Finite element analysis shows areas of increased stress on stent struts during many physiologic body motions such as walking and bending of the knee and hip joints. These motions create axial compression and elongation, segmental bending, and repetitive compression of the stent, which predispose the strut to fracture. Further in-depth finite element analysis has shown that stress on the stent material during cyclical bending is proportional to the accuracy of the radius of the vein—the smaller the radius of the bend, the higher the stress. Focal compression of the stent appears to increase the stress especially during cyclic compression and bending. These findings suggest that stents should be fully dilated when deployed and in locations subject to cyclical bending such as in the common femoral vein. In addition to the stent location, stent material, surface finish, and geometric design have also been implicated in stent refracture. Similar forces in the veins may result in stent fracture, but those forces in the arterial system may have a similar effect on the stents in the venous system, although to a variable degree. While the iliac veins are not as mobile as the superficial femoral artery, they are subject to repetitive cyclic compression by the adjacent artery. Extension of stents into the common femoral vein can predispose the stent to similar stress forces described earlier. Residual narrowing in the stent in the segment of the common femoral vein may further increase stress and the risk of fracture. Stent migration is an uncommon problem, with the majority of studies either reporting no migration or only a very few cases of stent migration. In general stent migration is a function of stent location, sizing, type of stent, deployment mechanism, and familiarity of the operator with all of the earlier factors. Stent embolization is an extremely rare phenomenon and is most likely related to mis-sizing of the stent.

Correct Answer   **B** 21%–25%

Reference
Ye, K., Lu, X., Li, W., et al. (2012). Long-term outcomes of stent placement for symptomatic nonthrombotic iliac vein compression lesions in chronic venous disease. *J Vasc Interv Radiol*, *23*(4), 497–502. PMID: 22342482

33. **RATIONALE**

The main reason to adopt the strategy of thrombus removal is the severe morbidity associated with post-thrombotic syndrome following iliofemoral venous thrombosis. Early removal of the thrombus from the iliofemoral venous segment improves long-term results and reduces venous pressures often to normal levels. Anticoagulation alone in the management of iliofemoral DVT may result in late development of symptoms of venous claudication in up to 40% of patients. The aim of the procedure is to remove all the thrombus, restore patency of the operative veins, and maintain unobstructive flow from the iliofemoral venous segment into the inferior vena cava. This is achieved by opening the thrombosed infrainguinal venous segments, correcting any underlying venous lesions or compression, and preventing rethrombosis by constructing an arterial venous fistula followed by adequate anticoagulation, often using catheter-directed technique into the thrombectomized veins. With preoperative imaging studies the proximal and distal aspect of the DVT should be clearly defined. The routine use of inferior vena cava filters is not necessary except in patients with nonocclusive thrombus in the inferior vena cava. Heritable thrombophilia workup is not required, as the risk of recurrence is governed by the extent of DVT rather than by thrombophilia. The procedure is associated with relatively few complications, and long-term iliac vein patency in 80% of patients has been reported following venous thrombectomy.

Correct Answer D Multiple trauma, intracranial bleeding, and in pregnancy

Reference
Hartung, O., Benmiloud, F., Barthelemy, P., et al. (2008). Late results of surgical venous thrombectomy with iliocaval stenting. *J Vasc Surg*, *47*(2), 381–387. PMID: 18241761

34. RATIONALE

The aim of open iliofemoral venous thrombectomy is to remove all thrombus, restore patency to the operated veins, and maintain unobstructed flow from the iliofemoral venous segment into the vena cava and is best achieved by opening the thrombosed infrainguinal venous segments, correcting any underlying venous lesions or compression, and preventing deep thrombosis by constructing an arteriovenous fistula and providing adequate anticoagulation, often by catheter-directed techniques, into the thrombectomized veins. The long-term patency of the iliac vein in 80% of patients has been reported following iliofemoral venous thrombectomy with arteriovenous fistula. Routine use of IVC filters is not necessary except in patients with a free-floating thrombus in the inferior vena cava. After completion of iliofemoral venous thrombectomy, intraoperative venography and intravascular ultrasound are performed to detect any iliac vein stenosis and should be corrected by iliac vein angioplasty and stenting. An end-to-side AV fistula is constructed by anastomosing the amputated end of the proximal great saphenous vein or a large proximal branch of the great saphenous vein to the side of the superficial femoral artery with an anastomotic diameter of 3.5–4 mm. The purpose of AVF is to increase venous velocity but not the venous pressure.

Correct Answer C 80% of patients

Reference
Comerota, A., & Ruiz-Gamboa, R., (2018). Operative venous thrombectomy. In S. Hans, Shepard, A., Weaver, M., et al. (Ed.), *Endovascular and open vascular reconstruction: a practical approach* (pp. 383–388). Boca Raton, FL: Taylor & Francis/CRC Press.

35. RATIONALE

Oral anticoagulation is started when the patient resumes oral intake after open thrombectomy. Heparin infusion followed by direct-acting oral anticoagulants and, in some cases, warfarin is continued for an extended period, generally for 1 year or longer. Intermittent pneumatic compression garments are used on both legs postoperatively when the patient is not ambulating. Before discharge, the patient is fitted with a 30–40 mmHg ankle gradient below the knee compression stockings for walking in the morning until bedtime. Randomized trials have demonstrated at least a 50% reduction in post-thrombotic morbidity with the use of 30–40 mmHg ankle gradient compression stockings.

Correct Answer D 50%

Reference
Prandoni, P., Lensing, A. W., Prins, M. H., et al. (2004). Below-knee elastic compression stockings to prevent the post-thrombotic syndrome: a randomized, controlled trial. *Ann Intern Med*, *141*(4), 249–256. PMID: 15313740

36. RATIONALE

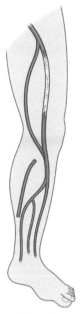

Saphenopopliteal bypass. Note the distal GSV disconnected from the GSV used for the bypass.

Saphenopopliteal bypass (SPB) involves transplantation of the ipsilateral great saphenous vein to bypass a femoral vein occlusion. It can be used to treat unilateral occlusion of the femoral vein, especially if the profunda femoris vein (PFV) is an inadequate collateral conduit. Preoperative venogram and imaging with duplex ultrasound, including superficial vein mapping, are obtained. Usually, profunda femoris vein flow compensates for femoral vein occlusion. Saphenopopliteal bypass may be indicated if there is evidence of unilateral occlusion of the femoral vein with a patent iliac venous system and occlusion of the profunda femoris vein or the profunda femoris is small in caliber. Appropriate candidates for this procedure must have preserved inflow and outflow, including a popliteal vein, great saphenous vein, saphenofemoral junction, and patent proximal iliocaval venous outflow. The decision to include a distal arteriovenous fistula to augment inflow is made intraoperatively by assessment of the flow through the bypass and is performed between the popliteal artery and vein distal to the anastomosis or an interposition graft using a 1- to 2-cm segment from a side branch, or a distal segment of the great saphenous vein is harvested. A side-biting clamp is applied to the popliteal artery distal to the saphenopopliteal anastomosis. An arteriotomy is created and then extended with an arterial anastomosis and then completed in an end-to-end manner with 6-0 polypropylene suture. A side-biting clamp vascular clamp is then applied, and an end-to-side anastomosis is performed. Arteriovenous fistula should be assessed for a thrill. Primary patency of saphenopopliteal bypass is 53%; primary assisted patency rates of 69% and 75% have been reported.

Correct Answer   **C** Unilateral occlusion of the femoral vein with a patent iliac venous system and occlusion of the profunda femoris vein

Reference
Coleman, D. M., Rectenwald, J. E., Vandy, F. C., & Wakefield, T. W. (2013). Contemporary results after sapheno-popliteal bypass for chronic femoral vein occlusion. *J Vasc Surg Venous Lymphat Disord*, *1*(1), 45–51. PMID: 26993893

37. RATIONALE

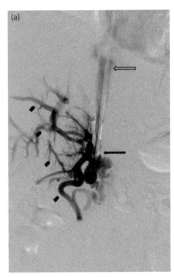 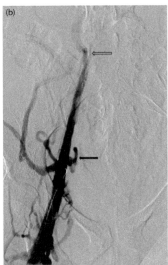 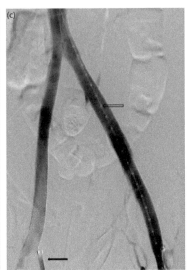

(a) Inferior venocavogram from right IJ vein access. Large network of retroperitoneal and hepatic caudate vein collaterals are seen. (b) Antegrade right common femoral digital subtraction venogram shows contrast in the diminutive right EIV and CIV. (c) Bilateral iliofemoral venogram show widely patent reconstructed iliofemoral veins with robust outflow into IVC.

Inferior venocavogram through a 9 Fr, 30-cm sheath from the right internal jugular vein access with the tip of the sheath placed in the suprarenal inferior vena cava. Antegrade right common femoral digital subtraction venogram through a 6 Fr, 30 cm great saphenous vein sheath, which is upsized to 10 Fr. Only retroperitoneal and pelvic collateral veins are visible in patients with no visualization of the external iliac vein or common iliac vein. Using the great saphenous vein as access with the wire advanced into the inferior vena cava using access from the contralateral side. Final placement of two kissing wall stents (12 mm) and an 18-mm wall stent in the suprarenal inferior vena cava with a short 5-cm (approximately) segment of inferior vena cava at renal veins was not intentionally stented to preserve renal vein outflow. The patient was discharged on low molecular weight heparin, clopidogrel, and aspirin. Staged procedures for a complex case with acute thrombosis below the groin and chronic occlusive lesions of external iliac veins, common iliac veins, and inferior vena cava are more appropriate.

Correct Answer   **B** Venography with thrombolysis, balloon angioplasty, suction thrombectomy from above the knee popliteal veins to external iliac veins followed by bilateral iliofemoral recanalization with bilateral overlapping wall stents from the common iliac vein, external iliac vein, and rostral femoral vein 6 months later

Reference
Williams D. M. (2014). Iliocaval reconstruction in chronic deep vein thrombosis. *Tech Vasc Interv Radiol*, *17*(2), 109–113. PMID: 24840966.

38. RATIONALE
Creation of arteriovenous fistula is an important adjunct if there is concern for poor inflow. Postoperatively patients are started on low molecular weight heparin followed by oral anticoagulation, and in some cases antiplatelet medications are added. These medications alone are

not sufficient to prevent thrombosis in a crossover femoro-femoral venous bypass. Therefore, creation of an arteriovenous fistula is a necessary adjunct. The 5-year primary patency of femoro-femoral venous bypass is 70%, and a secondary patency rate of 78% has been reported. Complications of crossover femoro-femoral venous bypass includes surgical site infection, hematoma, and early graft occlusion.

Correct Answer **D** Creation of arteriovenous fistula

Reference
Garg, N., Gloviczki, P., Karimi, K. M., et al. (2011). Factors affecting outcome of open and hybrid reconstructions for nonmalignant obstruction of iliofemoral veins and inferior vena cava. *J Vasc Surg, 53*(2), 383–393. PMID: 21146346

39. RATIONALE

Popliteal vein aneurysms are a rare entity that necessitate repair because of the associated high risk of pulmonary embolism. Up to 71% of patients with venous aneurysms develop venous thromboembolism. Several methods of repair have been described. If there is a redundant length of the vein associated with the aneurysm, resection and end-to-end anastomosis to the proximal and distal segments of the vein can be performed.[1,2] If additional length of the vein is required for tension-free anastomosis, resection with an interposition graft of the great saphenous vein or femoral vein should be performed. Alternatively, surgical aneurysmectomy and lateral venorrhaphy can be considered. In the presence of thrombosis, open thrombectomy before plication should be performed. Preoperative evaluation includes duplex ultrasound and MRV. Posterior approach for popliteal vein aneurysm is preferable than medial approach.

Correct Answer **C** To prevent pulmonary embolism

References
1. Sessa, C., Nicolini, P., Perrin, M., et al. (2000). Management of symptomatic and asymptomatic popliteal venous aneurysms: a retrospective analysis of 25 patients and review of the literature. *J Vasc Surg, 32*(5), 902–912. PMID: 11054222
2. Teter, K. A., Maldonado, T. M., & Adelman, M. A. (2018). A systematic review of venous aneurysms by anatomic location. *J Vasc Surg Venous Lymphat Disord, 6*(3), 408–413. PMID:29661366

40. RATIONALE

The largest single-institution series of popliteal venous aneurysm consists of 25 patients who underwent surgical repair (n19). The reported complications were 8% hematoma, 8% transient peroneal nerve palsy, 4% local infection, and 12% early thrombosis. A recent meta-analysis summarizes the complications reported in the literature and reveals that 20% (5/25) had early thrombosis from the procedure, 4% had late thrombosis, and 12% had aneurysm recurrence. The varying rates of early thrombosis likely reflect differing practice patterns in anticoagulation, ranging from the use of low molecular weight heparin for a limited time to varying treatment lengths of oral anticoagulation ranging from 3 months to lifelong. In the setting of thrombus and recurrence of pulmonary embolism, open thrombectomy with an adjunct procedure to correct the cause of the nidus for thrombus formation should be considered.

Correct Answer C 20%

Reference
Maldonado-Fernandez, N., Lopez-Espada, C., Martinez-Gamez, F. J., et al. (2013). Popliteal venous aneurysms: results of surgical treatment. *Ann Vasc Surg, 27*(4), 501–509. PMID: 23522443

41. RATIONALE

Nutcracker syndrome describes a phenomenon that occurs when the left renal vein is compressed between the aorta and the superior mesenteric artery. Posterior nutcracker syndrome is another variant of this condition, which occurs when a retroaortic left renal vein is compressed between the aorta and vertebral body. Many patients are symptomatic. The most common symptom is hematuria followed by abdominal or flank pain. Hematuria is secondary to left renal vein compression. Increased intraluminal pressure within the left renal vein results in the development of hilar varices around the renal pelvis and the ureter, and rupture of thin-walled veins within the collecting system may result in both macroscopic and microscopic hematuria. Other symptoms include orthostatic proteinuria, pain in the left flank or left upper quadrant of the abdomen, left-sided varicocele, and fatigue. Conservative treatment of nutcracker syndrome is successful in up to 30% of patients. For patients with more severe symptoms, distal transposition of the left renal vein directly into the inferior vena cava should be considered. Other open surgical options include gonadal vein reimplantation, ectopic kidney transplantation, and even nephrectomy. Endovascular stenting is being increasingly utilized, but long-term outcome data is lacking. The preferred open technique for treating nutcracker syndrome is left renal vein transposition 3–5 cm below the formal opening of the left renal vein. Adjunct procedures using great saphenous vein interposition should be considered in select cases to avoid narrowing of the left renal vein and to decrease the tension between the left renal vein and inferior vena cava when the length of the left renal vein is too short to reach the inferior vena cava comfortably. Primary patency of 74% has been reported at 2 years. A reintervention rate of 10% within 30 days after open venous procedure has been reported, most often due to left renal vein stenosis as detected by intravascular ultrasound.

Correct Answer A Hematuria

Reference
Velasquez, C. A., Saeyeldin, A., Zafar, M. A., Brownstein, A. J., & Erben, Y. (2018). A systematic review on management of nutcracker syndrome. *J Vasc Surg Venous Lymphat Disord, 6*(2), 271–278. PMID: 29292117

42. RATIONALE

Pelvic congestion syndrome occurs in premenopausal women secondary to venous drainage obstruction causing multiple varicose veins and painful venous congestion in the pelvis, perineum, and vulva. Pain becomes worse on standing, walking, and factors increasing intraabdominal pressures such as lifting and pregnancy. The pain is relieved on lying down. Vessel diameter alone is only accurate in 56% for reflux identification. Venous reflux can be divided into three grades:

- Grade I – When the retrograde flow is limited to ovarian vein
- Grade II – When the retrograde flow is present in the parauterine veins
- Grade III – Retrograde flow crossing the midline passing to the parauterine plexus of the contralateral side

CT and MRI provide accurate anatomical visualization. Venography remains the gold standard for diagnosis of pelvic congestion syndrome. It should be reserved for patients who had prior noninvasive imaging while the interventional therapy is being planned. Minimally invasive intervention in the form of ovarian vein embolization and embolization of the branches of the internal iliac vein should be considered. All venous outlets should be closed, and when multiplication of ovarian veins is present, embolization of each branch should be performed.

Correct Answer   B 71.2% at 5 mm, 83.3% at 6 mm, 81.1% at 7 mm, and 75.8% at 8 mm

Reference
Bałabuszek, K., Toborek, M., & Pietura, R. (2022). Comprehensive overview of the venous disorder known as pelvic congestion syndrome. *Ann Med*, *54*(1), 22–36. PMID: 34935563

43. RATIONALE

Post-embolization syndrome occurs in 20% of patients characterized by increased pelvic pain, hyperthermia, and tenderness over the embolized vein. The use of nonsteroidal antiinflammatory drugs helps in resolution of symptoms. A potentially dangerous complication is coil or vascular plug migration to central veins and its eventual migration to the pulmonary artery. The endovascular approach is usually successful in the retrieval of coils or vascular plug if not in a desirable location.

Correct Answer   B 20%

Reference
Bałabuszek, K., Toborek, M., & Pietura, R. (2022). Comprehensive overview of the venous disorder known as pelvic congestion syndrome. *Ann Med*, *54*(1), 22–36. PMID: 34935563

44. RATIONALE

A systemic literature search including 1197 studies (45 trials) showed that compared with the low molecular weight heparin (LMWH)–vitamin K antagonist combination, a treatment strategy using ultra-fractionated heparin UFH–vitamin K antagonist combination was associated with an increased risk of recurrent venous thromboembolism (hazard ratio 1.42). The reported incidences of patients experiencing recurrent thromboembolism during 3 months of treatment were 1.84% for the UFH–vitamin K antagonist combination and 1.30% for the LMWH–vitamin K antagonist combination. Apixaban and rivaroxaban were associated with a lower risk of bleeding than the LMWH–vitamin K antagonist combination, with a lower proportion of patients experiencing a major bleeding event during 3 months of anticoagulation. The conclusion of this analysis was that there were no statistically significant differences for efficacy and safety associated with most treatment strategies used to treat acute venous thromboembolism compared with the LMWH–vitamin K antagonist combination. However, findings suggest that the UFH–vitamin K antagonist combination is the least effective strategy and that rivaroxaban and apixaban may be associated with the lowest risk for bleeding.

Correct Answer   A Oral apixaban

Reference
Castellucci, L. A., Cameron, C., Le Gal, G., et al. (2014). Clinical and safety outcomes associated with treatment of acute venous thromboembolism: a systematic review and meta-analysis. *JAMA*, *312*(11), 1122–1135. PMID: 25226478

45. RATIONALE

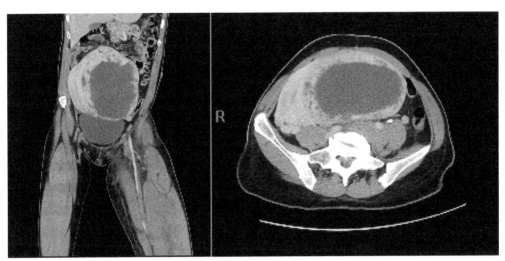

Left, CT coronal view, Right, CT axial view of 18.6 cm × 15.5 cm × 9.9 cm pelvic mass causing an effect on pelvic structures.

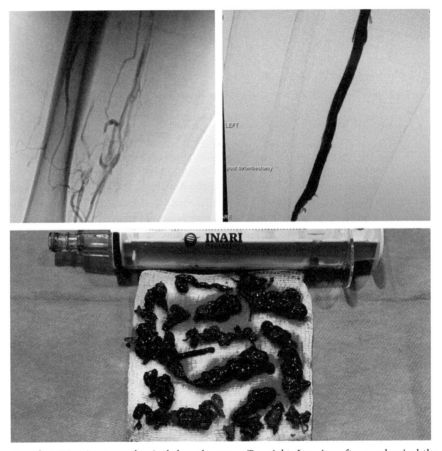

Top left, imaging after tPA prior to mechanical thrombectomy. Top right, Imaging after mechanical thrombectomy. Bottom, thrombus extracted using Inari device.

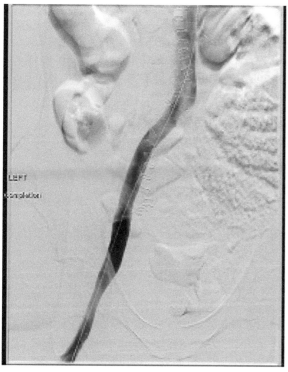

Left common iliac vein stent.

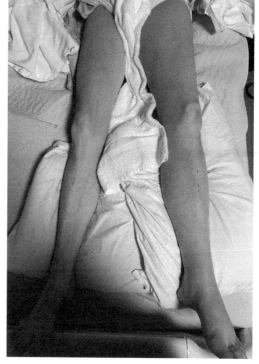

Left lower extremity on hospital discharge.

Phlegmasia cerulea dolens is a precursor of venous gangrene and is a limb life-threatening condition with a mortality of 20%–40%, and in approximately 30% of these, death is caused by pulmonary embolism. This is slightly more prevalent in men, with a male-to-female ratio of 1.5 to 1. The patients present with pain followed by significant swelling and cyanosis secondary to thrombosis in the main axial and collateral veins causing a massive fluid shift into the interstitium, obstructing arterial flow and causing venous gangrene. The patient described in this question developed compression of the left common iliac vein from a large uterine fibroid measuring 18×18 cm. The management of this serious condition is by elevation of the extremity, anticoagulation, catheter-directed mechanico-pharmacological thrombolysis, and left common iliac vein angioplasty/stenting in selected cases. In addition, removal of the cause – hysterectomy in this patient for a large uterine fibroid – will result in a satisfactory outcome in most instances.

Correct Answer   C Phlegmasia cerulea dolens

Reference
Ekkel, E., Chandran, T., Trpkovski, M., & Hans, S. (2022). Management of phlegmasia cerulea dolens caused by a giant leiomyoma. *J Vasc Surg Cases Innov Tech*, *8*(2), 240–243. PMID: 35493345

46. RATIONALE

May–Thurner syndrome results from the compression of the proximal segment of the left common vein by the crossing of the right common iliac artery. Autopsy studies have shown the prevalence of May–Thurner syndrome is 14%–32% in the general population, and some have suggested that iliac vein compression could be a normal anatomical pattern. The compression caused by the artery against the lumbar spine results in deposition of the collagen and venous spur formation with thrombosis, resulting from overlapping risk factors for DVT such as oral contraceptive use, postpartum status, scoliosis, and thrombophilia. Duplex venous imaging and CT venography are diagnostic, although duplex venous study can visualize the left common iliac vein in only 47% of instances. May–Thurner syndrome accounts for only 2%–5% of all patients presenting with DVT. In symptomatic patients, mechanico-pharmacological thrombectomy for associated iliofemoral venous thrombosis followed by venous angioplasty and stenting is recommended. Anticoagulation should be continued for at least 6–12 months following intervention for May–Thurner syndrome.

Correct Answer **B** 2%–5% of cases

Reference
Birn, J., & Vedantham, S. (2015). May–Thurner syndrome and other obstructive iliac vein lesions: meaning, myth, and mystery. *Vasc Med, 20*(1), 74–83. PMID: 25502563

47. **RATIONALE**

Vascular malformations, though uncommon (0.8%–1.1% of the general population), are often associated with significant morbidity. Vascular anomalies can be divided into two groups: Vascular tumors or vascular malformations. The most common vascular tumor is hemangioma, which is present at birth, is a proliferative lesion, and usually resolve spontaneously during childhood. Vascular malformations are also present at birth, with growth rates parallel with the patient, although they may not become clinically evident until later in life. Vascular malformations have normal endothelial cells and clinically do not regress, but rather continue to progress over the lifetime of the patient. Vascular malformations can be trivial to life threatening, from focal to extensive. They are classified based on the territory of vascular involvement, vascular structure (arterial, venous, lymphatic, or combined), and flow dynamics. The crucial distinction between high-flow and low-flow lesions should be ascertained because prognosis and treatment are dependent on the flow dynamics of the lesion. The utility of dynamic contrast-enhanced magnetic resonance imaging (DCE MRI) to distinguish between high-flow and low-flow vascular malformation was successful in 83.8% of patients, minimizing the need for invasive catheter-based arteriography.

Correct Answer **C** Dynamic contrast-enhanced MRI

Reference
Lidsky, M. E., Spritzer, C. E., & Shortell, C. K. (2012). The role of dynamic contrast-enhanced magnetic resonance imaging in the diagnosis and management of patients with vascular malformations. *J Vasc Surg, 56*(3), 757–764.e751. PMID: 22840741

48. **RATIONALE**

A reported 136 vascular malformations in 135 patients were classified as low-flow lesions in 105 and high-flow lesions in 31. Of 105 low-flow vascular malformations (77.2%), 23 (21.9%) were managed conservatively, 30 (36.2%) were treated with sclerotherapy (sodium tetradecyl sulfate, polidocanol, doxycycline, and/or ethanol), 19 (17.1%) were surgically resected, and 8 (7.6%) were managed with a combination of all three modalities. Of the 31 (22.8%) high-flow vascular malformations, 8 (25.8%) were managed conservatively, 8 (25.8) were treated with transcatheter embolization, 6 (19.4%) required embolization followed by sclerotherapy, and 5 (16.1%) underwent primary resection. Patients requiring sclerotherapy underwent a median of three sessions. Primary resection was performed in 23 (low- and high-flow lesions combined), of which 12 lesions (52.2%) were venous, 5 (21.7%) were lymphatic, and 1 (4.3%) was venolymphatic and 5 had an arterial component. Infection, ulceration, deep venous thrombosis, pulmonary embolism, and minor hemorrhage are reported complications.

Correct Answer   **D** All of the above

Reference

Lidsky, M. E., Spritzer, C. E., & Shortell, C. K. (2012). The role of dynamic contrast-enhanced magnetic resonance imaging in the diagnosis and management of patients with vascular malformations. *J Vasc Surg, 56*(3), 757–764.e751. PMID: 22840741

49. RATIONALE

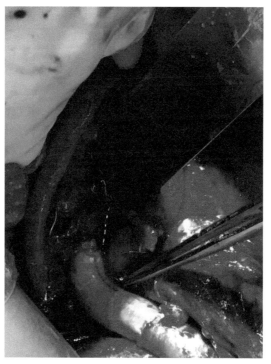

Left external iliac interposition 10-mm PTFE graft.

The patient underwent emergent bedside duplex venous ultrasound in the recovery room, which confirmed the absence of flow in the left common femoral and external iliac vein and minimal flow in the left femoral and popliteal vein. The patient was reexplored using midline infraumbilical incision extending from the symphysis pubis to 2 cm above the umbilicus. The left external iliac vein was found to be occluded, and a 10-mm PTFE graft was interposed from the external iliac vein just above the groin to the common iliac vein bifurcation, with complete relief of symptoms of swelling and discoloration. The left lower extremity regained its normal appearance. Follow-up duplex vein imaging 2 years following reconstruction showed a patent interposition graft. Patients with iatrogenic iliac vein injury diagnosed during the index operation should be repaired by lateral venorrhaphy and interposition graft if there is more than 30%–40% loss of circumference of the iliac vein. Patients should be monitored for deep venous thrombosis in the perioperative period. Major venous injury may occur during aortoiliac reconstruction, oncologic pelvic operations, and anterior lumbar spine surgery. Emergent vascular consultation is recommended for management of such serious injuries.

Correct Answer   **B** Left iliac vein occlusion

Reference
Hans, S. S., Vang, S., & Sachwani-Daswani, G. (2018). Iatrogenic major venous injury is associated with increased morbidity of aortic reconstruction. *Ann Vasc Surg, 47*, 200-204. PMID: 28887236.

50. RATIONALE

Portal vein thrombosis is a known complication of cirrhosis of the liver with portal hypertension and hypersplenism. Acute portal/superior mesenteric vein thrombosis will result in intestinal venous congestion, resulting in intermittent or continuous abdominal pain and diarrhea. Chronic portal vein thrombosis most often is asymptomatic. Portal vein thrombus is not an indication for splenectomy, liver transplant, or distal splenorenal shunt. Anticoagulation helps in recanalization of the portal vein with improved survival.

Correct Answer   **C** Anticoagulation

Reference
Kinjo, N., Kawanaka, H., Akahoshi, T., et al. (2014). Portal vein thrombosis in liver cirrhosis. *World J Hepatol, 6*(2), 64-71. PMID: 24575165

51. RATIONALE

The Caprini model of risk stratification for venous thromboembolism has been validated in a NSQIP study involving more than 8000 elective surgical procedures. Risk factors are scored from 1 to 5 points with stroke (less than 1 month), knee or hip arthroplasty, hip, pelvis, leg fracture, and spinal cord injury (less than 1 month) representing 5 points. A total risk score of 1 or less (low risk) means the incidence of deep venous thrombosis is 2%; a total risk score of 5 or more is the highest risk, with incidence of deep venous thrombosis as high as 40%–80% with up to 5% mortality. The use of this model to identify and grade the risk of venous thromboembolism aids in selecting suitable prophylaxis for venous thromboembolism.

Correct Answer   **D** Acute spinal cord injury

Reference
Caprini, J. A. (2010). Risk assessment as a guide for the prevention of the many faces of venous thromboembolism. *Am J Surg, 199*(1 Suppl), S3-10. PMID: 20103082

52. RATIONALE

Venous ulcer is a common condition, and its incidence increases with advanced age and in women. The ulcers are typically located just above the ankle on the medial side (occasionally on the lateral side) and are usually superficial. In a systemic review of 48 randomized controlled trials comparing compression dressings with no compression, compression dressings with multiple layers of elastic components were the most effective treatment method of increasing healing of the venous ulcers, unless the ulcer is infected with associated cellulitis and drainage causing significant discomfort. When the associated cellulitis is present, cultures and appropriate antibiotics should be administered depending on the sensitivity results. Routine use of antibiotics without any clinical evidence of infection in the ulcers is not indicated. If the venous ulcer does not respond to conservative treatment, venous reflux study should be performed to detect any perforator or great saphenous vein incompetence, which may be amenable to endovenous ablation or sclerotherapy. Though uncommon, iliocaval venous obstruction should be ruled out in patients who do not have a superficial or deep venous reflux in the femoral, popliteal, and tibial veins or perforator veins. The mere existence of either reflux or obstruction does not appear to be the complete pathology for venous ulcers, as activation of the inflammatory cascade may act as an inciting factor for the appearance of ulceration. In some cases, healing is impaired due to concomitant arterial obstruction, local trauma, lymphedema, autoimmune disease, and superimposed infection.

Correct Answer   **C** Graduated compression stockings with local wound care and management of dermatitis

Reference
O'Donnell, T. F., Jr, Passman, M. A., Marston, W. A., et al. (2014). Management of venous leg ulcers: clinical practice guidelines of the Society for Vascular Surgery ® and the American Venous Forum. *J Vasc Surg, 60*(2 Suppl), 3S–59S. PMID: 24974070.

SECTION 14: LYMPHOLOGY

MCQs 1–19

Q1. Female-to-male ratio in primary lymphedema is:
A. 2.5 to 1
B. 3.5 to 1
C. 4.5 to 1
D. 5.5 to 1

Q2. The most common form of lymphedema in developed countries is:
A. Congenital (Milroy disease)
B. Lymphedema praecox (Meigs disease)
C. Lymphedema tarda
D. Acquired lymphedema

Q3. Clinically significant edema of the upper extremity after axillary intervention in breast cancer survivors occurs in:
A. <6% of patients
B. 6%–30% of patients
C. 31%–35% of patients
D. 36%–40% of patients

Q4. In primary lymphedema, obstruction of proximal lymphatics or nodes with an absence of distal lymphatic involvement occurs in:
A. 20% of cases
B. 30% of cases
C. 40% of cases
D. 50% or more of cases

Q5. Staging of chronic lymphedema is based on:
A. Biopsy of subcutaneous tissue
B. Clinical exam
C. Lymphoscintigraphy
D. MRI

Q6. The following signs are associated with the diagnosis of lymphedema except:
A. Peau d'orange
B. Kaposi–Stemmer sign
C. Buffalo hump
D. Homans sign

Q7. The most common complication of lymphedema is:
A. Elephantiasis nostras verrucosa
B. Immunodeficiency and malnutrition
C. Infection
D. Malignant tumors

Q8. The incidence of post-mastectomy angiosarcoma (Stewart–Treves syndrome) varies from:
A. Less than 0.07%
B. 0.07%–0.45%
C. 0.46%–1%
D. 1.1%–1.5%

Q9. The 5-year survival of Stewart–Treves syndrome is:
A. 3%–8.4%
B. 8.5%–13.6%
C. 13.7%–15%
D. 15.1%–18%

Q10. Tropical lymphedema is most often caused by:
A. Podoconiosis
B. Lymphatic filariasis
C. Filamentous bacteria or true fungus causing mycetoma
D. Extensive burns of the extremity

DOI: 10.1201/9781003389897-14

Q11. Podoconiosis (mossy foot) is caused by:
A. True fungi (eumycetoma)
B. Filamentous bacteria (actinomycetoma)
C. Absorption of mineral microparticles into the soles of the bare foot exposed to red clay soil derived from alkalinic volcanic rock
D. CLOVES syndrome

Q12. For objective documentation of lymphatic dysfunction, the best study is:
A. Direct lymphography
B. Near-infrared fluorescent imaging
C. Magnetic resonance imaging
D. Isotopic lymphoscintigraphy

Q13. Typical abnormalities observed in lymphedema using isotopic lymphoscintigraphy include:
A. Dermal backflow and crossover filling with retrograde backflow
B. Absent or delayed transport of tracer
C. Delayed or absent visualization of lymph nodes
D. Dermal backflow, crossover filling and retrograde backflow, delayed or absent transport of tracer, delayed or absent visualization of lymph nodes

Q14. The advanced imaging modality of choice for diagnosis and management of lymphedema is:
A. CT
B. MRI
C. PET/MR lymphography
D. Ultrasound

Q15. Lifestyle changes for the management of early stage of lymphedema include:
A. Daily hygiene and skin care
B. Weight loss
C. Aerobic exercises
D. Daily hygiene and skin care, weight loss, and aerobic exercises

Q16. Complex decongestive therapy should be the first line of treatment for which stage of lymphedema:
A. Stage II lymphedema
B. Stage III lymphedema
C. Stage I lymphedema
D. Stage II and III lymphedema

Q17. The goals of compression therapy for management of lymphedema include:
A. Improvement of the lymphatic flow and venous return
B. Reduction of the accumulated protein debris and sustained volume control
C. Maintenance of skin integrity and protection of the limb from potential trauma
D. Improvement of the lymphatic flow and venous return, reduction of accumulated protein debris and decreased volume, and maintenance of skin integrity

Q18. Surgical approaches for lymphedema are best reflected by which statement:
A. Physiologic procedures such as microscopic lymphovenous anastomosis (LVA) and vascularized lymph node transfer (VLNT) are effective only in later stages of lymphedema
B. Debulking procedures or reductive procedures are useful in the early stages of lymphedema
C. Conservative therapy can be stopped after surgical approaches to lymphedema
D. LVA and VLNT are effective in early stages of lymphedema and debulking procedures in the later stages, with a combination of conservative therapy immediately after any surgical procedure

Q19. Debulking procedures for more advanced stages of lymphedema include all of the following except:
A. Liposuction
B. Charles procedure
C. Sistrunk procedure
D. Groin lymph node dissection

RATIONALE 1–19

1. RATIONALE

Of 125 patients treated at the Mayo Clinic, 97 (78%) were women and 28 (22%) were men, with a higher ratio in women of 3.5 to 1. The ratio of unilateral to bilateral lymphedema was 3 to 1. Lymphedema primarily affects girls near menarche. Primary lymphedema affects 1 of every 6000–10,000 live births and is present in 1.15 per 100,000 people under 20 years of age. The influence of estrogen and inflammation are thought to be important etiological factors in primary lymphedema. In congenital lymphedema, skin is roughened; becomes hyperkeratotic; and develops verrucous cobblestone-like papules, plaques, and nodules with woody fibrosis. Subcutaneous tissue is filled with watery fluid and abundant fat lobules. The deep tissues and muscles are never affected by primary lymphedema.

Correct Answer **B** 3.5 to 1

Reference
Smeltzer, D. M., Stickler, G. B., & Schirger, A. (1985). Primary lymphedema in children and adolescents: a follow-up study and review. *Pediatrics, 76*(2), 206–218. PMID: 4022694

2. RATIONALE

Lymphedema can be primary or secondary. Primary lymphedema results from a developmental abnormality, lack of an offending injury, and often with a positive family history. This form of lymphedema may present at birth, during adolescence, or later in life. Primary lymphedema can be further subdivided into congenital lymphedema, lymphedema praecox, and lymphedema tarda. Congenital lymphedema or Milroy disease (10%–25% of primary lymphedema) manifests within the first 2 years of life. It usually affects women (2 to 1 female-to-male ratio), is bilateral, and involves a lower extremity. It is usually not progressive and may improve spontaneously over time. It is associated with the *FLT4* gene and is autosomal dominant. Lymphedema praecox (Meigs disease) constitutes 65%–85% of primary lymphedema and most commonly manifests at puberty but may appear any time before the age of 35. It predominately affects women (4 to 1 female-to-male ratio), is unilateral, and involves the lower extremities. The associated gene is *FOXC02*, and inheritance is autosomal dominant. Lymphedema tarda (10% of primary lymphedema) appears after the age of 35 years. Secondary lymphedema is the most common form of lymphedema encountered in the United States.

Correct Answer **D** Acquired lymphedema

Reference
Smeltzer, D. M., Stickler, G. B., & Schirger, A. (1985). Primary lymphedema in children and adolescents: a follow-up study and review. *Pediatrics, 76*(2), 206–218. PMID: 4022694

3. RATIONALE

The secondary (acquired) form of lymphedema is the most common form of lymphatic obstruction. In the United States, iatrogenic causes are predominant among the acquired form of lymphedema. Lymphatic trauma following surgery or radiation therapy for cancer is the next leading cause of acquired lymphedema. According to recent estimates 6%–30% of breast cancer survivors who have undergone axillary node dissection experience clinically significant lymphedema. The advent of sentinel lymph node biopsy has decreased the incidence to 5%–7%. Adjuvant radiation therapy for local treatment of nodal disease can lead to upper or lower extremity lymphedema. Other factors such as trauma, infection, and obesity contribute to secondary lymphedema. Worldwide the most common cause of secondary lymphedema is infection by the microfilaria *Wuchereria bancrofti*, which is transmitted by various mosquito vectors. Adult filarial worms reside in and obstruct lymphatic channels causing irreversible scarring and fibrosis and resulting in massive edema. Eosinophilia is present in peripheral blood smear and microfilaria can be demonstrated in peripheral nocturnal blood, centrifuged urine sediment, or lymphatic fluid. Other types of lymphatic vascular trauma include burns and larger circumferential wounds to the extremity. Other causes of acquired lymphedema include bacterial or fungal infection, infection after snake or insect bites, pregnancy, contact dermatitis, and rheumatoid arthritis.

Correct Answer   **B** 6%–30% of patients

Reference
Brayton, K. M., Hirsch, A. T., O'Brien, PJ. (2014). Lymphedema prevalence and treatment benefits in cancer: impact of a therapeutic intervention on health outcomes and costs. *PLoS ONE, 9*(12), e114597. PMID: 25470383

4. RATIONALE

It has been suggested that a morphological classification of primary lymphedema provides more useful information in regard to prognosis than classification by age at onset. This classification relies on an anatomical description of the lymphatic vasculature.

A. *Aplasia* – no lymphatic vessels can be identified
B. *Hypoplasia* – a diminished number of lymphatic vessels
C. *Numerical hyperplasia* – an increased number of lymphatic vessels
D. *Hyperplasia* – in addition to an increase in number, the vessels have valvular incompetence and display tortuosity and dilatation (mega lymphatics, lymphangiectasia)

Mega lymphatics and lymphatic hyperplasia are less common than hypoplasia or aplasia. These patients often have unilateral edema involving the entire lower extremity. Mega lymphatics are associated with a great extent of involvement and a worse prognosis. Aplasia and hypoplasia have a different natural history depending on whether they involve the distal or proximal portion of the leg. Distal obstruction – approximately one-third of all cases – results from agenesis, hypoplasia, or obstruction of the distal lymphatic vessels with relatively normal proximal vessels. In these cases, the swelling is usually bilateral and mild, and women are affected much more frequently than men. The prognosis is good. Familial occurrence, female preponderance, and indolent progression characterize this pattern of lymphatic disturbance. Proximal obstruction occurs in more than half of the cases and involves obstruction of the proximal lymphatics or nodes with an absence of distal lymphatic involvement. Pathologic findings reveal intranodal fibrosis. The finding is unilateral and severe with a slight female preponderance. Because of progression with associated severe abnormality, patients may require surgical intervention if there is isolated obstructive hypoplasia with worsening of the edema of the entire limb.

Correct Answer   **D** 50% or more of cases

Reference
Rockson, S. G. (2003). Syndromic lymphedema: keys to the kingdom of lymphatic structure and function? *Lymphat Res Biol, 1*(3), 181–183. PMID:19642940

5. RATIONALE

The 10th International Society of Lymphology suggests staging of chronic lymphedema regardless of cause into four stages (grades) and subclassified as mild, moderate, or severe based on clinical examination.

- *Stage 0* – Latent phase: Excessive fluid accumulates and fibrosis develops around the lymphatics, but no edema is apparent clinically with only mild discomfort
- *Stage 1* – Swelling relieved by elevation, including pitting edema, with no clinical evidence of fibrosis
- *Stage 2* – Swelling not relieved by limb elevation, moderate to severe fibrosis
- *Stage 3* – Irreversible edema caused by repeated bouts of inflammation, fibrosis, and sclerosis of skin and subcutaneous tissue, also called lymphostatic elephantiasis

This classification allows for the evaluation of treatment effectiveness and the comparison of different treatment modalities. The drawback is that in some cases staging based on clinical examination may be difficult without a biopsy of the subcutaneous tissue.

Correct Answer   B Clinical exam

Reference
Greene, A. K., & Goss, J. A. (2018). Diagnosis and staging of lymphedema. *Semin Plast Surg, 32*(1), 12–16. PMID: 29636648

6. RATIONALE

Lower extremity lymphedema occurs as the interstitial space is expanded by an excess accumulation of protein-rich fluid and usually manifests as swelling in the dorsal surface of the foot with a characteristic blunt "squared-off" appearance of digits of the lower extremity. Initially there is preferential swelling of the distal extremity and there is progression proximally. Pitted or dimpled texture of the skin (peau d'orange) and the Kaposi–Stemmer sign (an inability to pinch the fold of the skin on the dorsal aspect of the base of the second toe) are characteristics of lymphedema. The dorsum of the forefoot is often involved, giving a typical appearance of a "buffalo hump." In advanced stages the skin over the affected area becomes hyperkeratotic and develops verrucous cobblestone-like papules, plaques, and nodules with underlying woody fibrosis. Primary lymphedema may be associated with yellow discoloration of the nails. Intense pain is rare, although heaviness or aching of a limb is a frequent complaint. If a patient with lymphedema complains of marked pain, infection, or neurotic pain in the area, scar tissue should be suspected. Unlike the skin changes in venostasis, lymphedema patients maintain a high degree of hydration and elasticity, and ischemic changes due to high skin tension and disruption of the circulation to the skin and subcutaneous tissue are rare. Homans sign is associated with deep venous thrombosis in the calf.

Correct Answer   D Homans sign

Reference
Grada, A. A., & Phillips, T. J. (2017). Lymphedema: diagnostic workup and management. *J Am Acad Dermatol, 77*(6), 995–1006. PMID: 29132859

7. RATIONALE

Recurrent soft tissue infection is one of the most common and difficult aspects of long-standing lymphedema. Accumulated fluid and proteins provide a good substrate for bacterial growth. Lymphatic dysfunction impairs local immune responses, which plays a permissive role in the propagation of bacterial and fungal invasion. With recurrent infection, there is progressive damage of lymphatic capillaries, and a reported infection rate of up to 31% has been reported. Recurrent episodes of cellulitis can damage the existing percutaneous lymphatics, exacerbate the skin disease, and worsen the edema. Lymphangiectasia with protein-losing enteropathy may result in loss of proteins, long-chain triglycerides, cholesterol, and calcium. Loss of cytokines and lymphocytes may result in immunodeficiency. In rare cases, chronic lymphedema may be complicated by development of lymphangiosarcoma, which manifests as multicentric lesions with bluish nodules and sclerotic plaques. The other malignant tumors, including Kaposi sarcoma, squamous cell carcinoma, and malignant lymphoma and melanoma, may occur.

Correct Answer   **C** Infection

Reference
Burian, E. A., Karlsmark, T., Franks, P. J., et al. (2021). Cellulitis in chronic oedema of the lower leg: an international cross-sectional study. *Br J Dermatol*, *185*(1), 110–118. PMID: 33405247

8. RATIONALE

Long-standing chronic lymphedema may result in deadly cutaneous angiosarcoma, also known as Stewart–Treves syndrome (STS), which is classically associated with radical mastectomy. However, STS can be associated with any long-standing primary or secondary lymphedema. The incidence of post-mastectomy STS of the arm varies from 0.07% to 0.45%. It manifests as painless, reddish-purple skin nodules that gradually increase in size and number. The primary lesion tends to form satellite lesions and telangiectasia. The tumor cells have a predilection for local ulceration and pulmonary metastasis via the hematogenous route. The diagnosis is often delayed.

Correct Answer   **B** 0.07%–0.45%

Reference
Sharma, A., & Schwartz, R. A. (2012). Stewart–Treves syndrome: pathogenesis and management. *J Am Acad Dermatol*, *67*(6), 1342–1348. PMID: 22682884

9. RATIONALE

An extensive investigation in the form of CT scan of the chest and abdomen and PET scan should be performed to determine the extent of metastatic disease and whether an aggressive treatment program is justified for the management of Stewart–Treves syndrome. The most common treatment is a limb disarticulation or forequarter amputation. When discovered early, however, a combination of radiation therapy and chemotherapy can help, resulting in temporary remission. The 5-year survival rate ranges from 8.5% to 13.6%. The median survival of STS patients is approximately 19 months after diagnosis. Prognosis is poor; therefore, multiple deep biopsy specimens of suspicious lesions in the affected extremity should be obtained and examined at the earliest.

Correct Answer   **B** 8.5%–13.6%

Reference

Schiffman, S., & Berger, A. (2007). Stewart-Treves syndrome. *J Am Coll Surg, 204*(2), 328. PMID: 17254938

10. RATIONALE

There are two main causes of tropical lymphedema. The most common cause is lymphatic filariasis, commonly known as elephantiasis, which is caused by infestation with the parasitic nematode *Wuchereria bancrofti* (and in Asia by *Brugia malayi* and *B. timori*) transmitted by mosquitoes as vectors. The second main cause is podoconiosis. Manifestations of acute filariasis include lymphangitis and orchitis. Chronic filariasis causes lymphedema with associated skin changes. If filariasis is suspected, a blood smear should be collected at night (between 11 PM and 3 AM stained with Giemsa or hematoxylin-eosin stain to look for microfilaria under the microscope). In the United States, filariasis has been reported in Hawaii. For active filariasis, diethylcarbamazine (DEC) is the treatment of choice.

Correct Answer   **B** Lymphatic filariasis

Reference

Molyneux, D. H. (2012). Tropical lymphedemas – control and prevention. *N Engl J Med, 366*(13), 1169–1171. PMID: 22455411

11. RATIONALE

Podoconiosis, also known as "mossy foot," is the second main cause of tropical lymphedema. It is an endemic non-filarial elephantiasis caused by the absorption of mineral microparticles in the soles of bare feet exposed to red clay soil derived from alkalinic volcanic rock. It has a genetic predisposition in the HLA class 11 region. This condition causes chronic lymphedema and usually manifests as bilateral swelling and disfigurement of the feet and legs. Treatment consists of avoidance of prolonged contact between the skin and the irritant soils by wearing robust footwear, avoiding exposure to the irritant soil, or by change in occupation. Maintaining foot hygiene through daily washing with soap and water or antiseptics is recommended. Using compression bandages and limb elevation above the level of the hip can both help promote venous and lymphatic return and reduce swelling.

Mycetoma is an uncommon chronic infection of the skin and subcutaneous tissues of the foot usually seen in tropical countries and is caused by true fungi (eumycetoma) or filamentous bacteria (actinomycetoma). The disease is characterized by the triad of tumefaction, draining sinuses, and presence of colonial grains in the exudates. CLOVES syndrome is characterized by congenital lipomatous overgrowth, vascular malformations, epidermal nevi, and skeletal anomalies. Skeletal abnormalities such as enlarged bony structure of the legs with superficial phlebectasia and capillary malformations are also present.

Correct Answer   **C** Absorption of mineral microparticles into the soles of the bare foot exposed to red clay soil derived from alkalinic volcanic rock

Reference

Davey, G., Tekola, F., & Newport, M. J. (2007). Podoconiosis: non-infectious geochemical elephantiasis. *Trans R Soc Trop Med Hyg, 101*(12), 1175–1180. PMID: 17976670

12. RATIONALE

Isotopic lymphoscintigraphy is an accurate and reproduceable method for confirming the diagnosis of lymphedema. It involves the injection of a filtered colloid, technetium 99, subdermally within one of the interdigital spaces of the affected limb. The lymphatic transport of the radiolabeled macromolecule is tracked with a gamma camera, thus providing a semi-quantifiable assessment of major lymphatic trunks and lymph nodes. The normal study shows several lymph vessels as the tracer is visualized along the anteromedial aspect of the leg. Many lymph channels in the calf may be identifiable. But lymph channels run close to each other, and separate activity in each larger channel is usually not visualized. Tracer activity clears in the groin lymph nodes in the range of 15–60 minutes. The qualitative interpretation of images shows moderate sensitivity and excellent specificity of the diagnosis of lymphedema. Quantitative lymphoscintigraphy may improve detection of early disease but cannot reliably distinguish primary from secondary lymphedema.

Correct Answer **D** Isotopic lymphoscintigraphy

Reference

Szuba, A., Shin, W. S., Strauss, H. W., & Rockson, S. (2003). The third circulation: radionuclide lymphoscintigraphy in the evaluation of lymphedema. *J Nucl Med*, *44*(1), 43–57. PMID: 12515876

13. RATIONALE

Typical abnormalities using isotopic lymphoscintigraphy include delayed or absent dermal backflow, absent or delayed transport of tracer, crossover filling with retrograde backflow, and either absent or delayed visualization of lymph nodes. Dermal backflow suggests the presence of lymphatic hypertension and valvular incompetence. In most patients with primary lymphedema, lymph channels are either absent or obliterated, and occasionally they may be incompetent and ectatic. The delayed appearance or asymmetrical appearance of radiocontrast material in the proximal nodal tissue can be useful to semi-quantitatively measure the severity of lymphatic insufficiency. The density of subcutaneous accumulation of radiotracer as a marker of dermal backflow can also be quantified. The ratio of radioactivity in ipsilateral versus contralateral nodal tissue can also be quantified in a patient with unilateral limb edema. Quantitation is of great value in predicating successful response to therapeutic intervention. The findings in lymphangiectasia consist of dilated lymph channels with virtually no delay in lymph transport.

Correct Answer **D** Dermal backflow, crossover filling and retrograde backflow, delayed or absent transport of tracer, and delayed or absent visualization of lymph nodes

Reference

Cambria, R. A., Gloviczki, P., Naessens, J. M., & Wahner, H. W. (1993). Noninvasive evaluation of the lymphatic system with lymphoscintigraphy: a prospective, semiquantitative analysis in 386 extremities. *J Vasc Surg*, *18*(5), 773–782. PMID: 8230563

14. RATIONALE

Lymphedema is typically confined to the epifascial space of the skin and subcutaneous tissue, sparing muscle. With CT or MRI imaging, a characteristic honeycomb distribution of edema within the epifascial structures, with thickening of the skin is seen. In edema due to other causes, both epifascial and subfascial compartments are affected. In lipedema there is fat accumulation without fluid. MRI also helps in identification of lymph nodes and enlarged lymphatic trunks and aids in differentiating various possible causes of lymphatic obstruction in secondary lymphedema. Magnetic resonance imaging lymphography (MRL) with intracutaneous administration of an MR contrast agent allows for assessment of both superficial and deep lymphatic channels. However, interpretation of MRL may be compounded by venous uptake of a gadolinium-based agent. The differential diagnosis includes lipedema, a type of lipodystrophy which results in uniform and symmetrical enlargement in both lower extremities but there is sparing of the feet. Systemic causes such as hepatic failure, renal failure, congestive heart failure, constrictive pericarditis, hypoproteinemia, malnutrition, and myxedema can also lead to leg swelling. Chronic venous insufficiency with venous stasis manifests as hemosiderin deposits in the skin, which leads to brownish pigmentation near the ankle. In contrast to lymphedema, which is painless (unless there is an associated infection), venous hypertension results in significant pain and venous claudication manifested as throbbing pain when walking. Chronic inflammation in subcutaneous tissue in patients with venous insufficiency may cause destruction of lymph channels with a mixed picture of venous and lymphatic edema.

Correct Answer   B MRI

Reference
Mills, M., van Zanten, M., Borri, M., et al. (2021). Systematic review of magnetic resonance lymphangiography from a technical perspective. *J Magn Reson Imaging*, *53*(6), 1766–1790. PMID: 33625795

15. **RATIONALE**

Conservative management of lymphedema can be burdensome, and the main reason for failure is the need for lifelong treatment which can lead to noncompliance. Attention to daily skin hygiene on the part of patient i.e., washing limbs regularly with soap and avoiding trauma, as this can be a potential source of infection. Patients with a history of fungal infection such as *Candida* and *Tinea* should be treated with topical antifungal medications like miconazole cream or clotrimazole cream. Walking and performing exercises such as aerobic exercises augment lymphatic flow. Exercise helps to decrease the swelling from lymphedema. During muscle contraction, the lymph flow is propelled to an alternative lymph node via the lymphatic vessels. Lymphatic circulation is not driven by a central pump such as the heart. Exposure to cold or heat should be avoided. Diuretics have a very limited role in the management of lymphedema, as they can worsen the condition by increasing the concentration of interstitial proteins.

Correct Answer   D Daily hygiene and skin care, weight loss, and aerobic exercises

Reference
Baddour, L. M. (2000). Cellulitis syndromes: an update. *Int J Antimicrob Agents*, *14*(2), 113–116. PMID: 10720800

16. **RATIONALE**

Complex decongestive therapy should be the first line of therapy for stage II and stage III lymphedema. It is a multimodal approach for the management of lymphedema. The program combines four main elements: Compression therapy, manual lymphatic drainage (MLD), exercise, and skin care. CDT can acutely reduce limb volume and provide long-term benefits through the acceleration of lymph drainage in the edematous limb and the dispersal of accumulated protein. CDT is administered in two phases: An intensive initial reductive phase and a maintenance phase. CDT is labor intensive and is effective for both primary and secondary lymphedema and can be used in both children and adults. Manual lymphatic drainage is safe and beneficial when combined with compression bandaging. Its benefit is more pronounced in patients with mild-to-moderate lymphedema. Each session usually takes 40–60 minutes and should be performed by a physical therapist with specialized training. Massaging techniques using low pressure (30–40 mmHg) and low frequency are intended to enhance lymphatic contractility and redirect lymph flow through the non-obstructed cutaneous lymphatics. During the initial phase of CDT, non-elastic, high-grade (40–80 mmHg) compressive wrappings should be applied after each session of manual lymphatic drainage to prevent reaccumulation of fluid and to promote lymph flow.

Correct Answer **D** Stage II and III lymphedema

Reference
Finnane, A., Janda, M., & Hayes, S. C. (2015). Review of the evidence of lymphedema treatment effect. *Am J Phys Med Rehabil, 94*(6), 483–498. PMID: 25741621

17. RATIONALE

In the initial phase of CDT a multilayer low-stretch bandage can be left on the affected area overnight for 24 hours. The multilayer bandage consists of a single protective layer of cotton bandage next to the skin and a soft synthetic wool (or foam) underpadding. Compression is provided by an outer layer of at least two short-stretch extensible bandages. The compression garment must be continuously used during the day and removed at night as long as the legs are kept elevated. They should have graduated compression that increases from the distal to proximal segment. A minimum pressure of 40 mmHg is required for compression. Garments should preferably be custom fit and need to be replaced in 3–6 months, as they may lose their elasticity. Pneumatic compression devices surround the limb with a sleeve containing air-filled chambers. The chambers are gradually filled with air to provide active sequential compression from distal to proximal and should be used for at least 2 hours daily. The advanced pneumatic compression device (APCD) delivers programmable external pneumatic compression though multiple inflatable compartments. APCDs are designed for home use and are intended to stimulate the labor-intensive MLD performed by the physical therapist.

Correct Answer **D** Improvement of the lymphatic flow and venous return, reduction of accumulated protein debris and decreased volume, and maintenance of skin integrity

Reference
Karaca-Mandic, P., Hirsch, A. T., Rockson, S. G., & Ridner, S. H. (2015). The cutaneous, net clinical, and health economic benefits of advanced pneumatic compression devices in patients with lymphedema. *JAMA Dermatol, 151*(11), 1187–1193. PMID: 26444458

18. RATIONALE

In lymphovenous anastomosis (LVA), subdermal lymphatics are anastomosed to adjacent venules using indocyanine green near-infrared lymphangiography to visualize fluorescent images and mark visible lymphatic pathways and incision sites. Lymphazurin is injected into the web spaces in the extremity (feet); the next step is to take down the subdermal post-obstruction dissection down to venous and lymphatic channels. Use of microsurgical connection to reestablish lymph flow with end-to-end anastomosis is next. End-to-side anastomosis can be used when veins are larger than the lymphatic channels. The patency of the shunt is confirmed by the presence of Lymphazurin into the vein. In a series of 100 patients undergoing LVA, improvement of symptoms was noted in 96% of patients with improvement in volume deferential in 74%.

The effectiveness of vascularized groin lymph node transfer (VLNT) is based on: The lymphatic "wick" of the bridge of proximal and distal lymphatic vessels in the recipient site and lymphangiogenesis is stimulated by growth factors produced by the lymph nodes; and the lymphatic "pump" which stems from lymphovenous communication with the lymph nodes of the transferred flap. During vascularized groin lymph node transfer, an elliptical skin paddle from the lateral to femoral pulse is harvested with the superficial circumflex iliac vessels at the recipient site using a transverse incision, and a microvascular anastomosis to the recipient artery and vein is performed. VLNT results in improvement in swelling in 86%–90% of patients with volume difference on an average of 22%.

Correct Answer **D** LVA and VLNT are effective in early stages of lymphedema and debulking procedures in the later stages with a combination of conservative therapy immediately after any surgical procedure

Reference
Campisi, C., & Boccardo, F. (2004). Microsurgical techniques for lymphedema treatment: derivative lymphatic-venous microsurgery. *World J Surg, 28*(6), 609–613. PMID: 15366754

19. **RATIONALE**

Surgical circumferential liposuction has been introduced during the last 3 decades for postmastectomy lymphedema and is useful in addressing large adipose tissue deposits. It is safe and quick and allows for immediate decrease in volume and pressure of the lymph fluid, thus promoting better lymphatic flow. It is usually indicated when excess volume is greater than 500 mL. Contraindications include metastatic disease, open wound, presence of more than pitting edema, and coagulation disorders. Risks include lidocaine toxicity, fat emboli, hematoma, and seroma. Excess volume reduction of 96.6% has been reported.

The Charles procedure is an aggressive approach including radical excision of the skin and subcutaneous tissue down to muscle fascia. The excised skin is used for grafting on the fascia, or other donor sites can be used. This approach is indicated for severe cases and carries a high risk of complications including infection, ulceration, hyperpigmentation, and unstable scar.

The Sistrunk procedure is a planned, staged excision of the affected subcutaneous tissue and involves burying dermal flaps within the skin flaps. Long-term results indicate a reduction of at least half of the affected tissue in 76% of patients. Groin lymph node dissection can result in secondary lymphedema.

Correct Answer **D** Groin lymph node dissection

Reference
Chang, D. W., Masia, J., Garza, R., et al. (2016). Lymphedema: surgical and medical therapy. *Plast Reconstr Surg, 138*(3 Suppl), 209s–218s. PMID: 27556764

SECTION 15: DIALYSIS ACCESS

MCQs 1–34

Q1. According to the Centers for Medicare and Medicaid Services, the percentages of patients using a tunneled hemodialysis catheter as their primary vascular access is approximately:
- **A.** 10%
- **B.** 15%
- **C.** 20%
- **D.** 25%

Q2. The desired blood flow rate for hemodialysis treatment with a hemodialysis catheter is:
- **A.** 200–250 cc
- **B.** 250–300 cc
- **C.** 300–500 cc
- **D.** Greater than 500 cc

Q3. The hemodialysis nurse reports an inadequately functioning tunneled catheter placed 6 weeks earlier. Cath flow (tPA) was unsuccessful. The next best option is:
- **A.** Chest X-ray to determine the position of the tip of the catheter and to rule out a kink in the catheter
- **B.** Insert a new catheter on the contralateral side
- **C.** Reverse the blood lines
- **D.** Schedule a tunneled hemodialysis catheter exchange in the intervention suite

Q4. The suboptimal rates of blood flow in tunneled hemodialysis catheters have been reported in:
- **A.** 20% of patients
- **B.** 25% of patients
- **C.** 30% of patients
- **D.** 35% of patients

Q5. The incidence of hemodialysis access infection per 100 patients is highest in:
- **A.** Autologous fistula
- **B.** Prosthetic graft
- **C.** Non-tunneled hemodialysis catheter
- **D.** Tunneled hemodialysis catheter

Q6. The National Kidney Foundation Kidney Disease Outcomes Quality Initiative (NKFKDOQI) states all of the following except:
- **A.** Arteriovenous fistulas have the lowest rate of thrombosis and require the fewest interventions
- **B.** Cost of AV fistula use and maintenance is the lowest
- **C.** Fistulas have the highest rates of infection
- **D.** Fistulas are associated with the highest survival and lowest hospitalization rates

Q7. Vascular hemodialysis access is implicated in what percentage of all bacteremias in patients on hemodialysis:
- **A.** 20%–33%
- **B.** 30%–40%
- **C.** 40%–63%
- **D.** 48%–73%

Q8. Management of catheter-related bacteremia is initial empiric antimicrobial therapy followed by:
- **A.** Catheter removal with immediate replacement
- **B.** Catheter exchange over a guide wire in the same tunnel
- **C.** Catheter exchange over a guide wire with creation of a new tunnel
- **D.** Catheter removal with delayed replacement after defervescence in patients with severe clinical symptoms

DOI: 10.1201/9781003389897-15

Q9. The incidence of 30-day graft infection rate with use of a PTFE conduit for an AV graft is:
A. Less than 1%
B. 1%–3%
C. 4%–5%
D. 6%

Q10. Diagnosis of dialysis access (fistula/graft) infection is usually made by:
A. Tagged leukocyte scan
B. Duplex ultrasound
C. CT scan
D. Clinical exam

Q11. Autologous AV access infection localized to the access site in patients undergoing hemodialysis should initially be treated with:
A. Removal of AV access and immediate tunneled hemodialysis catheter insertion
B. Removal of AV access and delayed (2–3 days) placement of tunneled hemodialysis catheter
C. Antibiotics
D. Conversion of autologous AV access to AV graft

Q12. The HeRO graft is relatively contraindicated in patients with all of the following except:
A. Inflow artery diameter less than 3 mm
B. Systolic blood pressure less than 100 mmHg or ejection fraction less than 20%
C. Active infection
D. Prior multiple upper extremity access procedures

Q13. A radial artery-cephalic vein direct wrist access fistula (Brescia Cimino) has a 2-year patency of:
A. 50%–60%
B. 55%–89%
C. 60%–95%
D. 65%–95%

Q14. The most common cause of failure of arteriovenous fistula and arteriovenous grafts for hemodialysis access is:
A. Low ejection fraction
B. Arterial inflow occlusive disease
C. Venous outflow obstruction
D. Use of inadequate vein for fistula creation

Q15. The most common site of stenosis in the dialysis circuit is:
A. At the needle insertion
B. Central outflow tract
C. Arterial inflow tract
D. Venous outflow tract adjacent to the anastomosis

Q16. The best test for the diagnosis of a stenosis in a hemodialysis circuit is:
A. Duplex ultrasound
B. Fistulogram/shuntogram
C. CTA
D. Catheter-based arteriography

Q17. The most prevalent time for neointimal hyperplasia in dialysis access fistula/graft occurs in:
A. Within a few weeks of index operation
B. Within 3 months of index operation
C. Within first year of index operation
D. Within first 2 years of index operation

Q18. The most important reason for thrombosis of the hemodialysis access-fistula/graft is:
A. Hypercoagulability
B. Vessel injury resulting in endothelial dysfunction
C. Patients with diabetes mellitus
D. Significant stenosis secondary to neointimal hyperplasia at the venous anastomosis

Q19. The following statement best reflects the results of percutaneous versus open surgical thrombectomies for thrombosed hemodialysis access:
A. Percutaneous thrombectomies have a higher rethrombosis rate but better assisted primary patency rate than open surgical thrombectomies
B. Percutaneous thrombectomies have a lower rethrombosis rate but worse assisted primary patency rate than open surgical thrombectomies
C. Percutaneous thrombectomies have a lower rethrombosis rate and better assisted primary patency rate than open surgical thrombectomies

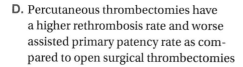

D. Percutaneous thrombectomies have a higher rethrombosis rate and worse assisted primary patency rate as compared to open surgical thrombectomies

Q20. Pseudoaneurysms at the anastomotic site of the AV fistula/graft are most often due to:
A. Poor surgical technique with inadequate depth of sutures
B. Excessive tension at the anastomotic site
C. Infectious complications
D. Inadequate depth of sutures at the anastomotic site, excessive tension at the anastomotic site, and infectious complications

Q21. The incidence of upper extremity ischemia in dialysis patients is up to:
A. 1%
B. 2%
C. 4%
D. 5%

Q22. Ischemic Rest pain in the hand as a symptom of steal syndrome following hemodialysis arteriovenous access reconstruction is graded as:
A. Stage I
B. Stage II
C. Stage III
D. Stage IV

Q23. The diagnosis of dialysis access–associated steal syndrome (DASS) is confirmed by:
A. Catheter-based arteriography
B. EMG and nerve conduction velocity study
C. Doppler ultrasonography with digital pressures and tracings with and without AV access compression
D. Clinical examination with and without AV access compression

Q24. Treatment of symptomatic steal syndrome (stage IV and selected patients with stage III) is:
A. Ligation of the access
B. Banding
C. Endoluminal-assisted revision
D. Distal revascularization with interval ligation (DRIL) procedure

Q25. There are several causes of peripheral neuropathy in patients on hemodialysis; the most serious is:
A. Entrapment causing peripheral nerve compression
B. Uronic neuropathy
C. Diabetic polyneuropathy
D. Ischemic monomelic neuropathy

Q26. Ischemic monomelic neuropathy differs from ischemic syndrome in all except it is:
A. Reversible
B. Exhibits no tissue necrosis
C. Warm hand
D. Palpable pulse or audible Doppler signal

Q27. What percentage of patients have central venous stenosis/occlusion (CVS) detected on venography for failing access and edema of the extremity?
A. Less than 5%
B. 5%–10%
C. 11%–16%
D. 17%–26%

Q28. During balloon angioplasty for venous stenosis near the distal anastomosis of the AV graft, there is a residual stenosis of approximately 30%. The next best option is:
A. Covered stent
B. Open patch angioplasty
C. Cutting balloon or high-pressure balloon angioplasty
D. Bare-metal stent

Q29. Treatment of symptomatic venous hypertension secondary to central venous stenosis/occlusion (CVS) is:
A. Open surgical management
B. Endovascular angioplasty
C. Bare-metal stent
D. Covered stent

Q30. Tapered arteriovenous grafts in upper extremity dialysis access over non-tapered grafts provide:
A. Better patency protection against ischemic steal syndrome
B. Less arm swelling
C. Similar primary patency
D. Less endovascular operative reintervention

Q31. The optimal treatment of bleeding in the dialysis patient with platelet dysfunction is:
A. Maintenance of hematocrit >36
B. Change the permanent access to tunneled dialysis catheter
C. Tranexamic acid
D. Desmopressin

Q32. A 74-year-old woman on hemodialysis with AV graft in the left upper arm not on any anticoagulation medication for the past 18 months presents to the ER with pulsatile bleeding from the needle puncture site during dialysis, which could not be controlled by local pressure by the dialysis access team. The optimal management is:
A. Immediately take the patient to the OR and perform a new interposition graft through healthy tissues
B. Immediate shuntogram
C. Compression Ace bandage
D. Direct pressure for 30–40 minutes; if bleeding persists, place a suture over the bleeding site and administer desmopressin; then evaluate the shunt by shuntogram followed by the appropriate management strategy

Q33. Access flow in patients with high-output heart failure as a complication of arteriovenous fistula/graft is greater than:
A. 1000 mL/min
B. 1200 mL/min
C. 1500 mL/min
D. >2000 mL/min

Q34. The advantages of arterio-arterial grafts as a prosthetic loop are:
A. No change in cardiac output
B. No change in peripheral perfusion
C. Axillo-axillary loop grafts are preferred to femoral artery loop grafts
D. No change in cardiac output or peripheral perfusion with preference for axillo-axillary loop grafts

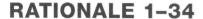

RATIONALE 1–34

1. RATIONALE

In the United States, most patients (75%) begin hemodialysis treatment with a central venous catheter as their initial vascular access. Most patients will have a tunneled hemodialysis catheter inserted into the internal jugular vein. According to the Centers for Medicare and Medicaid Services, the percentage of patients using a tunneled hemodialysis catheter as their primary vascular access was 29% in 2007 and 24% in 2010. The majority of patients who begin hemodialysis treatment using a central venous catheter will transition to an arteriovenous fistula or a prosthetic graft as their permanent vascular access. According to the National Kidney Foundation Kidney Disease Outcomes Quality Initiative (DOQI) guidelines, each patient should have a graft within 90 days of starting chronic hemodialysis treatment. However, a significant number of patients will continue to use a tunneled hemodialysis catheter for the first 6–12 months after start of the hemodialysis treatment.

Correct Answer **D** 25%

Reference
Vesely, T. (2013). The challenge of hemodialysis catheter use. *Endovasc Today*, 60–62.

2. RATIONALE

Hemodialysis catheter dysfunction is commonly defined as the inability to aspirate blood, a blood flow rate of less than 300 mL/min, and increased arterial or venous pressure or inability to deliver an adequate hemodialysis. Catheter dysfunction has been reported during 7% of hemodialysis sessions, and the median time to the first episode of catheter dysfunction was 95 days. Sixty-three percent of patients had at least one episode of catheter dysfunction, and 30% of patients had ≥1 episode of catheter dysfunction per month. If the desired flow rate is not achieved, the underlying cause needs to be determined. Early dysfunction is usually associated with kinking of the catheter or a poor position, while late dysfunction is more commonly associated with thrombosis or a fibrin sheath around the distal end of the catheter with or without thrombi.

Correct Answer **C** 300–500 cc

Reference
Frankel, A. (2006). Temporary access and central venous catheters. *Eur J Vasc Endovasc Surg, 31*(4), 417–422. PMID: 16360326

3. RATIONALE

In an inadequately functioning non-tunneled hemodialysis catheter, the patient's position should first be altered. The catheter should then be flushed with normal saline using a 10-cc syringe; obtaining a chest X-ray in tunneled hemodialysis catheter dysfunction helps in determining the position of the tip of the catheter. It also rules out a kink in the catheter. Several clinical studies have demonstrated that the performance and durability of hemodialysis catheters are improved if the tip is positioned within the right atrium. The majority of hemodialysis catheters are inserted in the anterior chest wall via the right internal jugular vein while the patient is in a supine position. When the patient moves to the standing position, the anterior chest wall will move inferiorly due to gravity. In the supine position, the mediastinal structures, including central veins, are compressed by the abdominal contents. When the patient moves to the upright position, the abdominal contents descend, the central veins lengthen, and the right atrium expands. This lengthening of the mediastinal structure will result in upward retraction of the catheter into the superior vena cava. A correctly placed catheter tip usually undergoes a 2- to 3-cm movement between the superior vena cava and the upper right atrium.[1] It has been reported that left-sided catheters terminating in the SVC or pericavoatrial junction had significantly more catheter-related dysfunction and infection as compared to right-sided catheters.[2]

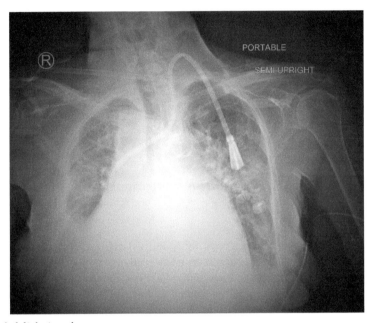

Kink in left IJ tunneled dialysis catheter.

Correct Answer A Chest X-ray to determine the position of the tip of the catheter and to rule out a kink in the catheter

References
1. Kowalski, C. M., Kaufman, J. A., Rivitz, S. M., Geller, S. C., & Waltman, A. C. (1997). Migration of central venous catheters: implications for initial catheter tip positioning. *J Vasc Interv Radiol, 8*(3), 443–447. PMID: 9152919
2. Engstrom, B. I., Horvath, J. J., Stewart, J. K., et al. (2013). Tunneled internal jugular hemodialysis catheters: impact of laterality and tip position on catheter dysfunction and infection rates. *J Vasc Interv Radiol, 24*(9), 1295–1302. PMID: 23891045

4. RATIONALE

A prospective study of 102 patients with tunneled hemodialysis catheters reported that 35% of catheters have suboptimal rates of blood flow, leading to reversal of the arterial and venous blood lines, which often improves the rate of blood flow though the catheter. However, this maneuver may be associated with significant access recirculation. Access recirculation occurs when dialyzed blood exiting the outflow lumen directly re-enters the inflow lumen, thereby bypassing the systemic circulation. Recirculation reduces the effective clearance of the solute by diluting the inflow concentration, thereby reducing the driving force of diffusion across the dialyzer membrane. A hemodialysis catheter recirculation rate of >10% reduces the adequacy of hemodialysis treatment. The arterial and venous end holes, located at the distal tip of the catheter, are separated (1–3 cm) to minimize recirculation of blood during hemodialysis treatment. The average recirculation for a tunneled hemodialysis catheter with distal tip position in the upper right atrium should be <5%.

Correct Answer   D 35% of patients

Reference
Depner, T. A. (2001). Catheter performance. *Semin Dial, 14*(6), 425–431. PMID: 11851927

5. RATIONALE

The major complication of hemodialysis catheters is infection. Numerous studies have confirmed that the risk of both local and blood-borne infection is highest in non-tunneled hemodialysis catheters. Catheter-associated infection can result in septic central vein thrombosis, infective endocarditis, osteomyelitis, and septic arthritis. The incidence of access infections per 100 patient months was reported with the type of access: Fistula 0.56, prosthetic graft 1.35, tunneled dialysis catheter 8.42, and non-tunneled dialysis catheter 11.98. The high rate of infection not only increases morbidity and mortality but also has a significant economic implication, as infection is the most common reason for admission of a patient on chronic hemodialysis to the hospital.

Correct Answer   C Non-tunneled hemodialysis catheter

Reference
Frankel, A. (2006). Temporary access and central venous catheters. *Eur J Vasc Endovasc Surg, 31*(4), 417–422. PMID: 16360326

6. RATIONALE

Arteriovenous fistula for hemodialysis access has the lowest rate of thrombosis requiring the least number of interventions at the lowest cost. Patients with fistulas are associated with the highest survival and lowest hospitalization rates, with the lowest rate of infection. The literature review indicates that there are growing numbers of studies reporting that creating an arteriovenous fistula in some patients is less likely to be successful in the presence of certain comorbidities. In addition, certain patient groups may have less incremental benefit from an AV fistula relative to an AV graft. By adjusting the fistula rates for patient characteristics and comorbidities associated with low AV fistula success rate, this measure accounts for some patients where an AV graft or even a tunneled dialysis catheter may be a more appropriate option.

Correct Answer   C Fistulas have the highest rates of infection

Reference
Lok, C. E., Huber, T. S., Lee, T., et al. (2020). KDOQI clinical practice guideline for vascular access: 2019 update. *Am J Kidney Dis, 75*(4 Suppl 2), S1–S164. PMID: 32778223

7. RATIONALE

Numerous reports implicate the vascular access in up to 48%–73% of all bacteremias in the hemodialysis population. The majority of these bacteremias are caused by staphylococcal organisms that are associated with high rates of mortality (8%–25%), recurrence (14%–44%), and serious metastatic complications. The incidence of infection is highest when the patient has a central venous catheter and lowest when it is a native arteriovenous fistula. An arteriovenous graft (PTFE, W.L. Gore, Newark, DE) is used when fistula creation is not feasible and is often plagued by infection. Infection or colonization at the exit site is followed by spread down the site of the catheter, resulting in a tunnel infection. Colonization of the inner wall of the catheter is a frequent occurrence and is usually accompanied by the presence of biofilm. This is produced by a combination of host factors (fibrinogen and fibrin) and microbial products (glycocalyx). Within the biofilm the colonizing bacteria convert to a sessile form and live in symbiosis with the patient. Among local factors, poor personal hygiene, use of occlusive transparent dressing, and accumulation of moisture around the exit site have been described as risk factors for catheter-related bacteremia. Nasal and skin colonization with *Staphylococcus aureus* as well as bacterial colonization of hemodialysis catheters has been reported as a risk factor for systemic infection. Systemic factors such as immunosuppression, diabetes mellitus, low albumin, and high ferritin have been found to be associated with increased risk of catheter-related bacteremia.

Correct Answer   D 48%–73%

Reference
Nassar, G. M., & Ayus, J. C. (2001). Infectious complications of the hemodialysis access. *Kidney Int,* *60*(1), 1–13. PMID: 11422731

8. RATIONALE

Management of catheter-related bacteremia in hemodialysis patients has two aspects. The first relates to antimicrobial therapy. Initial empiric antibiotic therapy should take into consideration the frequency of the bacterial isolates in such settings. Staphylococcal species are usually the most prevalent (60%–100%) bacterial isolates in hemodialysis patients with catheter-related bacteremia. The prevalence of *Staphylococcus aureus* and coagulase-negative staphylococcal bacteremia is similar in most series, along with enterococci in 11%–19% and Gram-negative rods are reported in up to 33% cases. Therefore, empiric antibiotic therapy should target both Gram-positive and Gram-negative organisms. The other aspect of management is related to the removal of the hemodialysis catheter, as it poses certain practical problems in patients whose vascular access sites have been exhausted. A prospective evaluation of 114 patients treated with appropriate antibiotics for catheter-related bacteremia were evaluated for a more conservative approach. Patients with severe clinical symptoms had catheter removal with delayed replacement after defervescence (86.5% cure rate). Patients with minimal symptoms but with a terminal or exit site infection had a catheter exchange over a guide wire with creation of a new tunnel (75% cure rate). Patients with minimal symptoms and a normal-appearing tunnel and exit site had a catheter exchange over a guide wire within 48 hours of antibiotic initiation (87.8% cure rate). Cure rates were defined as a 45-day, symptom-free interval after antibiotic therapy was complete.

Correct Answer   D Catheter removal with delayed replacement after defervescence in patients with severe clinical symptoms

Reference
Beathard, G. A. (1999). Management of bacteremia associated with tunneled-cuffed hemodialysis catheters. *J Am Soc Nephrol, 10*(5), 1045–1049. PMID: 10232691

9. RATIONALE

The risk of PTFE infection starts at the time of surgical placement. An initial 30-day graft infection rate of 6% has been reported. The femoral location of (thigh) PTFE graft is associated with a higher postoperative wound infection rates caused by moisture accumulation in between the overlying skin folds. The incidence of infection of autologous arteriovenous fistulas is approximately 0.56%–5%, and 4%–20% with AV grafts with staphylococcus species account for 30%–50% of infections, and infections with enterococcus and coagulase-negative staphylococcus occur in 20%–30% cases. Early microbial infections with Gram-negative bacteria account for 10%–20%. Coagulase-positive staphylococcus, especially MRSA and *Pseudomonas* infection, may lead to anastomotic disruption. Typical symptoms of graft infections include erythema; induration; drainage with sinus tracts; and systemic signs such as fevers, chills, and malaise. AV graft infections usually present with local symptoms as opposed to catheter-related infections, which present with systemic symptoms. Differential diagnosis include pneumonia, osteomyelitis, endocarditis, urinary tract infection, septic arthritis, and intrabdominal sources. Cellular immunity and polymorphonuclear neutrophil function are markedly diminished in patients with end-stage renal disease.

Correct Answer   D 6%

Reference
Padberg, F. T., Jr., Calligaro, K. D., & Sidawy, A. N. (2008). Complications of arteriovenous hemodialysis access: recognition and management. *J Vasc Surg, 48*(5 Suppl), 55s–80s. PMID: 19000594

10. RATIONALE

The diagnosis of dialysis access infection remains largely clinical. The utility of a tagged leukocyte scan in the diagnosis of AV fistula/graft infection can provide useful information in the presence of active infection; many false-negative scans are due to indolent or chronic infections with patients on antibiotic therapy. CT scans have low sensitivity in differentiating between prosthetic infection and postoperative changes in the acute setting. Contrast-enhanced CT scans may produce false-negative results in chronic low-grade and very late infections, and more than 80% show inconclusive findings.

Correct Answer   D Clinical exam

Reference
Erba, P. A., Leo, G., Sollini, M., et al. (2014). Radiolabelled leucocyte scintigraphy versus conventional radiological imaging for the management of late, low-grade vascular prosthesis infections. *Eur J Nucl Med Mol Imaging, 41*(2), 357–368. PMID: 24142027

11. RATIONALE

Autologous AV access site infections are usually localized to the access site and will respond to antibiotics provided the overlying skin is healthy. Prosthetic graft infections usually require total removal of the graft in patients with infections caused by organisms such as MRSA or *Pseudomonas*. Presence of a pseudoaneurysm in the graft with overlying skin breakdown or even superficial necrosis requires urgent removal of the graft. Occasionally low-grade localized prosthetic graft infections with coagulase-negative staphylococcus can be managed with segmental excision and jump graft reconstruction. Antibiotics for 4–6 weeks are usually necessary when attempting to salvage the graft in localized infections with satisfactory condition of the overlying skin.

Correct Answer **C** Antibiotics

Reference

Padberg, F. T., Jr., Calligaro, K. D., & Sidawy, A. N. (2008). Complications of arteriovenous hemodialysis access: recognition and management. *J Vasc Surg, 48*(5 Suppl), 55s–80s. PMID: 19000594

12. RATIONALE

The HeRO® graft has two components: A graft component with titanium connector and venous outflow component. The graft component has a 6-mm inner diameter, 7.4-mm outer diameter, and is 53-cm-long, inclusive of the connector. It consists of an expanded PTFE hemodialysis graft with PTFE beading to provide kink resistance near the proprietary titanium connector. The titanium connector attaches the arterial graft component. It has radiopaque silicon with braided nitinol reinforcement, a 5-mm inner diameter, and is 40 cm long. Patients with HeRO® graft placement usually have undergone multiple tunneled dialysis catheters and upper extremity access procedures previously. It is very important to evaluate their entire venous and arterial anatomy to identify the reason for failure. Besides physical exam, noninvasive vascular testing and venography should be performed. If the central venous stenosis or occlusion is the reason for failure, the HeRO® graft is a good option. Relative contraindications include inflow artery diameter less than 3 mm, systolic blood pressure less than 100 mmHg, ejection fraction less than 20%, and active infection. The HeRO® graft appears to provide similar patency, adequacy of dialysis, and bacteremia rates to those of conventional AV grafts.

Correct Answer **D** Prior multiple upper extremity access procedures

Reference

Nassar, G. M., Glickman, M. H., McLafferty, R. B., et al. (2014). A comparison between the HeRO graft and conventional arteriovenous grafts in hemodialysis patients. *Semin Dial, 27*(3), 310–318. PMID: 24428351

13. RATIONALE

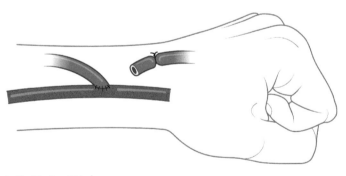

End to side: Radial-Cephalic Cimino Fistula.

Current Kidney Disease Outcomes Quality Initiative guidelines stipulate that all patients should be referred for creation of autologous access when the disease has progressed to stage 4 CKD (GFR <30 mL/min/1.73 m²). A native arteriovenous fistula (AVF) is the preferred access. A radial artery-cephalic vein direct wrist access fistula (Brescia Cimino Fistula) has a 2-year patency of 55%–89%. Other autologous options include radial artery branch cephalic vein direct access (snuffbox fistula); ulnar artery-basilic forearm transposition; brachial-cephalic vein upper arm direct access (antecubital venous brachial artery); and brachial artery-basilic upper arm transposition. Prosthetic options are constructed by interposing a PTFE graft between an artery and vein in a straight or a "C-shaped" or loop fashion. Maturation of fistula is defined by a flow of greater than 600 mL per minute, greater than 6 mm in diameter, less than 6 mm below the skin, at least 6 cm of vein available for cannulation, and expected maturation in 6 weeks.

Correct Answer   **B** 55%–89%

Reference
Gabel, J., & Neville, R.F. (2022). Surgical fistula creation. Techniques for ensuring maturation and long-term utility. *Endovasc Today*, *21*(6), 50–52.

14. RATIONALE

A venous outflow obstruction from stenosis, either peripherally or centrally, accounts for the most common reason of failure of fistulas and arteriovenous grafts. Venous stenosis most likely results from exposure of the outflow vein to the stress of significantly high arterial flow velocities and turbulent blood flow. Venous stenosis leads to stasis and eventual thrombosis of the vascular access. Neointimal hyperplasia (NIH) is the most common cause of stenosis. In NIH, fibroblasts, smooth muscle cells, and extracellular matrix accumulate in the intima and narrow the vessel lumen and has been histologically confirmed from collected tissue samples removed during surgical revisions showing the presence of smooth muscle cells, extracellular matrix, platelet-derived growth factor, and vascular endothelial growth factor expressed by macrophages. Due to repeated trauma of large-bore needles into the fistula/graft and circulating inflammatory markers in uremic states, NIH becomes accelerated.

Correct Answer   **C** Venous outflow obstruction

Reference
Reyna, M., & Tonia, K. (2014). Hemodialysis vascular access complications: recognition and management. *Hosp Med Clin*, *3*(4), 504–530.

15. RATIONALE

These stenoses may result in thrombosis of the fistula or its failure to mature. The problems with hemodialysis manifest in many ways such as increased venous pressures, difficulty of access, and prolonged bleeding after removal of the needle. The patient often complains of pain, swelling, and decreased fistula flow. In patients with obstruction due to central vein stenosis/occlusion, clinical features include edema involving the arm, shoulder, breast, supraclavicular region, neck, and face depending on the location and extent of the venous stenosis.

Correct Answer   **D** Venous outflow tract adjacent to the anastomosis

Reference
Collins, M. J., Li, X., Lv, W., et al. (2012). Therapeutic strategies to combat neointimal hyperplasia in vascular grafts. *Expert Rev Cardiovasc Ther*, *10*(5), 635–647. PMID: 22651839

16. RATIONALE

The sonographic variables that best reflect fistula formation are volume flows in the brachial artery and the caliber of and presence of stenosis in the outflow vein. Volume flows in the brachial artery in a successfully functioning arteriovenous fistula range from 500 to

1500 mL/min and a lower than 500 mL/min flow rate is associated with significant risk of thrombosis. A diagnosis of a stenosis is best made by fistulogram/shuntogram which additionally provides the ability to intervene if indicated. The main indication for percutaneous transluminal angioplasty is greater than 50% stenosis or thrombosis of the AV fistula/graft. Primary patency within the first year after balloon angioplasty is greater than 50%, while primary assisted patency is 80%–90% in the same time period. CTA and catheter-based arteriography are usually not necessary for the diagnosis of venous stenosis.

Correct Answer   **B** Fistulogram/shuntogram

Reference
Pietura, R., Janczarek, M., Zaluska, W., et al. (2005). Colour Doppler ultrasound assessment of well-functioning mature arteriovenous fistulas for haemodialysis access. *Eur J Radiol, 55*(1), 113–119. PMID: 15950108

17. RATIONALE

Graft surveillance with duplex ultrasound is most frequently performed within the first 2 years of index operation, as this is the most common time for development of neointimal hyperplasia. Early detection of a developing stenosis before the eventual thrombosis of the fistula/graft allows the feasibility of early intervention. Following angioplasty for stenosis in the hemodialysis circuit fistula, the flow rate was significantly better in native AV fistulas after angioplasty (88.4% flow increase) than in AV grafts (9.2% flow increase). Increase in fistula flow rate was greatest for valvular lesions (42.6% flow increase) followed by lesions at the needling site (40.1%). Peripheral outflow vein stenosis (29%), central outflow vein stenosis (28.9%), and at the anastomosis (19.9%) reflect the site stenosis.

Correct Answer   **D** Within first 2 years of index operation

Reference
Mohiuddin, K., Bosanquet, D. C., Dilaver, N., et al. (2018). Predicting technical success after fistuloplasty: an analysis of 176 procedures. *Ann Vasc Surg, 51*, 141–146.e142. PMID: 29522875

18. RATIONALE

Hemodynamically significant stenosis secondary to neointimal hyperplasia causes flow disturbances and changes, beginning the cascade that results in access thrombosis in 85% of cases. Hypercoagulability, stasis, and vessel injury with endothelial dysfunction are other common causes of thrombosis. Factors contributing to early failure include prior history of access surgery and absence of a thrill in the fistula or graft at the time of operation. Early thrombosis is associated with female gender, forearm fistula, and smaller diameter of the inflow artery and smaller diameter of the vein (2–3 mm). The literature remains conflicted in the role of antiplatelet and anticoagulant therapy for prevention of thrombosis in the hemodialysis access fistulas/grafts.

Correct Answer   **D** Significant stenosis secondary to neointimal hyperplasia at the venous anastomosis

Reference
Korn, A., Alipour, H., Zane, J., et al. (2018). Factors associated with early thrombosis after arteriovenous fistula creation. *Ann Vasc Surg, 49*, 281–284. PMID: 29477675

19. RATIONALE

Treatment of a thrombosed fistula/graft is thrombectomy via open surgical versus percutaneous methods. During open thrombectomy, shuntogram/fistulogram should be obtained after Fogarty balloon thrombectomy to detect the possible cause of thrombosis and managed accordingly with patch angioplasty or a balloon angioplasty. For percutaneous mechanical thrombectomy, proximal and distal access in the dialysis circuit is obtained and 6 Fr sheath towards the arterial end and 7 Fr sheath for the venous end. Aspiration thrombectomy (Angio-jet), with or without tPA, and balloon angioplasty after venography (to visualize central veins and the venous anastomosis) are performed during percutaneous intervention according to the findings detected at the time of venography. Percutaneous thrombectomies have better outcomes in terms of a lower rethrombosis rate and better primary assisted patency than surgical thrombectomies. However, percutaneous thrombectomies have a lower intervention-free patency and more frequently need additional procedures to maintain patency. Surgical revision procedures significantly increase the success rate of access thrombectomies. Approximately 56% of fully matured upper extremity AV fistulas require at least one intervention to maintain functional patency, with a mean time to first reintervention of 12.6 months. From a cost-effective standpoint, continued percutaneous intervention over open thrombectomies is preferable.

Correct Answer   C Percutaneous thrombectomies have a lower rethrombosis rate and better assisted primary patency rate than open surgical thrombectomies

Reference
Lambert, G., Freedman, J., Jaffe, S., & Wilmink, T. (2018). Comparison of surgical and radiological interventions for thrombosed arteriovenous access. *J Vasc Access*, *19*(6), 555–560. PMID: 29512417

20. RATIONALE

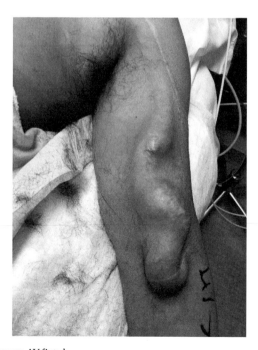

Large aneurysm in left upper arm AV fistula.

Two types of aneurysms occur in hemodialysis access circuits: True aneurysms and pseudoaneurysms. While pseudoaneurysms can occur in both arteriovenous grafts and fistulas, true aneurysms occur only in the fistula vein downstream from an obstruction. True aneurysms develop in 5%–10% of autologous upper extremity hemodialysis fistulas. The risk of rupture with the resulting catastrophic hemorrhage remains a major concern. Clinically, the most significant aneurysms are pseudoaneurysms that commonly occur at the site of needle punctures or at the anastomotic site due to infection or a poor surgical technique. The incidence of aneurysm development in hemodialysis circuits is higher in both proximal AV fistulas and more commonly involve the cephalic vein than the basilic vein. The presence of aneurysm should entail obtaining the contrast fistulogram/shuntogram for evaluation of anastomotic sites, outflow vein, and identification of ideal sites of cannulation. For significant aneurysmal disease, if the circuit is inappropriate for attempted revision or bypass, ligation and creation of a new access should be considered. The principles of treatment of both true and false aneurysms are similar. Repair should only be considered for clinically significant-sized aneurysms with risk of rupture. Clinically significant aneurysms are those that are rapidly enlarging and involve the anastomosis, overlying skin compromise, or in association with outflow venous stenosis or a large amount of intraluminal thrombosis or those associated with steal syndrome. For localized aneurysms, resection with end-to-end anastomosis after mobilization may occasionally be feasible. Plication and interposition grafts for more complex reconstructions with skin compromise may be necessary. Pseudoaneurysms can occasionally be treated with stent grafts, but there is an increased risk of late infection at the site of covered stent deployment.

Correct Answer **D** Inadequate depth of sutures at the anastomotic site, excessive tension at the anastomotic site, and infectious complications

Reference
Hossny, A. (2014). Partial aneurysmectomy for salvage of autogenous arteriovenous fistula with complicated venous aneurysms. *J Vasc Surg, 59*(4), 1073–1077. PMID: 24360585

21. RATIONALE

Ischemia is a serious complication of arteriovenous access. Both arteriovenous fistulas and grafts create a large amount of arterial venous pressure gradient that augments blood flow into the venous outflow circulation. There is shunting of a high volume of blood from the arterial into venous system, and distal ischemia develops as blood does not reach the most distal aspects of the extremity. By definition, physiologic steal results with arteriovenous access creation; pathological steal occurs when the patient experiences ischemic symptoms, and its incidence is up to 5% and is highest in proximal fistulas (10%–25%) brachiocephalic and brachiobasilic (4.3%), forearm grafts (6%), and radiocephalic AV fistulas (1%–1.8%). The larger the caliber of the artery, the higher the velocity and blood flow through arteriovenous access, the greater the likelihood of symptomatic distal ischemia. Due to collateral circulation, some patients may not experience ischemic symptoms.

Correct Answer **D** 5%

Reference
Tordoir, J. H., Dammers, R., & van der Sande, F. M. (2004). Upper extremity ischemia and hemodialysis vascular access. *Eur J Vasc Endovasc Surg, 27*(1), 1–5. PMID: 14652830

22. RATIONALE

Steal syndrome is a graded complication with four stages to classify the symptoms and assist in management, with stage I with pale, blue, or cold hand without pain; stage II pain during exercise or during hemodialysis; stage III rest pain; and stage IV ulcer necrosis and gangrene. Symptoms may occur within days to months of the creation of hemodialysis access. Approximately 50%–66% of patients who develop steal syndrome occur within 30 days after access has been performed. Steal syndrome is primarily a clinical diagnosis, and a complete history and physical exam is important for its recognition. Unilateral neurological complaints associated with digital tissue necrosis pallor/cyanosis of a distal portion of the extremity include reduced distal flow beyond the distal anastomotic site with flow reversal. A noninvasive Doppler arterial study of the manual compression of the fistula/graft should restore almost normal flow to the distal portion of the extremity, including hand, digit, and forearm.

Correct Answer   **C** Stage III

Reference

Bucktowarsing, B. (2019). An Overview of Dialysis Access-Associated Steal Syndrome. Retrieved from https://www.renalfellow.org/2019/06/30/an-overview-of-dialysis-access-associated-steal-syndrome/

23. RATIONALE

Diagnosis of DASS can be made by clinical examination but may be difficult in patients who have associated arterial occlusive disease of the extremity, which should be evaluated prior to construction of an AV access by clinical examination and Doppler study. Predicting ischemic steal syndrome can be challenging, but in patients age above 60 years, with diabetes mellites, prior several access procedures in the same extremity, and use of brachial artery inflow are at increased risk of access associated steal syndrome. On Doppler ultrasonography, digital pressures of less than 50 mmHg, digital-brachial index (DBI) less than 0.6, and TcPO$_2$ less than 20–30 mmHg are markers of steal pathology. Relief of symptoms and normalization of finger (digital) blood flow as assessed by digital pressures, waveforms, and improvement in TcPO$_2$ are confirmatory.

Correct Answer   **C** Doppler ultrasonography with digital pressures and tracings with and without AV access compression

Reference

Tordoir, J. H., Dammers, R., & van der Sande, F. M. (2004). Upper extremity ischemia and hemodialysis vascular access. *Eur J Vasc Endovasc Surg, 27*(1), 1–5. PMID: 14652830

24. RATIONALE

Most patients with steal syndrome (stage I, II, and selected patients with mild rest pain) will improve with conservative treatment such as keeping the hand warm with hand exercises as collaterals develop with the passage of time. However, in patients with neurological symptoms (paresthesia in the hand with severe rest pain or stage III or tissue loss, stage IV) should be treated urgently, as failure to improve the arterial flow may result in permanent loss of function. Treatment varies according to the underlying cause of arterial steal. If arterial stenosis exists proximal to access, PTA with stenting of the arterial stenosis and the occlusion artery is the initial treatment of choice. Banding is not usually recommended due to the high complication rate of thrombosis of the access. The minimally invasive limited ligation, endoluminal-assisted revision, is a hybrid technique using an endoluminal balloon with a small 1- to 2-cm incision. The initial results were satisfactory, but subsequent studies have not confirmed its role in the treatment of steal syndrome. Distal revascularization and interval ligation is a two-step procedure and consists of ligation of the artery just distal to its anastomosis with creation of an arterial bypass from the artery proximal to the arterial anastomosis and of the arterial bypass distal to the ligated site of the artery to provide satisfactory flow to the distal extremity beyond the distal anastomosis. Either great saphenous vein or a PTFE graft is used as a conduit for the bypass. Symptomatic relief is reported in 83%–100% of patients with steal syndrome, with secondary patency of the access in 73%–98%. Complications ranged up to 70% and were mostly surgical site infection and thrombosis. Revision using distal inflow (RUDI) is accompanied by ligating the original upper arm AV outflow near the anastomosis and creating a new anastomosis with a smaller-caliber, more distal artery such as the proximal radial or ulnar artery for the inflow using a graft. The original venous outflow is maintained. Another procedure referred to as proximalization of arterial inflow entails moving the arterial supply to a more proximal brachial artery level or axillary artery using an interposition graft. In severe cases of steal, ligation of the fistula may be warranted to restore blood flow to the distal extremity emergently with obvious loss of access.

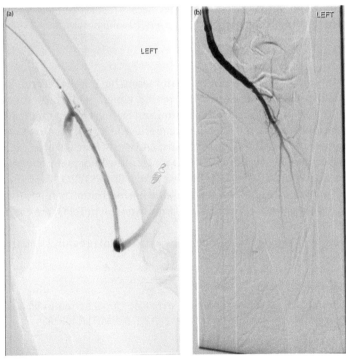

(a) Left upper arm AV graft with DRIL procedure using GSV as a bypass with origin from midbrachial artery and ligation of the brachial artery distal to the proximal anastomosis of the AV graft (coils are seen from remote procedure to embolize the side branch of the fistula). (b) Distal anastomosis of the GVS vein bypass to the distal brachial artery.

Correct Answer   **D** Distal revascularization with interval ligation (DRIL) procedure

Reference
Knox, R. C., Berman, S. S., Hughes, J. D., et al. (2002). Distal revascularization-interval ligation: a durable and effective treatment for ischemic steal syndrome after hemodialysis access. *J Vasc Surg*, *36*(2), 250–255; discussion 256. PMID: 12170205

25. RATIONALE

Neuropathy in some form occurs in patients on hemodialysis with an incidence of 70%. Ischemic monomelic neuropathy (IMN) is a rare and specific type of ischemia affecting only the nerves. This condition causes arterial insufficiency involving a single extremity (monomelic) and causing selective dysfunction (neuropathy) of multiple peripheral nerves. After hemodialysis access procedures, there is a steal that results in hypoperfusion of the vasa nervosum causing damage to the distal nerve fibers and resulting in severe acute neurological symptoms such as pain; paresthesias; and numbness in the distribution of the median, radial, and ulnar nerves including muscle weakness or paralysis. This devastating complication can result in permanent disability, even if the fistula or graft is ligated immediately after surgery.

Correct Answer   **D** Ischemic monomelic neuropathy

Reference
Sheetal, S., Byju, P., & Manoj, P. (2017). Ischemic monomelic neuropathy. *J Postgrad Med, 63*(1), 42–43. PMID: 27853044

26. RATIONALE

IMN differs from ischemic syndrome in that it is irreversible, exhibits no tissue necrosis, and the hand is warm with a palpable pulse. Risk factors include female gender, long-standing diabetes mellitus, and pre-existing peripheral neuropathy. As sensory impairment and motor weakness progress, resulting in claw hand deformity, significant loss of function and severe neurogenic pain occur. Electromyography aids in confirming the diagnosis as it shows axonal loss, low amplitude, or absent responses to sensory and motor nerve stimulation with relatively preserved conduction velocities. Besides IMN, uremic polyneuropathy has been estimated to be present in 60%–100% of patients on hemodialysis. Uremic polyneuropathy targets large-diameter axons in most distal nerve trunks causing distal segmental demyelination and axonal degeneration with proximal nerve sparing. Nerve biopsy helps in establishing these patterns. Diabetic polyneuropathy is bilateral and correlates with chronicity of the disease with loss of vibration sense and sensory loss in a "glove and stocking" distribution.

Correct Answer   **A** Reversible

Reference
Krishnan, A. V., & Kiernan, M. C. (2007). Uremic neuropathy: clinical features and new pathophysiological insights. *Muscle Nerve, 35*(3), 273–290. PMID: 17195171

27. RATIONALE

CVS has been identified in 17%–26% of patients undergoing venography for failing access or edema of the extremity. CVS stenosis or occlusion is often not diagnosed prior to access placement, as the patient may not have any significant signs or symptoms of CVS. The patient may demonstrate symptoms after the access has been placed. The presumed etiology of CVS is chronic endothelial trauma during cardiac and respiratory cycles, caused most likely by a previously placed tunneled dialysis catheter, central venous catheters, pacemaker wires, and defibrillator wires. A study of 150 patients undergoing PICC-line placement with venography before and after insertion revealed a 7% incidence of stenosis/occlusion centrally, especially in those patients with a longer catheter dwell time. Sources of peripheral venous stenosis include NIH in the outflow anastomosis, cephalic vein stenosis, incompetent valves, or feeding branches. Symptoms of venous hypertension include fullness in the chest, swelling of the upper extremity, and collateral veins seen in the chest wall.

Correct Answer **D** 17%–26%

Reference
Schwab, S. J., Quarles, L. D., Middleton, J. P., et al. (1988). Hemodialysis-associated subclavian vein stenosis. *Kidney Int, 33*(6), 1156–1159. PMID: 2969991

28. RATIONALE
Significant stenosis at the venous anastomosis off the hemodialysis graft responds favorably to standard balloon angioplasty. Primary patency within the first year after angioplasty is greater than 50% while primary assisted patency is 80%–90%. If the suboptimal result is obtained with a standard balloon angioplasty, high-pressure balloon or a cutting balloon angioplasty should be considered as a second-line method of relieving the stenosis. Covered stent and bare-metal stents are reserved for the management of complications and for central outflow stenosis. PTA is the treatment of choice for stenosis caused by an obstruction of the fistulas. Repeated PTA may be required for better long-term patency.

Correct Answer **C** Cutting balloon or high-pressure balloon angioplasty

Reference
Bountouris, I., Kritikou, G., Degermetzoglou, N., & Avgerinos, K. I. (2018). A review of percutaneous transluminal angioplasty in hemodialysis fistula. *Int J Vasc Med, 2018*, 1420136. PMID: 29785307

29. RATIONALE

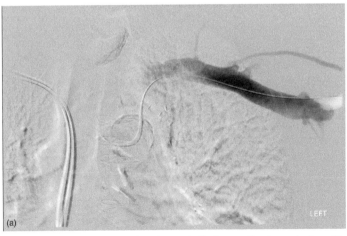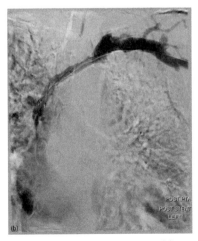

(a) Venography demonstrates brachiocephalic (central) vein occlusion—Defibrilator wires in the right IJ vein. (b) Post Angioplasty and stenting across the brachiocephalic vein with reconstitution of blood flow.

Angioplasty for CVS may not be as effective in vessels with increased elasticity and recoil. Angioplasty has even been shown to accelerate restenosis, with recurrent lesions showing a more aggressive neointimal hyperplasia. PTA is the first-line approach as recommended by KDOQI, with stenting reserved for angioplasty failure. However, an excellent early result but a poor long-term patency of 50% at 6 months and 25% at 12 months has been reported with angioplasty alone. Stent grafts have shown better outcomes over bare-metal stents with improved primary and assisted patency rates. A covered stent may jail important collaterals of a central vein leading complications for the future. In the setting of wires from the pacemaker/defibrillator, it may be prudent to place a contralateral access for hemodialysis at the time of the index permanent arteriovenous access procedure. Open surgical management is considered a last remaining option for recurrence of failed endovascular management and includes internal jugular vein transposition, axillo-jugular bypass, axillo-axillary crossover bypass, and axillo-atrial bypass. Hybrid alternatives such as the Hemoaccess Reliable Outflow (HeRO) vascular access device (Hemosphere, Inc., Minneapolis, MN) should be considered.

Correct Answer   D Covered stent

Reference
Agarwal, A. K. (2013). Central vein stenosis. *Am J Kidney Dis, 61*(6), 1001–1015. PMID: 23291234

30. RATIONALE

A review of a vascular quality initiative database of 3608 patients compared tapered with non-tapered grafts. Tapered grafts had similar rates of ischemic steal at 3 months (4.1% vs. 4.6%) and on multivariate analysis did not affect primary patency or reintervention rates of both open as well as endovascular interventions. Therefore, tapered arteriovenous grafts for hemodialysis do not provide any additional advantage as compared to non-tapered grafts for hemodialysis access.

Correct Answer   C Similar primary patency

Reference
Roberts, L., Farber, A., Jones, D. W., et al. (2019). Tapered arteriovenous grafts do not provide significant advantage over nontapered grafts in upper extremity dialysis access. *J Vasc Surg, 69*(5), 1552–1558. PMID: 30583896

31. RATIONALE

Several factors contribute to the increased risk of bleeding in a patient on hemodialysis. A common etiology is anemia of chronic disease secondary to end-stage renal disease. As hematocrit declines, there is reduced clearance of nitric oxide causing platelet inhibition and vasodilation, and ultimately coagulopathy. Maintenance of hematocrit greater than 30% is the key, with an inverse relationship between packed red cells and bleeding times. Uremia-induced platelet dysfunction with ineffective adhesion to sub-endothelium from reduced expression of Gp1b receptors and a reduced affinity for Von Willebrand factor (vWF) is associated with increased risk of bleeding in a patient on hemodialysis. Treatment with desmopressin immediately acts on endothelial vasopressin receptors, and CAMP-mediated signaling decreases bleeding time. Maximal effect is seen at 1 hour lasting 4–6 hours. Infusion of other blood products to replenish clotting factors may also be necessary.

Correct Answer   D Desmopressin

Reference
Kim, J. H., Baek, C. H., Min, J. Y., et al. (2015). Desmopressin improves platelet function in uremic patients taking antiplatelet agents who require emergent invasive procedures. *Ann Hematol, 94*(9), 1457-1461. PMID: 25933676

32. RATIONALE

Most ESRD patients do not have kidney failure in isolation, with associated comorbidities requiring antiplatelet or anticoagulant therapy being quite common such as history of deep venous thrombosis, atrial fibrillation, and coronary artery disease, and the use of medications increases bleeding risk in an already predisposed population towards coagulopathy. Physical trauma of large-size needles during hemodialysis causes a continuous risk of bleeding. Pulsatile bleeding with or without rapidly expanding hematoma should be temporarily controlled with constant, direct pressure at the bleeding site for 30–40 minutes or until bleeding resolves. Tourniquet application is rarely feasible, as most AV fistulas/AV grafts are placed in the upper arm. If bleeding persists despite pressure, a suture may be placed through the skin and subcutaneous tissue but not through the underlying fistula/graft using proximal and distal manual pressure to visualize the area of bleeding. Persistent pulsatile bleeding is concerning for venous outflow stenosis, graft infection, and pseudoaneurysm. The patient will likely require a shuntogram. If there is skin comprise, including thinning/ulceration, with exposed access, an interposition graft tunneled in healthy tissue planes and sutured to a well-incorporated segment of a previously placed graft near the arterial and the venous end anastomosis is recommended. Skin breakdown over the graft needs emergent operation.

Correct Answer   D Direct pressure for 30–40 minutes; if bleeding persists, place a suture over the bleeding site and administer desmopressin, then evaluate the shunt by shuntogram followed by the appropriate management strategy

Reference
Inui, T., Boulom, V., Bandyk, D., et al. (2017). Dialysis access hemorrhage: access rescue from a surgical emergency. *Ann Vasc Surg, 42*, 45–49. PMID: 28341509

33. RATIONALE

Development of high-output heart failure is an underappreciated complication of permanent dialysis access in patients with a proximal access and with a history of compensated heart failure. Flow in a well-functioning access fistula is approximately 700–1500 mL/min. This may result in left ventricular hypertrophy, reduced ejection fraction, and heart failure. Symptoms include tachycardia, elevated pulse pressure, and jugular venous distention. On examination the fistula appears large with rapid flow and aneurysmal growth, often referred to as a "mega fistula." Characteristic findings include pulmonary hypertension with normal pulmonary vascular resistance and high cardiac output with low-normal systemic vascular resistance. In patients with high cardiac output heart failure, intraoperative access flow monitoring demonstrates flow >2000 mL/min. Treatment involves reduction of flow as described in the rationale for management of dialysis-associated steal syndrome (DASS).

Correct Answer   D >2000 mL/min

Reference
Stern, A. B., & Klemmer, P. J. (2011). High-output heart failure secondary to arteriovenous fistula. *Hemodial Int, 15*(1), 104–107. PMID: 21223485

34. RATIONALE

An arterio-arterial graft for hemodialysis is rarely indicated. The main indications are that all large four deep veins (femoral and internal jugular vein) are occluded or are not suitable due to septic complications; the patient in heart failure is refractory to therapy so that standard arterial venous access will have a negative effect on heart failure. To guarantee a sufficient flow for effective dialysis access, always insert a loop graft in the course of an artery. A large size artery with high flow is selected. The physiological advantage of arterio-arterial interposition grafts includes their lack of effect on cardiac output or peripheral perfusion. The flow rate in these grafts is typically around 150–250 cc/minute, which is much lower than the standard AV fistula or graft; the time required for dialysis sessions is longer (5–6 hours). Large surface area dialyzers increase the efficiency of hemodialysis. Primary patency rates range from 67% to 94.5% at 6 months to 54% to 61% at 36 months with secondary patency rates from 83%–93% at 6 months to 72%–87% at 36 months.

Correct Answer   **D** No change in cardiac output or peripheral perfusion with preference for axillo-axillary loop grafts

Reference

Grima, M. J., Vriens, B., Holt, P. J., & Chemla, E. (2018). An arterioarterial prosthetic graft as an alternative option for haemodialysis access: a systematic review. *J Vasc Access*, *19*(1), 45–51. PMID: 29148001

SECTION 16: AMPUTATIONS

MCQs 1–9

Q1. The most common indication for below the knee amputation is:
A. Trauma
B. Failed arterial reconstruction for chronic limb ischemia
C. Sarcoma involving lower leg
D. Critical limb ischemia in patients with diabetes mellitus presenting as infected gangrene

Q2. In patients undergoing transmetatarsal amputation (TMA) for diabetic foot ulceration, the risk of reulceration during a follow-up time of 4 years is:
A. 15%–20%
B. 21%–30%
C. 31%–40%
D. 41% or higher

Q3. Contraindications to transmetatarsal amputation (TMA) include all of the following except:
A. Forefoot infection, cellulitis
B. Dependent rubor involving the dorsal forefoot proximal to the metatarsal phalangeal crease
C. Gangrenous changes in the plantar skin extending proximal to the metatarsal phalangeal crease
D. Patients above age 75

Q4. The conversion rate of below the knee amputation to above the knee amputation is approximately:
A. <5%
B. 6%–9%
C. 10%–15%
D. 16%–20%

Q5. The most common complication following below the knee and above the knee amputations are:

A. Cardiac
B. Wound infection
C. Pneumonia
D. Hematoma

Q6. The following statement best reflects the energy expenditure in patients with lower extremity amputation:
A. An estimated 50% more energy is expended to walk on an AKA prosthesis compared to 20% on a BKA prosthesis
B. An estimated 60% more energy is expended to walk on an AKA prosthesis compared to 30% on a BKA prosthesis.
C. An estimated 70% more energy is expended to walk on an AKA prosthesis compared to 40% on a BKA prosthesis

Q7. All are potential complications of above the knee amputation except:
A. Hematoma
B. Wound complications and stump ischemia
C. Deep venous thrombosis
D. Arteriovenous fistula involving the femoral artery and vein

Q8. Energy requirements with use of a prosthesis following hip disarticulation is:
A. 50% of normal ambulation
B. 100% of normal ambulation
C. 150% of normal ambulation
D. 200% of normal ambulation

Q9. The incidence of wound complications following hip disarticulation is:
A. Less than 10%
B. 10%–15%
C. 16%–20%
D. 20%–50%

DOI: 10.1201/9781003389897-16

RATIONALE 1–9

1. RATIONALE

A large proportion of amputations (82%) are performed for critical limb ischemia in patients with diabetes mellitus presenting as infected gangrene despite prior attempts at repeated arterial reconstructions for limb salvage. Some patients with diabetes mellitus with chronic ulcers in the feet present to the ER with gas gangrene and require emergent guillotine amputation above the ankle to be followed by definitive amputation after source control, usually in 5–7 days after guillotine amputation. Motor vehicle accidents are the leading cause of traumatic amputations. Combat and terrorist attacks are other causes of traumatic amputations. Terrorist attack are also common causes of below the knee amputation. In cases of severe infection, acute cellulitis needs to be controlled prior to amputation. The level of amputation should be decided after assessing the type of pathology, potential for rehabilitation, and presence of adequate perfusion. Clinical condition of the skin below the knee is an important determinate in the healing of the BK stump.

Correct Answer **D** Critical limb ischemia in patients with diabetes mellitus presenting as infected gangrene

Reference
McIntyre, K. E. (2014). Below knee amputation. In J. C. Stanley, F. Veith, & T. W. Wakefield (Eds.), *Current therapy in vascular and endovascular surgery* (pp. 647–648). Elsevier Health Sciences.

2. RATIONALE

Among 83 transmetatarsal amputations for diabetic foot ulcers over a 4-year period, reulceration occurred in 44% of patients with transmetatarsal amputation at a mean follow-up of 15 months after surgical healing. Successful transmetatarsal amputation is defined as one which had clinical healing 1 year after surgery. Mean follow-up in the forementioned study was 4 years and mean time to surgical healing was 109.8 days. Patients with reulceration were younger, with a significantly higher preprocedure Hb1Ac.

Correct Answer **D** 41% or higher

Reference
Tokarski, A. R., Barton, E. C., Wagner, J. T., et al. (2022). Are transmetatarsal amputations a durable limb salvage option? A single-institution descriptive analysis. *J Foot Ankle Surg, 61*(3), 537–541. PMID: 34794876

3. RATIONALE

TMA is indicated for trauma, tissue loss, infection, and gangrene limited to the toes. TMA requires shoe modification and inserts with forefoot space replacement. Amputation may be done for gangrene extending a short distance on the dorsal skin past the metatarsal phalangeal crease, provided plantar skin is healthy and arterial inflow is adequate. In patients with arterial occlusion and dependent rubor, endovascular or open surgical reconstruction should be considered prior to transmetatarsal amputation. Previous revascularization attempts, ABI equal to or less than 0.4, insulin-dependent diabetes mellitus, low albumin level (less than 3.0 g/dL), and high C-reactive protein are the important factors associated with poor transmetatarsal amputation outcomes.

Well-padded dressing with short-leg plaster cast will control edema and prevent stump trauma immediately after TMA. Early ambulation after TMA should be avoided. A rigid dressing is used until the transmetatarsal flap is well healed, which usually occurs 3–4 weeks following surgery. Transmetatarsal amputation is not contraindicated in patients above 75 years of age.

Correct Answer   **D** Patients above age 75

Reference
Aljarrah, Q., Allouh, M. Z., Husein, A., et al. (2022). Transmetatarsal amputations in patients with diabetes mellitus: a contemporary analysis from an academic tertiary referral centre in a developing community. *PLoS ONE, 17*(11), e0277117. PMID: 36327256

4. RATIONALE

The below the knee amputation site may not heal and may require further debridement, skin grafts, and intensive wound care. In spite of all the available treatment modalities, approximately 9.4%–12% with below the knee amputation need to be converted to above the knee amputation. There is no ideal test available to predict satisfactory healing of a below the knee stump. Doppler arterial evaluation, presence of popliteal pulse, transcutaneous oxygen measurements, and catheter-based arteriography are not completely reliable in predicting healing of a below the knee amputation. Clinical examination with satisfactory condition of the skin at the site of amputation are as important as any available test to determine the healing of a below the knee amputation site.

Correct Answer   **C** 10%–15%

Reference
Aulivola, B., Hile, C. N., Hamdan, A. D., et al. (2004). Major lower extremity amputation: outcome of a modern series. *Arch Surg, 139*(4), 395–399; discussion 399. PMID: 15078707

5. RATIONALE

From a study of 959 patients with lower extremity amputations (704 below the knee and 255 above the knee), the overall 30-day mortality was 16.5% for above the knee amputations and 5.7% for below the knee amputations ($P \leq 0.001$). Complications include cardiac (10.2%), wound infection (5.5%), and pneumonia (4.5%). Overall survival was 69.7% at 1 year and 34.7% at 5 years. Survival was significantly worse for above the knee amputations (50.6% at 1 year and 22.5% at 5 years) than below the knee amputation (74.5% at 1 year and 37.8% at 5 years, $p <0.001$). Survival in patients with diabetes mellitus and end-stage renal disease was significantly worse than those undergoing lower extremity amputations without diabetes mellitus or ESRD.

Correct Answer   **A** Cardiac

Reference
Aulivola, B., Hile, C. N., Hamdan, A. D., et al. (2004). Major lower extremity amputation: outcome of a modern series. *Arch Surg, 139*(4), 395–399; discussion 399. PMID: 15078707

6. RATIONALE

The ability to ambulate for patients who have undergone major amputations of the lower extremity is largely determined by the level of amputation. The energy expenditure in the case of transmetatarsal amputation is increased by 16%–33% at a comfortable walking speed. Transfemoral amputations require 65%–70% more energy, and in patients with above the knee amputation, an estimated 70% more energy is expended with use of a prosthesis as compared to 40% with a below the knee amputation prosthesis.

Correct Answer   **C**   An estimated 70% more energy is expended to walk on an AKA prosthesis compared to 40% on a BKA prosthesis

Reference

Chin, T., Sawamura, S., Shiba, R., et al. (2005). Energy expenditure during walking in amputees after disarticulation of the hip. A microprocessor-controlled swing-phase control knee versus a mechanical-controlled stance-phase control knee. *J Bone Joint Surg Br, 87*(1), 117–119. PMID: 15686251

7. RATIONALE

Deep venous thrombosis has been reported in up to 50% of patients following major lower extremity amputations and may result in mortality in a large proportion of such patients. Venous thromboembolic prophylaxis is essential in patients undergoing major amputation. Incidence of wound complication is 40%, most often secondary to ischemia and wound infection. Wound infections are more common when amputation is performed for infectious indications and in patients with diabetes mellitus, malnutrition, malignancy, wound hematoma, and prior prosthetic graft arterial reconstruction. Excisional debridement, systemic antibiotics, and nutritional optimization are essential. Vacuum-assisted dressings are very useful. Stump ischemia manifests as persistent pain with pallor and coolness of the stump with blister formation. Mortality following above the knee amputation ranges from 11% to 18%. The survival rate after 1 year is approximately 50%, and less than 10% of elderly patients can walk using an above the knee prosthesis.

Correct Answer   **D**   Arteriovenous fistula involving the femoral artery and vein

Reference

Nehler, M. R., Coll, J. R., Hiatt, W. R., et al. (2003). Functional outcome in a contemporary series of major lower extremity amputations. *J Vasc Surg, 38*(1), 7–14. PMID: 12844082

8. RATIONALE

Hip disarticulation is most often performed for treatment of high-grade diaphyseal tumors distal to the lesser trochanter, occasionally after massive trauma, severe infections, massive decubitus ulcers, severe arterial insufficiency, and congenital limb anomalies. Few patients are able to utilize a prosthesis, as energy requirements to use a prosthesis following disarticulation have been estimated to be 200% of normal ambulation. Mortality rates up to 44% have been reported following disarticulation of the hip.

Correct Answer   **D**   200% of normal ambulation

Reference

Sugarbaker, P. H., & Chretien, P. B. (1981). A surgical technique for hip disarticulation. *Surgery, 90*(3), 546–553. PMID: 7268632

9. RATIONALE

A review of 53 hip disarticulations performed for atherosclerotic arterial occlusive disease in 10, infection in 12, infection and ischemia in 14, and tumors 17 demonstrated an overall mortality of 20.8%, with 50% mortality in patients who underwent hip disarticulation due to arterial occlusive disease. No patient was able to use a prosthesis, but most were independent in wheelchairs. The incidence of wound complications following hip disarticulation is 20%–50%. In patients with gangrene of the extremity with prior failed revascularization attempts, hip disarticulation should not be delayed in those for whom above the knee or subtrochanteric amputation is not feasible. Prior above the knee amputation and urgent operation were associated with increased risk of wound complications following hip disarticulation. Both limb ischemia and wound infection substantially increase the morbidity and mortality of disarticulation of the hip.

Correct Answer   D 200% of normal ambulation

Reference

Endean, E. D., Schwarcz, T. H., Barker, D. E., et al. (1991). Hip disarticulation: factors affecting outcome. *J Vasc Surg, 14*(3), 398–404. PMID: 1880849

SECTION 17: ENDOVASCULAR RETRIEVAL OF FOREIGN BODIES

MCQs 1–4

Q1. The incidence of fragmentation or embolization of a central venous catheter is approximately:
- **A.** 1%
- **B.** 2%
- **C.** 3%
- **D.** 4%

Q2. The most optimal method to retrieve an intravascular foreign body is:
- **A.** Open surgical removal
- **B.** Endovascular removal with loop snare
- **C.** Endovascular using retrieval forceps and using internal jugular vein access
- **D.** Endovascular with retrieval forceps and using femoral vein access

Q3. A fragment of a mediport catheter broke and lodged in the right pulmonary artery branch. The best option for access in removing the foreign body is via:
- **A.** Right subclavian vein
- **B.** Right femoral vein
- **C.** Right internal jugular vein
- **D.** Open operative removal

Q4. Endovascular retrieval forceps are best used for:
- **A.** Cutting the struts of the IVC filter
- **B.** Removing an IVB with a free end
- **C.** Removing a spherical or an ovoid object (bullet)
- **D.** Removing an IFB without a free end

DOI: 10.1201/9781003389897-17

RATIONALE 1–4

1. RATIONALE

The overall complication rate of central venous catheter placement is approximately 15%, and the most common complications are hematoma, pneumothorax, infection, and iatrogenic arterial injury (carotid or subclavian artery). Embolization of a catheter or its fragmentation is a rare but serious complication. It comprises 1% of all complications but has an associated mortality of 71% and hence the need for early retrieval. The signs associated with fragment embolization in order of decreasing incidence are catheter malfunction, cardiac arrythmias, shortness of breath, and signs of sepsis. An upright chest z-ray should be obtained to confirm the location of the catheter, ensure the catheter in its entirety, and rule out embolized fragments. The common location of embolized material includes the right atrium, pulmonary artery, right ventricle, superior vena cava, and subclavian vein.

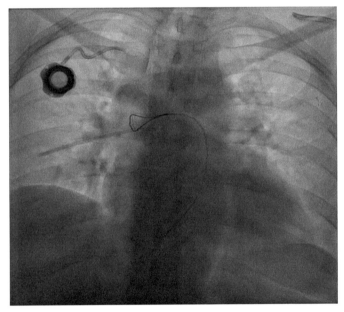

The gooseneck snare used to retrieve an IFB.

Correct Answer   **A** 1%

Reference

Surov, A., Wienke, A., Carter, J. M., et al. (2009). Intravascular embolization of venous catheter – causes, clinical signs, and management: a systematic review. *JPEN J Parenter Enteral Nutr, 33*(6), 677–685. PMID:19675301

2. RATIONALE

The rapid growth of endovascular interventions has led to the development of multiple devices used for the retrieval of intravascular foreign bodies (IFBs). It is designed to be flexible, facilitating navigation through the vasculature to reach the right atrium or pulmonary arteries. A disadvantage to its use is its weak grip strength, making chronic, adherent IFBs difficult to remove.

The snare can be a single loop, also referred to as an Amplatz Gooseneck Nitinol Snare (EV3, Inc., Plymouth, MN) or multiple loops such as EN Snare (Merrit Medical, Jordan, UT). When deployed, the loop emerges perpendicular to the catheter at a 90-degree angle, making placement of the loop around the IFB more feasible. The loop snare's design permits its use for removing a variety of IFBs, including fragmented central venous catheters, wires, stents, and IVC filters.

Correct Answer   **B** Endovascular removal with loop snare

Reference
Schechter, M. A., O'Brien, P. J., & Cox, M. W. (2013). Retrieval of iatrogenic intravascular foreign bodies. *J Vasc Surg*, *57*(1), 276–281. PMID: 23140798

3. RATIONALE

Various techniques using the loop snare device have been described to remove intravascular foreign bodies. The proximal capture technique is the most basic of all approaches described in the literature. In order to use this method, there must be a free end of the IFB that is accessible. The venous system is accessed through one of the major veins, preferably the right common femoral vein. In certain situations, such as patients with inferior vena cava filters or with bilateral iliac vein thrombosis, the IJV or subclavian vein is the preferred access site. The catheter is advanced under fluoroscopic guidance into the desired vessel to a point just before the IFB. Once in position, the outer catheter is withdrawn deploying the snare, then the entire system is advanced until the loop is around the free end of the IFB. Once the loop encompasses the IFB, the snare is tightened around the IFB by advancing the catheter. After the snare is tightened, the IFB should be oriented parallel to the vessel, which reduces the likelihood of vessel damage during retrieval. The entire system, including the snare, is removed through the 8 Fr sheath. Care must be taken that the loop is around the free end of the IFB. Success rates have been reported to be in excess of 92%.

Correct Answer   **B** Right femoral vein

Reference
Schechter, M. A., O'Brien, P. J., & Cox, M. W. (2013). Retrieval of iatrogenic intravascular foreign bodies. *J Vasc Surg*, *57*(1), 276–281. PMID: 23140798

4. RATIONALE

Endovascular forceps are not used as much as the loop snare for foreign body retrieval. Their design typically employs side-opening jaws, which allow for greater grip strength. The access is obtained through the IJV or femoral vein. They come in a variety of sizes ranging from 3 Fr to 12 Fr and can be passed through a guiding catheter. The Vascular Retrieval Forceps (Cook Medical, Bloomington, IN) are used in larger vessels and can be used to retrieve IFBs from central veins and the right atrium. The Alligator Retrieval Device (Covidien, Mansfield, MA) can be used in small vessels and is often used to remove coils from the cerebral circulation. The greatest advantage of endovascular forceps is the ability to remove IFBs without a free end. Drawbacks to using the forceps are their high risk of iatrogenic injuries and a rigid design leading to difficult navigation. Endovascular forceps have been used to facilitate the removal of stents, coils, and IFBs that are adherent to the endothelium of the vessel. If excessive force is used with endovascular forceps, there could be damage to the lining of the vessel and even a risk of perforation. Once access is obtained, the guiding catheter is then directed to the desired location. The forceps are passed through the catheter and gently advanced until the jaws emerge. The catheter and forceps are then manipulated to grasp the IFB. Once the IFB is in the jaws of the forceps, the guiding catheter and the forceps are gently removed as a single unit.

Correct Answer   **D** Removing an IFB without a free end

Reference
Schechter, M. A., O'Brien, P. J., & Cox, M. W. (2013). Retrieval of iatrogenic intravascular foreign bodies. *J Vasc Surg, 57*(1), 276–281. PMID: 23140798

SECTION 18: GRAFT INFECTIONS

MCQs 1–6

Q1. The mortality rate of extracavitary graft infection is:
A. 8%–10%
B. 11%–15%
C. 16%–18%
D. 19%–22%

Q2. A retroflexed gracilis muscle flap is best used for exposed graft in the groin in patients:
A. With a patent superficial femoral artery
B. When the sartorius muscle has been previously used as a muscle flap
C. When a large amount of tissue coverage is required
D. In patients with involvement of vascular anastomosis

Q3. Following femoral-infrapopliteal in situ bypass for ischemic toe gangrene, there is breakdown of the knee incision with exposure of the arterial bypass in its inferior portion. The best option for tissue coverage is:
A. Vastus medialis muscle flap
B. Soleus muscle flap
C. Medial head of gastrocnemius muscle flap
D. Retroflexed sartorius muscle flap

Q4. Following carotid endarterectomy in a patient with a prior history of radical neck dissection followed by radiation therapy for carcinoma of the oropharynx, the most optimal tissue coverage is provided by:
A. Full-thickness skin graft
B. Trapezius myocutaneous flap
C. Pectoralis major myocutaneous flap
D. Sternomastoid flap

Q5. The sternocleidomastoid flap has a high rate of:
A. Infection
B. Restriction of neck flexion
C. Prolonged operative time
D. Ischemic complications

Q6. A 78-year-old man undergoes open repair of a secondary aortoduodenal fistula with excision of the previously placed aortic graft and in situ reconstruction. The optimal management for coverage of the in situ repair is:
A. Retroflexed rectus abdominis flap
B. Fascial and peritoneal flap from posterior aspect of the anterior abdominal wall
C. Repair should be done by retroperitoneal approach so that no coverage of the reconstruction is necessary
D. Pedicled omental flap

DOI: 10.1201/9781003389897-18

RATIONALE 1-6

1. RATIONALE

Extracavitary vascular graft infections carry a mortality of 17% and a major amputation rate of up to 70%. Patients at high risk for wound complications or conduit infection may benefit from prophylactic measures such as local tissue coverage, flaps, or vacuum-assisted closure. Such techniques help in preventing surgical site infection at the time of index operation. *Staphylococcus epidermidis* is now the most common pathogen causing surgical site infection following vascular reconstructions. Other pathogens include *Staphylococcus aureus, Pseudomonas*, and other Gram-negative bacteria. There are bimodal peaks in the incidence of vascular graft infection either occurring in the first 2 months and late graft infection at least 4 months from the time of index operation. Early infection involving the graft is more often due to contamination at the time of surgery or direct extension of superficial infection to the graft. Late infection is due to seeding of the graft from bacteremia, either from a new infection or reactivation of a subclinical infection. Grafts remain susceptible to infection for up to 1 year from implantation while the pseudointima is developing. When vascular grafts are infected, the infection is likely to spread to the native vessel, causing inflammation, subsequent aneurysmal dilatation, hemorrhage, or occlusion. In cases where there is involvement of anastomosis, lifelong antibiotics are recommended, whereas in cases without an involved suture line, 6 weeks of antibiotic therapy is adequate. If vascular anastomosis is involved, removal of the graft is mandatory, as myocutaneous flaps will not be adequate in managing graft infection with involvement of the anastomotic site.

Correct Answer   **C** 16%–18%

Reference
Gharamti, A., & Kanafani, Z. A. (2018). Vascular graft infections: an update. *Infect Dis Clin North Am,* *32*(4), 789–809. PMID:30241716

2. RATIONALE

The gracilis muscle receives its segmental blood supply from the medial circumflex femoral artery – a branch of the deep femoral artery – and its innervation from the obturator nerve. A retroflexed gracilis muscle flap is preferable in cases where either the sartorius muscle has been previously used or is no longer available or a small amount of tissue coverage is required. An immediate split-thickness skin graft and vacuum-assisted closure device application to the groin wound in cases where no native tissue exists for primary closure are options. As the most superficial muscle in the medial thigh, it can be identified by its characteristically rope-like distal portion. Its blood supply does not rely on the superficial femoral artery, which is often occluded or compromised in patients with lower extremity arterial occlusive disease. Skip incisions are used to decrease the morbidity of the harvest site. The facial sheath extending superficially and anterior and medial edges of the gracilis muscle belly are bluntly dissected free, carefully preserving the perforating vascular bundles anteriorly. The muscle is retroflexed with a simple silk suture to the free end of the gracilis muscle and its vascular supply is checked with a Doppler probe. The retroflexed muscle covers the exposed area of the graft or the native artery in the groin, and a split-thickness skin graft can be applied over the muscle with vacuum-assisted closure.

Correct Answer **B** When the sartorius muscle has been previously used as a muscle flap

Reference
Ali, A. T., Rueda, M., Desikan, S., et al. (2016). Outcomes after retroflexed gracilis muscle flap for vascular infections in the groin. *J Vasc Surg, 64*(2), 452–457. PMID: 27189769

3. RATIONALE

The medial head of the gastrocnemius is supplied by the muscular branch of the popliteal artery. The medial head of the gastrocnemius can cover an area of the medial side of the knee. Use of this flap results in minimal morbidity from a slight decrease in knee flexion, which improves subsequently. The gastrocnemius muscle flap has a generous arc of rotations and can cover wounds of the anterior knee and popliteal fossa. The medial head of the gastrocnemius is carefully separated from the soleus muscle, and the sural nerve should be gently protected while the medial head is being separated from the lateral head of the gastrocnemius following along the fascial raphe. The flap is released distally with or without a portion of the tendon depending on the area that needs to be covered. The gastrocnemius muscle flap is not recommended as a myocutaneous flap due to difficulty in closure of the donor site. Instead, a split-thickness skin graft over the flap is recommended, with the wound vac left in place over the sutured skin graft for 3–5 days.

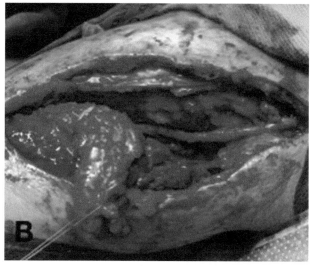

Suture through the distal end of the medial head of the gastrocnemius muscle.

Correct Answer **C** Medial head of the gastrocnemius muscle flap

Reference
Moebius, B., & Scheller, E. E. (2012). The pediculated gastrocnemius muscle flap as a treatment for soft tissue problems of the knee — indication, placement, and results. *GMS Interdiscip Plast Reconstr Surg DGPW, 1*, Doc07. PMID:26504691

4. RATIONALE

The pectoralis major muscle arises from the medial half of the clavicle and the anterior surface of the sternum. It has a generous blood supply with the myocutaneous flap based on the thoracoacromial artery, which is a branch of axillary artery. Additional blood supply arises medially from the internal mammary artery and laterally from the long thoracic artery. The initial skin incision is made from the lateral edge of the designed skin paddle toward the anterior axillary line and is above the nipple in men and below the breast in women. The incision is carried down to the pectoralis major muscle with identification of the medial and the inferior extents of the muscle. The muscle flap is elevated inferior to superior from the chest wall deep to the pectoralis major fascia, with care to elevate the vascular pedicle attached posteriorly to the muscle belly and can be done with blunt finger dissection. The flap is elevated superiorly carefully to control branches of the internal mammary artery and muscle perforators. The flap is tunneled over the clavicle into the neck. The donor site is closed primarily over a suction drain. An immediate split-thickness skin graft is recommended where a myofascial flap is used. The pectoralis major muscle flap does not lead to additional shoulder morbidity than that resulting from previous major head and neck surgery.

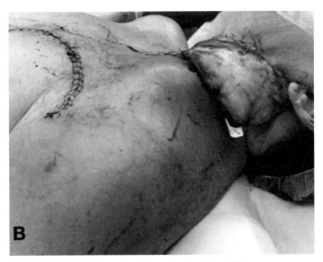

Immediate postoperative appearance of the left pectoralis major rotational flap.

Correct Answer **C** Pectoralis major myocutaneous flap

Reference
Fagan, J. (2023). Pectoralis major flap. In J. Fagan (Ed.), *Open access atlas of otolaryngology head and neck surgery*. Retrieved from http://www.entdev.uct.ac.za/guides/open-access-atlas-of-otolaryngology-head-neck-operative-surgery/

5. **RATIONALE**

The arterial supply of the sternocleidomastoid is based on three pedicles. The superior pedicle is the sternocleidomastoid branch of the occipital artery, the middle pedicle is usually a branch of the superior thyroid artery, and the inferior pedicle is from a branch of the suprascapular artery. Venous drainage reflects the arterial supply. Venous insufficiency is a major reason for flap failure. A complication rate of 10%–30% has been reported. Free flaps have a much greater success rate than sternocleidomastoid muscle flaps. Preserving both the occipital artery and superior thyroid artery branches may ensure that blood supply reaches the entirety of the muscle. The sternocleidomastoid flap remains an easy-to-use flap in a convenient location with a shorter operating time and should be considered as an alternative when a patient cannot tolerate a long operation and other muscle flap options are unavailable.

Correct Answer   D Ischemic complications

Reference
Jones, L. F., Farrar, E. M., Roberts, D., et al. (2019). Revisiting the sternocleidomastoid flap as a reconstructive option in head and neck surgery. *J Laryngol Otol*, *133*(9), 742–746. PMID: 31422777

6. RATIONALE

An omental pedicle flap is based on the right or left gastroomental artery, also known as the gastroepiploic artery, that forms an anastomosis along the greater curvature of the stomach. There is minimal morbidity from the procedure. In cases of intracavitary vascular reconstructions, the pedicle omental flap is a very reliable source of natural tissue coverage with the added benefit inherent to the omentum. For in situ reconstruction after excision of the mycotic aortic aneurysm or aortoiliac aneurysm, pedicle omental flaps are recommended to facilitate delivery of the immune system and phagocytosis of residual infectious particles and for the physical nature of a tissue bolster between the intraperitoneal organs and the new vascular conduit. In patients undergoing open repair of aortoenteric fistula, either with direct suture repair or excision and in situ reconstruction, pedicled omental flap coverage of the repair is recommended. A rectus abdominus and a peritoneal flap are not suitable choices. Retroperitoneal repair for aortoenteric fistula may not always be feasible.

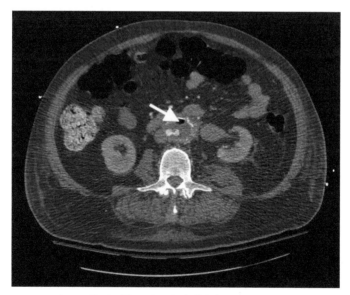

CTA showing gas in aneurysm sac in a patient with aortoenteric fistula.

Correct Answer   D Pedicled omental flap

Reference
Bartley, A., Scali, S. T., Patterson, S., et al. (2022). Improved perioperative mortality after secondary aortoenteric fistula repair and lessons learned from a 20-year experience. *J Vasc Surg*, *75*(1), 287–295.e283. PMID: 34303801

SECTION 19: VASCULAR CLOSURE DEVICE

MCQs 1–4

Q1. Vascular closure devices (VCDs) have shown improvement over manual compression in all of the following except:
- A. Patient's comfort and satisfaction
- B. Time to hemostasis
- C. Early ambulation
- D. Infections and thrombotic complications

Q2. Failure of a vascular closure device (VCD) as compared to successful deployment results in:
- A. Increased risk of MI
- B. Increased risk of true aneurysm at site of femoral access
- C. Increased mortality
- D. Increased risk of major vascular and minor vascular complications

Q3. The use of a vascular closure device (VCD) for antegrade femoral artery punctures is associated with:
- A. Increased risk of infection
- B. Increased risk of thrombotic complications
- C. Increased risk of operative treatment
- D. Lower odds of hematoma

Q4. Following atherectomy of the left superficial femoral artery using a right retrograde femoral access with a 45-cm-long 6 Fr right Pinnacle Sheath in place (Terumo Corporation Chicago, IL), the CELT closure device became dislodged in the right mid-superficial femoral artery in a 2-cm segment with 70% stenosis of the mid-superficial femoral artery, which was diagnosed 5 days after use of the closure device. The patient complains of right calf claudication. The next best step in the management is:
- A. Using left femoral access to snare the maldeployed CELT device
- B. Right femoral-popliteal bypass graft
- C. Use of antegrade access to snare the maldeployed CELT device
- D. Removal by direct incision near the mid-superficial femoral artery with superficial femoral endarterectomy and patch grafting

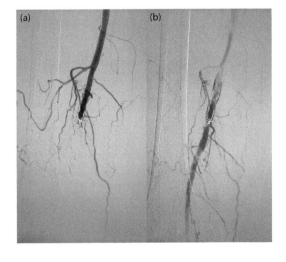

(a)　　　　(b)

RATIONALE 1–4

1. RATIONALE

From a literature review of 34 articles during the last 10 years for both diagnostic and therapeutic percutaneous interventions using femoral access, complication rates, safety, and efficacy were comparable between vascular closure devices (VCDs) and manual compression (MC): 12% for VCDs and 13% for manual compression. VCDs have a low incidence of major complications and a high success rate with faster turnover of patients. The risk of infectious complications was greater with VCDs (0.6% vs. 0.2%, $p = 0.002$%). The risk of thrombotic complications with VCD was 0.3% and none with MC. The interventionalist must be familiar with the device and its limitations to achieve hemostasis safely and effectively after femoral artery puncture. VCDs are only used in 30%–50% of catheter-based procedures performed worldwide to obtain hemostasis.

Correct Answer   D Infections and thrombotic complications

Reference
Noori, V. J., & Eldrup-Jørgensen, J. (2018). A systematic review of vascular closure devices for femoral artery puncture sites. *J Vasc Surg*, *68*(3), 887–899. PMID:30146036

2. RATIONALE

From a prospective registry of 9823 patients undergoing cardiac catheterization who received either a collagen plug (Angio-seal, Terumo, Inc., Somerset, NJ) or a suture (Perclose, Abbott Medical, Chicago, IL) in whom VCD failure was defined as unsuccessful deployment or failure to achieve homeostasis, a major vascular complication was defined as any retroperitoneal hemorrhage, limb ischemia, or any patient needing surgical repair. A minor vascular complication was defined as any groin bleeding, hematoma (equal to or greater than 5 cm), pseudoaneurysm, or AV fistula. "Any" vascular complication was defined as either a major or a minor vascular complication. Failure of VCD occurred in 268 (2.7%; 2.3% diagnostic vs. 3.0% PCI $p = 0.029$). Patients with VCD failures have a significantly increased risk of any complication (6.7% vs. 1.4%; $p < 0.0001$), major vascular complication (1.9% vs. 0.6% $p = 0.0006$), or minor complication (6% vs. 1.1%, $p < 0.0001$) compared with the group with no complication following successful deployment of the VCD. The increased risk of vascular complication was unchanged in a propensity score–matched cohort. Patients with VED failure should be closely monitored.[1]

From another study of 23,813 consecutive interventional coronary procedures in Massachusetts using a collagen-based plug in 18,533 or nitinol-based clip in 2,284 or suture-based in 2,996 between June 2005 and December 2007, VCD failed in 781 (3.3%) procedures. VCD failure was a significant predictor of subsequent vascular complications for both collagen-based plug VCD and nitinol-based clip VCD, but not for suture-based VCD.[2]

Correct Answer   D Increased risk of major vascular and minor vascular complications

References
1. Bangalore, S., Arora, N., & Resnic, F. S. (2009). Vascular closure device failure: frequency and implications: a propensity-matched analysis. *Circ Cardiovasc Interv*, *2*(6), 549–556. PMID:20031773
2. Vidi, V. D., Matheny, M. E., & Govindarajulu, U. S., et al. (2012). Vascular closure device failure in contemporary practice. *JACC Cardiovasc Interv*, *5*(8), 837–844. PMID: 22917455

3. RATIONALE

From a retrospective review of vascular quality initiative data, 11,562 patients undergoing antegrade femoral access were evaluated, with closure device used in 5869 and no closure device in 5693. Closure device cases were less likely to develop access site hematoma (2.55% vs. 3.53%, $p = 0.002$) or hematoma requiring intervention (0.63% vs. 1.62%, $p = 0.001$) and had no difference in access site stenosis or occlusion. It is to be noted that the use of a vascular closure device for antegrade access in the femoral arteries is not approved by the FDA.

Correct Answer   **D** Lower odds of hematoma

Reference
Ramirez, J. L., Zarkowsky, D. S., & Sorrentino, T. A. (2020). Antegrade common femoral artery closure device use is associated with decreased complications. *J Vasc Surg, 72*(5), 1610–1617.e1611. PMID:32165058

4. RATIONALE

Vascular closure devices can be classified into three main categories: (1) Vascular plug (Angioseal, Terumo, Chicago IL; Vasoseal Datascope Corp, Mahwah, NJ; Exoseal Cordis Corporation, Baer, Switzerland); (2) vascular clips (Star Close, Abbott Vascular, Chicago IL; Angiolink EVS, Angiolink Corporation, Tauton, MA; CELT ACD, Vesorum, Dublin, Ireland); and (3) suture closure (Perclose, Abbott Vascular, Chicago, IL). Immediate or early repuncture of the femoral artery is relatively contraindicated following application of a vascular closure device owing to the potential for local infection and the time required for collagen degradation at the puncture site. The CELT ACD device is deployed in three steps. The device is inserted into the lumen while the existing sheath and the distal wings are extended, then the device is then retracted to oppose the distal wings against the luminal wall, and the proximal wings are deployed to anchor the plug. The anchored stainless steel device is then released from the delivery handle. In this patient, because of associated superficial femoral artery occlusive disease, local removal with arteriotomy and endartectomy of the superficial femoral artery was the best option.

Correct Answer   **D** Removal by direct incision near the mid-superficial femoral artery with superficial femoral endarterectomy and patch grafting

Reference
Hart, B., & Hans, S. S. (2022). Maldeployment of Celt ACD vascular closure device. *J Vasc Surg Cases Innov Tech, 8*(1), 39–41. PMID: 35097246

SECTION 20: RARE VASCULAR ENTITIES

MCQs 1–25

Q1. Takayasu arteritis is a rare condition characterized by which of the following:
- **A.** Is a type of small vessel vasculitis
- **B.** Occurs predominantly in women
- **C.** Extracranial carotid artery aneurysms occur in 5%–15% of patients
- **D.** It affects the large joints

Q2. The most common artery involved in adventitial cystic disease is:
- **A.** External iliac artery
- **B.** Femoral artery
- **C.** Popliteal artery
- **D.** Brachial artery

Q3. A 69-year-old man was seen in the clinic with symptoms of intermittent claudication affecting the left calf on walking 50 yards for the past 3 months. Left dorsalis pulse and posterior tibial pulse are diminished as compared to the right. Ankle-brachial index on the right is 1.0 and on the left is 0.8. Left lower extremity arteriography shows:
- **A.** Entrapment syndrome affecting the popliteal artery
- **B.** Thrombosed pseudoaneurysm affecting the popliteal artery
- **C.** Adventitial cystic disease affecting the popliteal artery
- **D.** Focal atherosclerotic near occlusion of the popliteal artery

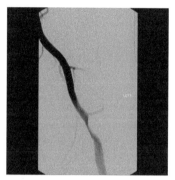

Q4. The optimal management of adventitial cystic disease of the popliteal artery is:
- **A.** Aspiration of the cyst
- **B.** Balloon angioplasty
- **C.** Complete excision of the cyst
- **D.** Covered stent followed by angioplasty

Q5. The incidence of bilateral popliteal artery entrapment syndrome is:
- **A.** Less than 10% of cases
- **B.** Less than 20% of cases
- **C.** 21%–40% of cases
- **D.** 22%–67% of cases

Q6. The diagnosis of popliteal artery entrapment syndrome is confirmed by:
- **A.** Absence of dorsalis pedis/posterior tibial pulse on active plantar flexion against resistance
- **B.** Duplex imaging on active plantar flexion
- **C.** CTA
- **D.** Catheter-based arteriography/MRA

DOI: 10.1201/9781003389897-20

Q7. The optimal management of popliteal artery entrapment syndrome resulting in thrombotic occlusion of the popliteal artery is:

A. Arterial repair with interposition graft

B. Supera stent

C. Myotomy of the medial head of the gastrocnemius or division of any abnormal musculotendinous band only

D. Arterial repair with interposition graft and myotomy of the medial head of the gastrocnemius band and abnormal musculotendinous bands

Q8. The functional entrapment syndrome is characterized by:

A. Abnormal popliteal artery anatomy

B. Resolution of symptoms with surgery in 50% of patients at 3-year follow-up

C. Resolution of symptoms with surgery in 65% of patients at 3-year follow-up

D. Resolution of symptoms with surgery in 78% at 3-year follow-up

Q9. The optimal management of functional popliteal artery entrapment syndrome consists of:

A. Percutaneous myotomy of the abnormal slip of the medial head of the gastrocnemius or any myofascial band

B. Medial approach for debulking the medial head of the gastrocnemius muscle

C. Fasciotomy of the posterior compartment muscles of the calf

D. Posterior approach for debulking the medial head of the gastrocnemius and removal of any fibrous band impinging on the popliteal artery

Q10. A 76-year-old man underwent resection of a thrombosed popliteal artery with adventitial cystic disease using a posterior approach. An interposition great saphenous vein graft

(non-reversed) was performed. The patient presented 8 months later with recurrent symptoms of intermittent claudication with thrombosis of the interposition graft. The next step in management consists of:

A. Open thrombectomy

B. Femoral-popliteal bypass using PTFE conduit

C. Pharmacologic thrombolysis using tPA with access from the contralateral femoral artery

D. Antegrade access of the left common femoral artery with thrombolysis using tPA

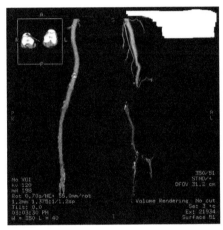

Occlusion after interposition vein graft (popliteal artery) for thrombosed popliteal artery due to adventitial cystic disease.

Q11. Following 24 hours of thrombolysis in the patient described in question 10, patency of the diffusely narrow vein graft is restored. The next best option is:

A. Open patch angioplasty

B. Self-expanding covered stent

C. Supera stent

D. Balloon angioplasty with drug eluting balloon

Q12. The vascular complications in Takayasu arteritis (TA) occur in:

A. 20% of patients

B. 28% of patients

C. 38% of patients

D. 48% of patients

Q13. The imaging study of choice for the diagnosis of Takayasu arteritis (TA) is:
A. Catheter-based arteriography
B. MRA
C. CTA
D. Aortic ultrasound with inflammatory markers assay

Q14. A 28-year-old woman was evaluated for symptoms of intermittent claudication involving both lower extremities in March 2022 with diminished bilateral femoral pulses. ABI on the right side was 0.67 and on the left was 0.76. Abdominal aortography showed long-segment stenosis of the infrarenal aorta. The most likely diagnosis is:
A. Marfan syndrome
B. Early onset of atherosclerotic occlusive disease of the infrarenal aorta
C. Mid-aortic syndrome caused by Takayasu arteritis (TA)
D. Extrinsic compression of the abdominal aorta from a retroperitoneal mass

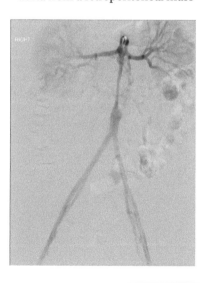

Q15. The 28-year-old woman described in question 14 is in remission and should be treated with:
A. Percutaneous angioplasty
B. Covered stent
C. Supraceliac aorta to distal abdominal aorta bypass using transperitoneal approach using PTFE graft

D. Supraceliac aorta to distal abdominal aorta bypass graft using left flank retroperitoneal approach through the eighth ICS

Q16. Out of the following arterial occlusive diseases, which one has the strongest association with tobacco exposure:
A. Arteriosclerotic disease
B. Buerger disease (thromboangiitis obliterans)
C. Takayasu's arteritis
D. Monckeberg medial sclerosis

Q17. The pattern of involvement of arteries in patients with thromboangiitis obliterans (TAO) is:
A. Origin of main trunks from aortic arch such as brachiocephalic, common carotid artery, and left subclavian artery
B. Abdominal aorta, iliacs, and femoral arteries
C. Occlusion of distal small arteries without involvement of veins of the lower extremities
D. Occlusion of distal small arteries and veins of lower and upper extremities

Q18. The characteristic findings on catheter-based contrast arteriography in patients with thromboangiitis obliterans are:
A. Occlusion of distal abdominal aorta and proximal common iliac arteries
B. Mid-superficial femoral artery occlusion 10–12 cm long
C. Occlusion of distal popliteal artery and tibial-peroneal trunk
D. Distal small- to medium-sized arteries involvement, segmental occlusions, and corkscrew-shaped collaterals

Q19. Patients with thromboangiitis obliterans undergoing bypass surgery have a primary patency rate at 5 years of:
A. 60%
B. 50%
C. 42%
D. 32%

Q20. The most prominent changes in the vasculature of patients with systemic sclerosis (Scleroderma) are:
A. Peripheral vascular disease
B. Pulmonary hypertension
C. Aortic dissection
D. Raynaud's phenomenon

Q21. Blisters and edema formation on the dorsum of the hand following cold exposure (frostbite) represents which degree of frostbite?
A. First degree
B. Second degree
C. Third degree
D. Fourth degree

Q22. Vascular complications occur in what percentage of patients with Behcet's disease:
A. 1%–6%
B. 7%–29%
C. 15%–35%
D. 20%–39%

Q23. A 34-year-old woman with a history of rheumatoid arthritis, inflammatory bowel disease, and lupus erythematosus presented with bruising of the volar aspect of her third finger with associated pain and swelling. She has no history of trauma. She had experienced three episodes of a similar nature in the past with complete resolution within 72 hours of onset. She has no history of tobacco abuse. Doppler digital waveform was dampened in the third finger. The most likely diagnosis is:
A. Raynaud's disease
B. Dermatitis artefacta
C. Achenbach syndrome (paroxysmal finger hematoma)
D. Embolic digital artery occlusion from arterial thoracic outlet syndrome

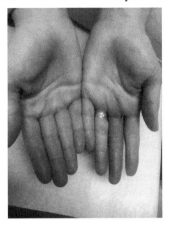

Q24. Fibromuscular dysplasia most often presents as:
A. Medial hyperplasia
B. Medial fibroplasia
C. Intimal fibroplasia
D. Perimedial fibroplasia

Q25. All of the following statements about fibromuscular dysplasia (FMD) are true except:
A. Result of atherosclerosis
B. Result of non-inflammatory cause
C. Primarily affects midsize vessels
D. Most often asymptomatic

RATIONALE 1–25

1. RATIONALE

Takayasu arteritis (TA) is a rare chronic granulomatous large vessel vasculitis occurring predominately in women in the second or third decades of life. Patients often present with clinical findings of absent or diminished pulses, loss of blood pressure, or bruits. Takayasu arteritis can result in carotid artery stenosis, occlusion, and aneurysmal degeneration. Common carotid artery dissection has also been reported in patients with Takayasu arteritis. Carotid artery involvement has been reported in 45%–84% of patients with Takayasu disease. Patients may have elevated C-reactive protein and sedimentation rates. Patients with active Takayasu disease should receive a course of steroid therapy, and surgical intervention should be limited for aneurysmal and occlusive disease when the disease is in the inactive stage (remission). Patients with carotid artery aneurysm in Takayasu arteritis have a risk of rupture even in the non-inflammatory stage. An autologous conduit should be used in repairing the aneurysmal segment.

Correct Answer **B** Occurs predominantly in women

Reference
Tabata, M., Kitagawa, T., Saito, T., et al. (2001). Extracranial carotid aneurysm in Takayasu's arteritis. *J Vasc Surg, 34*(4), 739–742. PMID: 11668332

2. RATIONALE

Adventitial cystic disease was first described in 1947 by Atkins and Key involving the external iliac artery; however, more than 85% of reported cases involve the popliteal artery—over 300 cases have been reported. Other arteries less commonly involved are the external iliac, femoral, brachial, axillary, and renal arteries. It is well established that this pathology occurs in arteries coursing adjacent to a joint space. There is no unifying consensus on the etiology of this disease process. Many hypotheses, including repetitive trauma theory, systemic disorder theory, and developmental theory, have been advocated. Adventitial cysts are filled with gelatinous mucoid material between the arterial adventitia and the medial layers. Popliteal artery adventitial cystic disease typically presents in males (5:1) in the third decade with sudden onset of symptoms of intermittent claudication when walking a short distance.

Correct Answer **C** Popliteal artery

Reference
Allemang, M. T., & Kashyap, V. S. (2015). Adventitial cystic disease of the popliteal artery. *J Vasc Surg, 62*(2), 490. PMID: 26211381

3. RATIONALE

The pathognomonic sign of adventitial cystic disease of the popliteal artery is scimitar sign (eccentric narrowing) or hourglass sign (concentric narrowing). Following duplex imaging, which can be diagnostic in uncomplicated adventitial cystic disease, catheter-based arteriography should be obtained. MRA or CTA is an alternative noninvasive imaging modality which can confirm the diagnosis of adventitial cystic disease. One-third of cases of adventitial cystic disease of the popliteal artery may have complete proximal popliteal artery occlusion.

The appearance of the lesion on arteriography is not consistent with the diagnosis of entrapment syndrome, atherosclerotic stenosis, or thrombosed pseudoaneurysm.

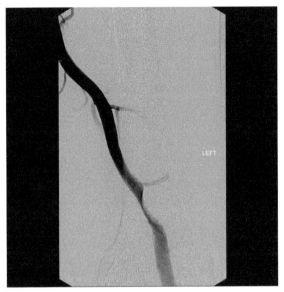

Arteriography showing scimitar sign diagnostic of adventitial cycstic disease.

Correct Answer   **C** Adventitial cystic disease affecting the popliteal artery

Reference
Lezotte, J., Le, Q. P., Shanley, C., & Hans, S. (2018). Adventitial cystic disease: complicated and uncomplicated. *Ann Vasc Surg, 46*, 370.e313–370.e315. PMID: 28911964

4. RATIONALE
Management of a popliteal adventitial cyst requires operative excision of the cyst with or without autologous graft placement. For most uncomplicated cysts, complete excision of the cyst containing multilocular gelatinous fluid is curative. The tense gelatinous fluid causes compression with narrowing of the lumen of the artery. After excision of the cyst, there is normalization of the arterial flow velocities throughout the popliteal artery with no evidence of obstruction on intraoperative duplex imaging. Patients presenting with complete occlusion of the popliteal artery require autologous vein bypass grafting following excision of the cysts containing a segment of the artery, which usually has a superimposed thrombus. The approach to the access to the popliteal artery for excision of the cyst depends on its location, with a medial approach for proximal popliteal artery adventitial cystic disease and a posterior approach for adventitial cystic disease behind the knee. A multi-institutional experience of adventitial cystic disease with operative intervention in 41 patients reported a reintervention rate of 18% over a mean follow-up of 20 months, with complete resection and interposition bypass most predictive of freedom from intervention.

Correct Answer   **C** Complete excision of the cyst

Reference
Motaganahalli, R. L., Smeds, M. R., Harlander-Locke, M. P., et al. (2017). A multi-institutional experience in adventitial cystic disease. *J Vasc Surg, 65*(1), 157–161. PMID: 27751735

5. RATIONALE

Popliteal artery entrapment syndrome affects young men (male-to-female ratio of 9:1) without atherosclerotic risk factors and is responsible for symptoms of intermittent claudication in 60% of young adults. Unilateral popliteal artery syndrome should prompt investigation of the contralateral limb, as the syndrome is bilateral in 22%–67% of patients. Popliteal artery entrapment syndrome is an embryologically developmental anomaly and results from aberrant relationship of the popliteal artery with the surrounding popliteal fossa myofascial structures. The patient complains of intermittent pain in the calves and feet after exercise, and the pain is relieved at rest. Recurrent popliteal artery compression by the adjacent myofascial band causes intimal damage, thrombosis, distal embolization, and post-stenotic dilation and may occasionally lead to development of an aneurysm. Unlike atherosclerosis, entrapment features neovascularization, inflammatory cell infiltrate vessel wall disruption, stimulating fibrosis, and collagenization.

Correct Answer   **D** 22%–67% of cases

Reference
Noorani, A., Walsh, S. R., Cooper, D. G., et al. (2009). Entrapment syndromes. *Eur J Vasc Endovasc Surg*, *37*(2), 213–220. PMID: 19046647

6. RATIONALE

Popliteal artery occlusion on stress maneuvers is reported on the order of 59%–85% of asymptomatic individuals, indicating a significant false-positive rate with duplex imaging on plantar flexion for diagnosis of popliteal artery entrapment syndrome. Arteriography with MRA-MRI is the best investigation for diagnosis of popliteal artery entrapment syndrome. MRI/MRA delineates the abnormal myofascial bands, and arteriography shows popliteal artery compression during plantar flexion. These findings strongly indicate the diagnosis of popliteal artery entrapment syndrome. In addition, one may see medial deviation of the popliteal artery, which is present in 24% of cases, indicative of type I popliteal artery entrapment syndrome with a normal medial head of the gastrocnemius; type II has a normal popliteal artery with a laterally displaced medial head of the gastrocnemius. Type III compression of the popliteal artery includes an additional slip of gastrocnemius. Type IV compression of popliteal artery includes the popliteus. Type V compression features the popliteal vein. Type VI is functional entrapment syndrome with no aberrant anatomy.

Correct Answer   **D** Catheter-based arteriography/MRA

Reference
Noorani, A., Walsh, S. R., & Cooper, D. G. (2009). Entrapment syndromes. *Eur J Vasc Endovasc Surg*, *37*(2), 213–220. PMID: 19046647

7. RATIONALE

Definitive management requires surgery to release the extrinsic compression and restore arterial flow. If arterial damage is minimal, myotomy of the medial head of the gastrocnemius or any other abnormal musculotendinous slips may be all that is required. In the most severe cases, arterial repair is required preferentially with an interposition graft. The complication rate with a thrombosed artery requiring patch grafting is much higher than with interposition grafting (45.5% versus 16.7% $p < 0.01$). Patency rates of 57%–65% at 10 years have been reported. The posterior approach is preferable for short occlusions in the popliteal artery behind the knee. Longer occlusions are preferably approached through a medial incision.

Correct Answer   **D**   Arterial repair with interposition graft and myotomy of the medial head of the gastrocnemius band and abnormal musculotendinous bands

Reference
Noorani, A., Walsh, S. R., & Cooper, D. G. (2009). Entrapment syndromes. *Eur J Vasc Endovasc Surg,* *37*(2), 213–220. PMID:19046647

8. RATIONALE

Functional popliteal artery entrapment syndrome (FPEAS) is a distinct entity where there is no obvious anatomical pathology and is most likely the result of compression from surrounding muscle with a repeated injury often seen in athletes. Following exercise stress testing with stress positional plethysmography and ankle-brachial index, a multiphasic CTA of the lower extremity is obtained on a 64-row CT scanner. In the relaxed state, the patient is placed in a supine position with their back supported by a 30-degree wedge pillow. Compression of the popliteal artery against the lateral femoral condyle in the stressed state is obtained by a sheet or a wrist strap that is wrapped around the metatarsophalangeal region of the patient's feet and the patient is instructed to use their arms to pull the sheet/wrist strap to simulate body weight while they plantar-flex their feet. A pulse oximeter is placed on the patient's toes. The diminished waveforms are used as an additional method to ensure adequate plantar flexion. The third stressed CTA is also performed with a slice thickness of 0.625 mm. The degree of popliteal artery narrowing with and without plantar flexion is described as well as any popliteal vein compression. Identification of any abnormal portion of the gastrocnemius muscle, compressive fibrous band, and accessory muscle slip of the medial head of the gastrocnemius is noted.

Correct Answer   **D**   Resolution of symptoms with surgery in 78% at 3-year follow-up

Reference
Lavingia, K. S., Dua, A., & Rothenberg, K. A., et al. (2019). Surgical management of functional popliteal entrapment syndrome in athletes. *J Vasc Surg, 70*(5), 1555–1562. PMID: 31327599

9. RATIONALE

Using a lazy-S popliteal incision and with deeper dissection, the popliteal artery is exposed with the leg and foot in a provocative position, confirming where the compression from the medial head of the gastrocnemius is pushing the popliteal artery against the lateral femoral condyle. A Liga-suture device is used to debulk the muscles immediately adjacent to the affected artery and is completed until there is no longer compression of the artery on passive flexion or extension of the leg and the foot. A Seprafilm Adhesion Barrier (Sanofi Aventis, Bridgewater Township, NJ) is wrapped around the artery to prevent scarring, and the leg is placed in the knee immobilizer with physical therapy after 1 week of operation to resume walking followed by active exercises in 4–6 weeks. Of 38 athletes (56 limbs), 78% returned to their sports activity. Fasciotomy has also been used successfully in treatment of functional popliteal artery entrapment syndrome.

Correct Answer   **D**   Posterior approach for debulking the medial head of the gastrocnemius and removal of any fibrous band impinging on the popliteal artery

Reference
Lavingia, K. S., Dua, A., & Rothenberg, K. A., et al. (2019). Surgical management of functional popliteal entrapment syndrome in athletes. *J Vasc Surg, 70*(5), 1555–1562. PMID: 31327599

10. RATIONALE

In patients with recent thrombosis of the bypass graft (4 weeks following index operation), thrombolysis using a contralateral femoral artery approach is preferable. From a study of 123 patients undergoing thrombolysis for acute graft occlusion in patients with 67% synthetic grafts and 23% vein grafts presenting with acute critical limb ischemia, a technical failure was reported in 28 patients. Synthetic grafts had a somewhat increased likelihood of technically successful thrombolysis as compared to vein grafts, but on the other hand, thrombolysis of synthetic grafts had a higher risk of amputation during late follow-up. Technical failure and advanced age were factors associated with major amputation. Presence of ischemic heart disease, older grafts, and synthetic grafts were associated with successful thrombolysis. In this patient with a short interposition graft in the popliteal artery, thrombolysis as an alternative to a new PTFE graft is a better option. Open thrombectomy can be considered but will require a repeat operation in the knee area, which could be technically challenging. In general, thrombolysis with a contralateral femoral approach is preferable than an antegrade approach.

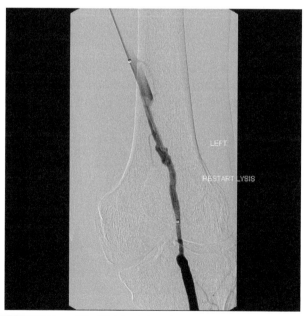

Diffuse stenosis of the interposition vein graft (popliteal artery) following thrombolysis treated with covered stent for management of adventitial cystic disease. (Viabhn W.L. Gore, Inc., Newark, DE.)

Correct Answer **C** Pharmacologic thrombolysis using tPA with access from the contralateral femoral artery

Reference
Koraen, L., Kuoppala, M., Acosta, S., et al. (2011). Thrombolysis for lower extremity bypass graft occlusion. *J Vasc Surg, 54*(5), 1339–1344. PMID: 21723070

11. RATIONALE

Covered stents (self-expanding) for exclusion of popliteal artery aneurysms are a safe and effective alternative to open surgical repair in high-risk patients. The Supera stent, because of its interwoven nitinol design, is useful in treating popliteal artery occlusive lesions. For vein graft stenosis behind the knee, a covered stent (Viabahn WL Gore) 6 mm in diameter was deployed following preangioplasty then followed by postangioplasty, and this was deemed preferable to repeat open repair. In this patient, a covered stent has remained patent for the past 10 years without requiring any secondary operation.

Correct Answer   **B** Self-expanding covered stent

Reference

Hans, S. S. (2020). Management of a patient with complicated adventitial cystic disease of the popliteal artery in challenging arterial reconstructions. In S. S. Hans (Ed.), *Challenging arterial reconstructions: 100 clinical cases* (pp. 259–262). Cham, Switzerland: Springer Nature Switzerland AG.

12. RATIONALE

From the French Takayasu Network, a retrospective multicenter study of characteristics and outcomes of 318 patients with Takayasu arteritis (TA) fulfilling American College of Rheumatology and Ishikawa criteria were analyzed. The median age at the time of diagnosis was 36 (25–47 years) and 276 (86.8%) were women. After a median follow-up of 6.1 years, relapses were observed in 43%, vascular complications in 38%, and death in 5%. A progressive clinical course was observed in 45%, carotidynia in 10%, and retinopathy in 4%. The 5-and-10-year event-free survival, relapse-free survival, and complication-free survival were 48.2% and 36.4%, 58.6% and 47.7%, and 69.9% and 53.7%, respectively. Progressive disease course ($p = 0.018$) and carotidynia ($p = 0.036$) were independently associated with event-free survival. Male sex ($p = 0.048$) and elevated C-reactive protein ($p = 0.013$) and carotidynia ($p = 0.003$) were associated with relapse-free survival. Progressive disease course ($p = 0.017$), thoracic aortic involvement ($p = 0.009$), and retinopathy ($p = 0.002$) were associated with complication-free survival. This nationwide study showed that 50% of patients with TA will relapse and will experience a vascular complication ≤10 years from diagnosis.

Correct Answer   **C** 38% of patients

Reference

Comarmond, C., Biard, L., Lambert, M., et al. (2017). Long-term outcomes and prognostic factors of complications in Takayasu arteritis: a multicenter study of 318 patients. *Circulation, 136*(12), 1114–1122. PMID: 28701469

13. RATIONALE

The basic pathologic features of TA are mural changes in the great vessels. Mural changes are often not satisfactorily evaluated by conventional angiography. Diagnosis during the early stage is often missed or delayed because of a non-specific clinical presentation and no luminal changes in the aorta or its branches but detectible by conventional arteriography, which often underestimates the extent of true disease extent even in a pulseless disease state. Among 85 patients undergoing carotid bifurcation to iliac bifurcation CTA, 81 (95%) had aortic involvement without or with aortic arch involvement; the left common carotid artery and left subclavian artery were most commonly involved: 77% and 76%, respectively.

The extent of disease assessed by mural changes was more extensive than that assessed by luminal changes in 52 (61%) patients. Arterial involvement was contiguous in 69 (81%) patients, and skipped lesions were identified in 16 (19%) patients. An analysis of mural findings revealed the coexistence of active and inactive lesions in 11% of patients. CT scans should be performed from the carotid bifurcation to the iliac bifurcation in order to adequately evaluate, diagnose, and manage TA.

Correct Answer   C CTA

Reference
Chung, J. W., Kim, H. C., Choi, Y. H., et al. (2007). Patterns of aortic involvement in Takayasu arteritis and its clinical implications: evaluation with spiral computed tomography angiography. *J Vasc Surg, 45*(5), 906–914. PMID: 17466787

14. RATIONALE

The patient's young age with angiographic findings are highly suggestive of mid-aortic syndrome cause by Takayasu arteritis. She should undergo CTA from carotid bifurcation to common femoral arteries. The patient should have genetic testing as well as blood tests for inflammatory markers such as C-reactive protein and sedimentation rate. The angiography is not consistent with the diagnosis of premature atherosclerotic disease, which can affect younger women from 30 to 40 years of age with a history of significant nicotine abuse, hypertension, and premature ovarian failure (menopause). The disease affects the distal aorta and proximal common iliac arteries, which are small in caliber. Inferior vena cava compression from a large retroperitoneal tumor may occur, but arterial occlusion from a retroperitoneal mass is extremely unlikely. Marfan syndrome usually causes ascending aortic aneurysm and may also cause an aneurysm in the aortic arch, descending thoracic, and abdominal aorta but is not a common cause of infrarenal aortic stenosis.

Correct Answer   C Mid-aortic syndrome caused by Takayasu arteritis (TA)

Reference
Delis, K. T., & Gloviczki, P. (2005). Middle aortic syndrome: from presentation to contemporary open surgical and endovascular treatment. *Perspect Vasc Surg Endovasc Ther, 17*(3), 187–203. PMID: 16273154

15. RATIONALE

The aim of treatment is to improve symptoms of intermittent claudication, reverse hypertension, and improve perfusion to the renal parenchyma and bowel. Medical control of hypertension and use of corticosteroids and immunosuppressive drugs is essential in the acute phase of the disease prior to surgical intervention. Balloon angioplasty of an aorta or covered stent is not indicated for mid-aortic syndrome. Patch angioplasty of the aorta can be considered in a shorter segment of involvement in mid-aortic syndrome. In most patients, aorto-aortic bypass, preferably using a left retroperitoneal approach through the eighth intercostal space, provides excellent exposure. Proximal anastomosis is performed to the supraceliac aorta and distal anastomosis to the distal aorta above its bifurcation. PTFE grafts are preferable to Dacron grafts, as the latter undergo aneurysmal dilatation over a period of years. Aortic bypass for mid-aortic syndrome is safe with an excellent long-term patency. The patient did not require renal artery reconstruction because of normal renal arteries.

Correct Answer **D** Supraceliac aorta to distal abdominal aorta bypass graft using left flank retroperitoneal approach through the eighth ICS

Reference
Delis, K. T., & Gloviczki, P. (2005). Middle aortic syndrome: from presentation to contemporary open surgical and endovascular treatment. *Perspect Vasc Surg Endovasc Ther, 17*(3), 187–203. PMID: 16273154

16. RATIONALE

Buerger disease or segmental thromboangiitis obliterans (TAO) is a non-atherosclerotic inflammatory arteritis that involves small- to medium-size arteries and veins of the extremities. Exposure to tobacco is central to the initiation, maintenance, and progression of TAO. The annual incidence of TAO is reported to be 12.6% per 100,000 in the United States and is much greater in the Middle East and Far East countries. Among in-hospital-treated patients with peripheral artery occlusive disease, the prevalence rate is 45%–63% in India and 16%–66% in Korea. The disease typically affects patients <45 years of age and is much more common in men. TAO is a vasculitis characterized by a highly cellular thrombus with relative splitting of the vessel wall. Patients with TAO have increased cellular immunity to types I and III collagen compared with those who have arteriosclerosis. The prothrombin gene mutation 20210 and the presence of anticardiolipin antibodies are associated with increased risk of disease. Hematocrit, red blood cell rigidity, and blood viscosity are increased in patients with TAO as compared to those with atherosclerosis. Nearly two-thirds of patients with TAO have severe periodontal disease and chronic anerobic periodontal infection. Polymerase chain reaction analysis demonstrated DNA fragments from anerobic bacteria in both arterial lesions and oral cavities of patients with TAO. TAO involves three phases: Acute, subacute, and chronic. In the acute phase, there is a highly cellular occlusive inflammatory thrombus with polymorphonuclear neutrophils (PMNs), microabscesses, and multinucleated giant cells. The chronic phase is characterized by organized thrombus and vascular fibrosis that may mimic atherosclerotic disease. However, in TAO there is preservation of the internal elastic lamina.

Correct Answer **B** Buerger disease (thromboangiitis obliterans)

Reference
Piazza, G., & Creager, M. A. (2010). Thromboangiitis obliterans. *Circulation, 121*(16), 1858–1861. PMID: 20421527

17. RATIONALE

Patients with TAO have involvement of distal small arteries and veins in both upper and lower extremities. Although symptoms may begin in the peripheral portion of a single limb, the disease frequently progresses proximally and involves multiple extremities. The initial presentation is that of symptoms of intermittent claudication of feet, legs, and hands. As the disease advances, rest pain, ulceration, and digital gangrene occur. Raynaud phenomenon is present in approximately 40% of patients with TAO and may be asymmetrical. Although most common in the extremities, the disease may involve the cerebral, coronary, renal, mesenteric, and pulmonary arteries. Superficial thrombophlebitis differentiates TAO from other vasculitides and atherosclerosis, although it may be observed in Behcet disease. Patients may describe a migratory pattern of tender nodules that follow the course of superficial veins. Neurological examination may document peripheral nerve involvement with sensory findings in up to 70% of patients.

Correct Answer   **D** Occlusion of distal small arteries and veins of lower and upper extremities

Reference

Piazza, G., & Creager, M. A. (2010). Thromboangiitis obliterans. *Circulation*, *121*(16), 1858–1861. PMID: 20421527

18. RATIONALE

TAO is a clinical diagnosis made by pertinent history and physical findings and diagnostic vascular abnormalities on imaging studies. Clinical criteria include age <45 years, current or recent history of tobacco use, exclusion of thrombophilia, autoimmune disease, diabetes mellitus, and a proximal source of emboli. Lab testing in patients suspected of TAO is used to exclude alternative diagnoses. Serological markers of autoimmune disease are negative in TAO. Catheter based arteriography provides the spatial resolution necessary to detect small artery pathology. Distal small-to-medium artery involvement, segmental occlusions, and "corkscrew-shaped collaterals" around the area of occlusions are diagnostic of TAO without involvement of the proximal limb arteries. Biopsy is rarely indicated and may result in non-healing of the incision.

Correct Answer   **D** Distal small- to medium-sized arteries involvement, segmental occlusions, and corkscrew-shaped collaterals

Reference

Piazza, G., & Creager, M. A. (2010). Thromboangiitis obliterans. *Circulation*, *121*(16), 1858–1861. PMID: 20421527

19. RATIONALE

The prognosis of patients depends largely on the ability to discontinue tobacco use. From the French Buerger Network, the study revealed that 34% of patients with thromboangiitis obliterans will experience an amputation within 15 years from the diagnosis. Surgical reconstruction is usually not feasible in patients with thromboangiitis obliterans because of the distant and diffuse nature of the disease. Arterial bypass may be considered in a few select patients with severe ischemia and suitable distal target vessels. Results of bypass surgery have suboptimal outcomes, with primary patency rates of 41%, 32%, and 30% and secondary patency rates of 54%, 47%, and 39% at 1, 5, and 10 years, respectively, and the patency rates are 50% lower in patients who continue to smoke after arterial bypass. Prostanoid vasodilator iloprost aids in the relief of ischemic rest pain, greater healing of ischemic ulcers, and a two-thirds reduction in the need for amputation. There is a limited role for intermittent pneumatic compression, spinal cord stimulation, and periarterial sympathectomy. Therapeutic angiogenesis has been attempted, but the results require further investigation and confirmation. From a nationwide multicenter study of 224 patients with TAO with a mean follow-up of 5.7 years, vascular events were noted in 58.9%, amputation in 21.4%, and death in 1.4%. A factor associated with amputation was limb infection. Patients who stopped their tobacco consumption had a lower risk of amputation.

Correct Answer   **D** 32%

Reference

Le Joncour, A., Soudet, S., Dupont, A., et al. (2018). Long-term outcome and prognostic factors of complications in thromboangiitis obliterans (Buerger's disease): a multicenter study of 224 patients. *J Am Heart Assoc*, *7*(23), e010677. PMID: 30571594

20. RATIONALE

One of the most important manifestations of patients with systemic sclerosis may present with symptoms of Raynaud phenomenon: A widespread form of vasospasm that is prodromal or concurrent with other changes in systemic sclerosis. Systemic sclerosis is characterized by three distinct pathological processes: Fibrosis, cellular/humoral, autoimmunity, and specific vascular changes. Although a mild vasculitis may sometimes be present, the vascular pathology of systemic sclerosis is best characterized as a vasculopathy. The injured cell type responsible for this vasculopathy is endothelium. The major evidence of this is serological. Systemic sclerosis is characterized by increased serum levels of von Willebrand factor, endothelium, and increased numbers of circulating viable and dead endothelial cells. A common feature of systemic sclerosis is capillary malformation; intimal hyperplasia and capillary rarefaction are responsible for Raynaud phenomenon. There is an inappropriate and exaggerated contraction of the small vessels in the fingers and toes in response to cold or emotional distress that is present in 80%–90% of cases of systemic sclerosis. Raynaud's phenomenon can be the presenting symptom in approximately 33% of patients. The frequency and severity of Raynaud's phenomenon in patients with systemic sclerosis are often worse than that observed in patients with primary Raynaud's phenomenon. The incidence of ulcerations and gangrene is increased, leading to amputation in some patients.

Correct Answer　**D** Raynaud's phenomenon

Reference
Fleming, J. N., & Schwartz, S. M. (2008). The pathology of scleroderma vascular disease. *Rheum Dis Clin North Am*, *34*(1), 41–55; vi. PMID: 18329531

21. RATIONALE

Frostbite classification is based on the severity and extent of tissue damage after thawing, with first-degree frostbite involving white patches of skin with edema and hyperemia, second-degree involving blisters, third-degree involving full skin necrosis with subcutaneous extension, and fourth-degree involving damage to muscle and bone and gangrene. Palpation can assist in differentiating superficial from deep frostbite. The affected area is stony hard or petrified when deeper layers are affected. The best treatment for frostbitten fingers/hands is rewarming in a warm (98–102°F) water bath. This is done until the affected part has become red and soft, and it takes about 15–30 minutes. During rewarming, there is actually more cellular injury. This is due to intimal damage in the small blood vessels. These changes are called reperfusion injury. Pain during rewarming may require narcotics. Aspirin, clopidogrel, and calcium blockers may be helpful. Additional treatment includes whirlpool baths, elevation of the effected part, and antiinflammatory medications. After frostbite, the fingers may become stiff, and physiotherapy may be necessary. Prevention is the best treatment. Many patients suffer from long-term sequelae such as vasomotor disturbances, neuropathic nociceptive pain, and damage to skeletal structures.

Correct Answer　**B** Second degree

Reference
(2020). Frostbite in hands. Retrieved from https://www.assh.org/handcare/condition/frostbite-in-hands.

22. RATIONALE

Behcet's disease is a chronic relapsing immunological syndrome. It occurs in the third or fourth decade of life and is prevalent in Mediterranean countries, the Middle East, and East Asia.

The disease is characterized by a classic triad of urogenital ulcerations, uveitis, retinal vasculitis, and erythema nodosum. The prognosis is determined by involvement of the cardiovascular, gastrointestinal, and central nervous system. Vascular complications occur in 7%–29% of patients and have a major effect on mortality. Vascular lesions are most common in the venous system; however, the arterial lesions are at greater risk. Involvement of a major artery is seen in 1.5%–2.2% of patients, often in the form of a rapidly expanding aneurysm. Pseudoaneurysm formation at the anastomosis or at the site of angiographic puncture is also possible. Histological examination of arterial lesions reveals leukocytoclastic arteritis, possibly responsible for ulceration and perforation of the arterial wall, and could explain the increased incidence of rupture despite their small size compared with atherosclerotic aneurysm. The suture line is reinforced with Teflon pledgets, and the intrabdominal prosthetic graft is wrapped with omentum. Recurrent deep vein thrombosis and superficial thrombophlebitis are common manifestations.

Correct Answer **B** 7%–29%

Reference
Iscan, Z. H., Vural, K. M., & Bayazit, M. (2005). Compelling nature of arterial manifestations in Behcet disease. *J Vasc Surg, 41*(1), 53–58. PMID: 15696044

23. RATIONALE

Paroxysmal finger hematoma (Achenbach syndrome) usually presents as recurring episodes of an unexplained sudden onset of painful swelling associated with deep ecchymosis of the volar aspect of the finger. The exact etiology remains unclear but is thought to be a vasomotor disorder. Owing to the self-limiting nature of this disease, invasive studies are not necessary and would be negative if performed. The condition is self-limiting, and skin discoloration resolves within an average of 4 days. The differential diagnosis is embolic digital artery occlusion from thoracic outlet syndrome and dermatitis artefacta, which presents as a superficial erosion in the hands of patients with chronic dermatitis. The diagnostic workup of a patient with purplish discoloration of a finger, with or without a diminished radial pulse, should include a Doppler arterial study and duplex ultrasound scan of the left subclavian artery to exclude a subclavian artery aneurysm in association with thoracic outlet syndrome. Raynaud's disease typically presents as episodes of a patient's fingers (unusually all) turning pale, followed by purplish discoloration. It is accompanied by paresthesias and cold sensation in both hands. The fingers will then turn warm and red as the vasospasm subsides. In contrast to Raynaud's phenomenon, systemic sclerosis in most instances is unilateral.

Correct Answer **C** Achenbach syndrome (paroxysmal finger hematoma)

Reference
Lehman, H., Acho, R., & Hans, S. S. (2021). Achenbach syndrome as a rare cause of painful, blue finger. *J Vasc Surg Cases Innov Tech, 7*(3), 589–592. PMID: 34541431

24. RATIONALE

Fibromuscular dysplasia is classified according to the affected segment of the arterial wall. The same classification is used for all the arteries affected by fibromuscular dysplasia. Medial fibroplasia is the most common (80%–90%) with a "string-of-beads" appearance secondary to alternating thinned and thickened medial ridges. This appearance on arteriography is secondary to stenotic webs that cause sequential stenosis and dilatations in the arterial wall.

These dilatations may lead to aneurysmal degeneration. Intimal fibroplasia is responsible for about 10% of cases of fibromuscular dysplasia, resulting in a long concentric stenotic lesion secondary to intimal collagen deposits. The differential diagnosis is atherosclerosis, vasculitis, and connective tissue disorder.

Correct Answer **B** Medial fibroplasia

Reference
Poloskey, S. L., Olin, J. W., & Mace, P. (2012). Fibromuscular dysplasia. *Circulation, 125*(18), e636–e639.
　PMID: 22566353

25. **RATIONALE**
Most patients with cerebrovascular FMD are asymptomatic middle-aged women who are otherwise healthy. The cause of FMD is unknown. Approximately 10% of patients with FMD have an affected family member as well. Patients may present with headaches or dizziness, and a carotid bruit may be detectable on physical examination. The incidence of ischemic cerebral events is quite low at long-term follow-up. Occasionally cerebral ischemia is secondary to a thromboemboli originating from a diseased arterial segment or from a low-flow state. Patients may present with arterial dissection. There is a higher incidence of intracranial aneurysms in patients with internal carotid artery or vertebral artery fibromuscular dysplasia. Duplex ultrasound is a standard first-line modality in diagnosing fibromuscular dysplasia. However, Doppler velocity diagnostic criteria applicable to atherosclerotic disease are not reliable in diagnoses of fibromuscular dysplasia. CTA and MRA of the neck are useful techniques in diagnosing fibromuscular dysplasia. CTA is preferable, but MRA may be helpful in diagnosing concurrent arterial dissection through simultaneously acquired T1-fat saturation images with time-of-flight or gadolinium-enhanced imaging. Low-dose aspirin is indicated. Duplex surveillance to rule out aneurysmal degeneration should be obtained on a yearly basis. In selected cases balloon angioplasty is indicated in patients who fail medical management and the lesion is progressive.

Correct Answer **A** Result of atherosclerosis

Reference
Kadian-Dodov, D., Gornik, H. L., Gu, X., et al. (2016). Dissection and aneurysm in patients with fibromuscular dysplasia: findings from the U.S. registry for FMD. *J Am Coll Cardiol, 68*(2), 176–185.
　PMID: 27386771

MCQs 1–11

Q1. Which of the following would be most likely to produce a selection bias in a sample:
- **A.** Only receiving a response from 60% of the people in the sample
- **B.** Biased wording in the questionnaire
- **C.** Interviews conducted on the phone in place of in-person interview
- **D.** Recruiting participants directly from clinics, who miss all the care who do not attend the clinic, or who seek care during the study

Q2. Which one of these statistic measures is unaffected by outliers:
- **A.** Mean
- **B.** Standard deviation
- **C.** Range
- **D.** Interquartile range

Q3. The regression line determines if:
- **A.** Any X values are outliers
- **B.** Any Y values are outliers
- **C.** To estimate the changes in Y for a unit change in X, this assumes that the relationship between X and Y is linear
- **D.** To determine if a change in X causes a change in Y, this assumes that the relationship between X and Y is linear

Linear Regression

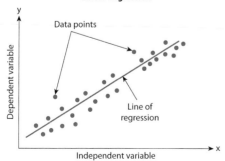

Q4. A Chi-square test of the relationship between the perception of emotional health and marital status leads to a rejection of the null hypothesis, indicating that there is a relationship between the two variables. The conclusion that can be drawn is:
- **A.** Better emotional health results in better marriage
- **B.** If one is more emotionally healthy, the more likely they are to be married
- **C.** There are likely to be confounding variables related to marital status as well as emotional health
- **D.** Marriage leads to better emotional health

Q5. Propensity score matching (PSM) is a statistical matching technique that:
- **A.** Is used in the analysis of contingency tables (Fisher exact) when sample sizes are small
- **B.** Statistical hypothesis used in the analysis of contingency tables when the sample sizes are large (Chi-square analysis)
- **C.** Step function illustrating the survival probability over time (Kaplan–Meier survival curve)
- **D.** Estimates the effect of the treatment policy by accounting for the covariates that predict receiving the treatment

Q6. If a p-value of a test statistic results estimates at 0.0596, what is the probability of falsely rejecting H_0 (null hypothesis)?
- **A.** 5.96%
- **B.** 5.09%
- **C.** 5.91%
- **D.** 5.06%

DOI: 10.1201/9781003389897-21

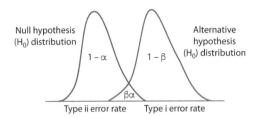

Null hypothesis (H₀) distribution — $1 - \alpha$ — β — Type ii error rate
Alternative hypothesis (H₀) distribution — $1 - \beta$ — α — Type i error rate

Q7. Type II error means:
- **A.** Rejecting the null hypothesis when it is false
- **B.** Rejecting the null hypothesis when it is true
- **C.** Not rejecting the null hypothesis when it is actually false
- **D.** Not rejecting the null hypothesis when it is true

Q8. If 17 smokers have lung cancer, 83 smokers do not have lung cancer, 1 non-smoker has lung cancer, and 99 non-smokers do not have lung cancer, the odds ratio (this hypothetical group of smokers) is:
- **A.** 10 times the odds of having lung cancer
- **B.** 15 times the odds of having lung cancer
- **C.** 20 times the odds of having lung cancer
- **D.** 25 times the odds of having lung cancer

Q9. A new noninvasive vascular test is to diagnose middle cerebral artery stenosis. All patients had a cerebral arteriogram, considered the "gold standard," as well as the new noninvasive vascular test. Out of 100 patients the cerebral angiogram reported 78 studies were positive and 22 studies were negative. Out of 78 patients reported by angiogram, 72 were reported positive by the new test and 6 were reported as negative. Out of the 22 patients reported as negative by the angiogram, 16 were reported as negative by the new test and 6 were reported as positive. The positive predictive value (PPV) and the negative predictive value (NPV) of the new test are:
- **A.** PPV 92.3   NPV 70.7
- **B.** PPV 90.3   NPV 70.7
- **C.** PPV 92.3   NPV 72.7
- **D.** PPV 95.3   NPV 74.7

Q10. In the aforementioned sample test (question 9), the sensitivity and specificity are:
- **A.** Sensitivity 81.8%   Specificity 72.7%
- **B.** Sensitivity 92.3%   Specificity 70.7%
- **C.** Sensitivity 92.3%   Specificity 72.7%
- **D.** Sensitivity 91.8%   Specificity 72.7%

Q11. The accuracy of the test in question 9 is:
- **A.** 88%
- **B.** 92%
- **C.** 96%
- **D.** 98%

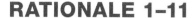

RATIONALE 1–11

1. RATIONALE

Selection bias is a distortion of association (such as a risk ratio) due to a sample selection that does not accurately affect the targeted population and proper randomization is not achieved. Selection bias can occur when investigators use improper procedures for selecting a sample population, but it can also occur because of factors that influence the continued participation of subjects in a study. In either case, the final study population is not representative of the targeted population. Selection bias occurs when the association between the exposure and health outcome is different for those who complete a study compared with those who are in the target population. Causes of selection biases are selective survival and losses to follow-up, volunteer and non-response bias, and hospital patient bias. Selection bias often occurs in observational studies where the selection is not random and is called undercoverage bias. In a case - control study of study of smoking and its possible relation to peripheral arterial disease, the association of exposure with disease will tend to be weaker if controls are selected from a hospital population (because smoking causes many diseases resulting in hospitalization) than if controls are selected from the community.

Correct Answer   D Recruiting participants directly from clinics, who miss all the care who do not attend the clinic, or who seek care during the study

Reference
Rothman, K. J., Greenland, S., & Lash, T. L. (2008). Validity in epidemiologic studies. In K. J. Rothman, S. Greenland, & T. L. Lash (Eds.), *Modern epidemiology* (3rd ed.). Philadelphia, PA: Lippincott Williams & Wilkins.

2. RATIONALE

Interquartile range (IQR) is a measure of statistical disposition, which is the spread of the data. The IQR may also be referred to as mid-spread/middle 50%, fourth spread, or H-spread and is defined as the difference between the 75th and 25th percentiles of the data. To calculate IQR the data set is divided into quartiles of four evenly ranked parts. These quartiles are denoted by Q1 (lower quartile), Q2 (the median quartile), and Q3 (upper quartile). The lower quartile corresponds with the 25th percentile and upper quartile with the upper 75th percentile.

Correct Answer   D Interquartile range

Reference
Dekking, F. M., Kraaikamp, C., Lopuhaä, H. P., et al. (2005). Testing hypotheses: elaboration. In *A modern introduction to probability and statistics: understanding why and how* (pp. 383–397). London: Springer London.

3. RATIONALE

A regression line indicates a linear relationship between the dependent variable in the Y axis and the independent variable in the X axis. The correlation is established by analyzing the data formed by the variable. The regression line is plotted closest to the data point in a regression graph. The formula for simple linear regression is $Y = mX + b$, where Y is the response (dependent) variable, m is the estimated slope, and b is the estimated intercept. You can calculate the regression line for two variables if their scatter plot shows a linear pattern and the correlation between the variables is very strong ($r = 0.98$). A regression line is simply a single line that best fits the data (smallest overall distance from the line to the points). Finding the best-fitting line is referred to as a simple linear regression analysis using the least squares method. The mean of the X values is denoted by x, the mean of the Y values is denoted by y, the standard deviation of the X values is Sx, and the standard deviation of the Y values is Sy. The correlation between the X and Y is denoted by r. The formula of the slope (m) of the best-fitting line is $m = r\frac{(Sy)}{Sx}$

where r is the correlation between x and y, and you simply divide Sy by Sx and multiply the result by r.

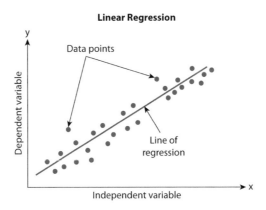

Linear Regression

Correct Answer C To estimate the changes in Y for a unit change in X, this assumes that the relationship between X and Y is linear

Reference
Rumsey, D. J. (2019). Correlation and regression. In *Statistics essentials for dummies* (pp. 113–126). Hoboken, NJ: Wiley.

4. RATIONALE

The null hypothesis defines the condition that the researchers need to discredit before suggesting an effect exists. Reject the null hypothesis when the p-value is less than or equal to your significance level. Conversely when the p-value is greater than your significance level, you fail to reject the null hypothesis. Failure to reject the null hypothesis is not the same as proving it. The null hypothesis varies by the type of statistic and hypothesis test. The t-test and ANOVA assess the difference between the group means. For these tests the null hypothesis states that there is no difference between the group means in the population. Null hypothesis Ho: Group proportions are equal in the population. Alternative hypothesis Ha: Group proportions are not equal in the population. Some studies assess the relationship between the two continuous variables rather than differences between the group. Analysis often uses correlation or regression analysis. For these tests, the null states that the correlation or regression coefficient is zero. As one variable increases, there is no tendency for the other variable to increase or decrease.

Correct Answer C There are likely to be confounding variables related to marital status as well as emotional health

Reference
Neyman, J., Pearson, E. S., & Pearson, K. (1933). IX. On the problem of the most efficient tests of statistical hypotheses. *Philos Trans R Soc London*. Series A, Containing Papers of a Mathematical or Physical Character, *231*(694–706), 289–337. doi:10.1098/rsta.1933.0009. Retrieved from https://royalsocietypublishing.org

5. RATIONALE

PSM attempts to reduce the bias due to cofounding variables that could be found in an esti-mate of the treatment effect obtained from simply comparing outcomes among units that received the treatment versus those that did not. In randomized trials, the randomization enables unbiased estimation of the treatment effect. Randomization implies that treat-ment groups will be balanced on an average by the law of large numbers. Making attempts to reduce the treatment bias and mimic randomization by creating a sample of units that receives the treatment – that is, comparable on all observed covariates to a sample of units that did not receive the treatment. Analysis of contingency tables for a small sample size is often done by the Fisher exact test, and for large samples by Chi-square analysis. The Kaplan–Meier survival curve is a non-parametric statistic used to estimate the survival function from lifetime data. It is often used to measure the fraction of patients living for a certain amount of time after treatment.

Correct Answer   **D** Estimates the effect of the treatment policy by accounting for the covari-ates that predict receiving the treatment

Reference
Austin, P. C. (2008). A critical appraisal of propensity-score matching in the medical literature between 1996 and 2003. *Stat Med*, *27*(12), 2037–2049. PMID: 18038446

6. RATIONALE

In statistical hypothesis testing, a type I error is the mistaken rejection of an actual true null hypothesis (false-positive finding), while a type II error is the failure to reject a null hypoth-esis that is actually false (false negative) – the alternative hypothesis is denoted by H1. In the aforementioned example there is a probability of 5.96% that we falsely reject Ho. If statistics are performed at a level like 0.05, then we can falsely reject Ho at 5%. Type II error is the mis-taken failure to reject the null hypothesis (false-negative test). In a clinical study you compare the symptoms of patients who received the new drug intervention to a controlled treatment. Using a t-test, you obtain a p-value of 0.035. This p-value is lower than your alpha of 0.05, so you consider your results statistically significant and reject the null hypothesis. However, the p-value means that there is 3.5% chance of your results occurring if the null hypothesis is true. Therefore, there is still a risk of making a type I error. To reduce the type I error probability, you can simply set a lower significant level.

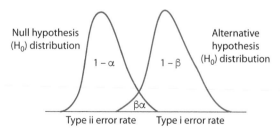

Correct Answer   **A** 5.96%

Reference
Bhandari, P. (2022). Type I & Type II Errors | Differences, Examples, Visualizations. Retrieved from https://www.scribbr.com/statistics/type-i-and-type-ii-errors

7. RATIONALE

A type II error means failing to conclude that there was an effect when there actually was. The study may have been underpowered. A power level of 80% or higher is usually considered acceptable. The risk of type II error is inversed related to the statistical power of a study. The higher the statistical power, the lower probability of making a type II error. By setting the type I error rate you inadvertently influence the size of the type II error rate. A type I error is usually worse and means going against the main statistical assumption of a null hypothesis. Based on the incorrect conclusion that the new drug is effective, many people may be prescribed the medication despite the risks of severe side effects, and other treatment options are rejected in favor of this intervention. In contrast with type II error, an intervention is considered ineffective when it can actually be useful.

Correct Answer **C** Not rejecting the null hypothesis when it is actually false

Reference
Bhandari, P. (2022). Type I & Type II Errors | Differences, Examples, Visualizations. Retrieved from https://www.scribbr.com/statistics/type-i-and-type-ii-errors

8. RATIONALE

Odds in the exposed group are calculated first as = smokers with lung cancer/smokers without lung cancer = 17/83 = 0.205.

Next, we calculate the odds for the non-exposed group. Odds in the non-exposed group = non-smokers with lung cancer/non-smokers without lung cancer = 1/99 = 0.01.

Finally, odds ratios are calculated:

$$\text{Odds ratio} = \frac{\text{Odds in exposed group}}{\text{Odds in nonexposed group}} = \frac{0.205}{0.01}$$

Thus, using the odds ratio, this hypothetical group of smokers had 20 times the odds of having lung cancer than non-smokers. The odds ratio confidence interval equals an alpha of 0.05, which means a confidence interval of 95% (1 – alpha). A 95% confidence interval is traditionally chosen in medical literature. The odds ratio should not be confused with relative risk.

Correct Answer **C** 20 times the odds of having lung cancer

Reference
Tenny, S., & Hoffman, M. R. (2022). Odds Ratio StatPearls. Retrieved from https://www.ncbi.nlm.nih.gov/books/NBK431098/

9. RATIONALE

In the aforementioned problem draw the Chi-square and populate the true-positive and false-positive and true-negative and false-negative square, with data considering the gold standard test (angiogram in this example) always assumed to be the correct result.

$$\text{PPV} = \frac{\text{True positives}}{\text{True positives and false positives}} = \frac{72}{72+6} = 92.3$$

$$\text{NPV} = \frac{\text{True negatives}}{\text{True negatives and false negatives}} = \frac{16}{16+6} = 72.7$$

Correct Answer   C PPV 92.3   NPV 72.7

Reference
Walker, N., Bryce, J., & Black, R. E. (2007). Interpreting health statistics for policymaking: the story
    behind the headlines. *Lancet, 369*(9565), 956–963. PMID: 17368157

10. RATIONALE

Sensitivity denotes the probability of a positive test result when the disease is present. A test
must be considered sensitive in general if it is positive for most individuals having the disease.

It is calculated as two positives divided by two positives plus false negatives equals:

$$\frac{72}{72+6} = \frac{72}{78} = 92.3$$

The specificity of a test determines the ability to diagnose an individual who does not have the
disease as negative. A highly specificity test means that there are few false-positive results.

It is calculated as true negatives divided by true negatives plus false positives equals:

$$\frac{16}{22} = 72.7$$

Correct Answer   C Sensitivity 92.3%   Specificity 72.7%

Reference
Parikh, R., Mathai, A., Parikh, S., et al. (2008). Understanding and using sensitivity, specificity, and
    predictive values. *Indian J Ophthalmol, 56*(1), 45–50. PMID:18158403

11. RATIONALE

The accuracy of the test is how well the test provides the correct answer, positive or negative.
The accuracy of a test is determined by:

$$\frac{\text{True positives} + \text{true negatives}}{\text{Total number of tests performed}\left(\text{true positive} + \text{false positive} + \text{false negative} + \text{true negative}\right)}$$

$$= \frac{72+16}{72+6+6+16} = \frac{88}{100} = 88\%$$

Correct Answer   A 88%

Reference
Zaborowska, L. (2022). Omni Accuracy Calculator. Retrieved from https://www.omnicalculator.com/
    statistics/accuracy

Index